AF179687

Silke Schicktanz, Andrew S. Gross, Richard Hölzl (eds.)
Infection and Injustice

Medical Humanities | 22

Editorial

Human beings are more than the sum of their organs and body parts: their roles in society, their (hi)stories, their living and economic conditions, but also their dreams, fears, and inventions impact their health.
The inter- and transdisciplinary edited series **Medical Humanities** will connect the perspectives of medicine, the humanities, and social sciences to gain new insights about how society, health, and the environment interact. Focusing on the living human body, the **Medical Humanities** series raises urgent questions on gender politics and bioethics, and mediates between care and health policies, technology and body images.

Silke Schicktanz, born in 1970, is a professor for Ethical and Cultural Studies of Biomedicine at the University Medical Center Göttingen, Germany. Her research focuses on cross-cultural bioethics, stakeholder engagement, as well as collectivity and responsibility.
Andrew S. Gross is a professor of American literature at Georg-August-Universität Göttingen, vice president of the German Association of American Studies, and editor-in-chief of the New American Studies Journal. He writes about American poetry and post-WWII American literature and culture.
Richard Hölzl is a researcher at Museum Fünf Kontinente in Munich and teaches at the Department of Medieval and Modern History at Georg-August-Universität Göttingen. His research focuses on environmental history, history of missions, and material cultures of colonialism.

Silke Schicktanz, Andrew S. Gross, Richard Hölzl (eds.)

Infection and Injustice

Narrative Dimensions in the Representation of Pandemics

[transcript]

Funded by the Georg-August-University Göttingen, Germany

GEORG-AUGUST-UNIVERSITÄT GÖTTINGEN IN PUBLICA COMMODA SEIT 1737

Bibliographic information published by the Deutsche Nationalbibliothek
The Deutsche Nationalbibliothek lists this publication in the Deutsche Nationalbibliografie; detailed bibliographic data are available online at https://dnb.dnb.de

This work is licensed under the Creative Commons License BY-NC-ND 4.0. For the full license terms, please visit the URL https://creativecommons.org/licenses/by-nc-nd/4.0/deed.de.
Creative Commons license terms for re-use do not apply to any content (such as graphs, figures, photos, excerpts, etc.) not original to the Open Access publication and further permission may be required from the rights holder. The obligation to research and clear permission lies solely with the party re-using the material.

2026 © Silke Schicktanz, Andrew S. Gross, Richard Hölzl (eds.)
transcript Verlag | Hermannstraße 26 | D-33602 Bielefeld | live@transcript-verlag.de

Cover design: Maria Arndt
Cover illustration: Nike Dietrich
Printing: Elanders Waiblingen GmbH, Waiblingen
https://doi.org/10.14361/9783839479735
Print-ISBN: 978-3-8376-8368-4 | PDF-ISBN: 978-3-8394-7973-5
ISSN of series: 2698-9220 | eISSN of series: 2703-0830

Printed on permanent acid-free text paper.

For Rebekka Habermas (1959–2023)

Contents

Literary Narratives and Metaphors

Social and Historical Narratives

Narratives and Morality

A Concluding Remark

Illustrations

Visually Narrating Disease? Syphilis in the German Public Sphere During the Early 20th Century – Victoria Morick

Injustice Narratives of Vaccine Critics. Insights from German Telegram Groups – Julia Brose

Acknowledgments

We thank Florian Zappe for his substantial support in editing and Victoria Morick for organizing and coordinating our interdisciplinary research project, as well as Valentina Jaensch and Sebastian Gross for their help with layout issues.

The Georg-August-Universität Göttingen co-financed the research project "Infection and Injustice. Narrative Responses to Pandemics" between August 2020 and September 2023 and made this collected volume possible.

Introduction: Narrating Pandemics

Andrew S. Gross, Richard Hölzl, Silke Schicktanz

Amidst the pain and suffering, the clashes and violence, the economic upheaval and political attempts at crisis management, a pandemic is also a crisis of social meaning.[1] The premise of this volume is that diseases are communicable in at least two ways: through contagion and narration. The modes of transmission reinforce and modulate each other even though they are distinct. Pathogens are not symbols, and diseases are not transmitted the way stories are. Nevertheless, people respond to pandemics, in part, by telling stories, and those stories motivate behaviors that directly impact the scope, rate, and trajectory of infection, for instance by encouraging or discouraging masking, social distancing, or vaccination.

In examining pandemics through the lens of narration and narratology, we follow the pioneering work of Priscilla Wald, whose 2008 *Contagious: Cultures, Carriers, and the Outbreak Narrative* explores how "[d]isease emergence dramatizes the dilemma that inspires the most basic of human narratives: the necessity and danger of human contact" (2). What Wald calls the "outbreak narrative" is a product of human efforts to understand, counter, and extrapolate from the spread of infectious diseases. The outbreak narrative is a storytelling paradigm that follows a familiar infectious pattern of contagion, spread, and containment to explain public health crises but also social crises more broadly. Wald notes that such "epidemiological stories" are socially productive: they inform state- and community-making, provide rationales for discipline and regulation, bolster experiences of exclusion and belonging, and even supply scientists with patterns for conducting medical research. The narrative paradigms – and metaphors – that have emerged through the human encounter with infectious disease are powerful, and outbreak narratives are, as Wald points out, widespread. However, other narrative paradigms counter epidemiological with social patterns of interaction, belonging and exclusion. Prominent among these is what we call the narrative of injustice.

1 We use the term "pandemic" broadly here – referring to major outbreaks of infectious diseases which cross social, political, and geographical boundaries – in order to stress the element of crisis, both as narrative element and social event.

"Narrative of injustice" is an umbrella term meant to invoke stories that counter the epidemiological metaphor operative in outbreak narratives with social and cultural metaphors stressing the validity of individual experience. Outbreak narratives represent communication in terms of contagion, and narratives of injustice invoke cultural, social, and personal registers to make sense of disease. The contrast might be said to involve a pathogenic version of the nature-culture debate: looked at it through the lens of contagion, meaning seems to spread like a disease; through the lens of injustice, sickness seems unfair, as do the means used to combat it. There are religious versions of the narrative of injustice that involve an angry or indifferent divinity. However, narratives of injustice can also be integrated into a secular "lessons learned" approach that helps make sense of the way people interact in the face of infection, for instance by wearing masks or practicing safe sex. The lessons learned can also involve paying attention to the unequal distribution of social cost when illness strikes. The point of the volume is to look at cases where communication in the face of contagion, rather than contagion itself, is the center point of narration, and personal stories stand at the center of what is communicated.

Though we often talk about messages "going viral," this is a metaphor. A narrative trajectory is not a vector of infection. Diseases do not spread through populations in the way stories circulate in the public sphere. Narratives move through a network of competing storylines, and each story draws on a variety of forms, contexts, rituals, traditions, temporalities (experience/precedence, the historical, or the unprecedented), registers (vernacular, traditional, religious, scientific), and voices (expert, populist, common sense). Narratives also move across overlapping and competing media platforms (from the newspaper, the book, to social media and chat groups and vice versa), sites (from a fine art gallery to an anti-vaccination demonstration), and modes (the textual, the visual, or the oral), creating their own publics and counterpublics that can coalesce or dissipate with the speed of breaking news.

Narration is a mode of expression, but it is also a field of social-political conflict: narratives of containment vie with counternarratives of destabilization, destruction, rebirth, and injustice as they circulate within – and define the boundaries of – the public sphere. Political positions ranging from socialism to libertarianism utilize narratives to motivate social action. These narratives are entangled with their respective material, spatial and temporal contexts. They change over time and in relation to the regional particularities of their production and distribution. Globalization facilitates the translation, transformation, and transregional adaptation of local narratives, just as local conditions transform international trends. This volume acknowledges the complexity by placing a number of historical and geographical narratives of infection in relation to each other.

Politics of Discourse and Material Pandemics

When considering the relation of infection to narration, it is important to acknowledge the work of Michel Foucault, who pioneered research into the discourse of disease. Foucault's work encouraged scholars in the humanities and social sciences to study disease *as* a discourse that could be organized into "disciplinary" structures of knowledge and power, for instance in his 1975 study on the development of prisons (*Discipline and Punishment*):

> The plague-stricken town, traversed throughout with hierarchy, surveillance, observation, writing; the town immobilized by the functioning of an extensive power that bears in a distinct way over all individual bodies – this is the utopia of the perfectly governed city. The plague (*envisaged as a possibility at least*) is the trial in the course of which one may define ideally the exercise of disciplinary power. In order to make rights and laws function according to pure theory, the jurists place themselves in imagination in the state of nature; in order to see perfect disciplines functioning, rulers dreamt of the state of plague. (Foucault 1995, 198–199, emphasis added)

Foucault's reservation, or hesitancy, is noteworthy – for him the plague is a "possibility," not necessarily a reality; imagination is cause enough for the exercise of total discipline. Foucauldian interpretations have been particularly important in the historiography of colonial health and disease regimes. There is an extensive pre-Covid scholarship demonstrating convincingly how "contagion" and "the contagious" have been formative in legitimizing oppressive and colonial regimes of border control, colonial governance, and global movement (Bashford/Hooker 2001, Bashford 2016, Amrith 2012, Tilley 2011, Anderson 2006, Ernst/Harris 1999, Marks/Worboys 1997, Arnold 1993, Bauche 2017).

Foucault's warnings against surveillance and control have been immensely influential in the humanities, but they resonate differently in the face of public health emergencies when the possibility of infection becomes a medical crisis. There is a difference between studying historical disease, represented by words on a page, and living through a pandemic. The need to counter the effects of disease but also the oppressive, sometimes colonial characteristics of disease control places both public health practitioners and theorists in a moral quandary.

The Swiss historian of science Paul Sarasin has noted the problems associated with approaching Covid-19 through a Foucauldian lens (Sarasin 2020). As he puts it, "We are in a different situation: we live in the midst of a pandemic and are subject to, or observe through the media, different modes of appearance of power and government" (Sarasin 2020, section 4). Sarasin calls for a differentiated reading of Foucault's models of governmental reactions to pandemics, a balanced approach to the sometimes conflicting demands of disease prevention and personal freedom. However, he stops short of posing a key theoretical question: How should historians, social anthropologists, philosophers, sociologists, and literary critics factor in the specific material qualities of disease and pandemics? The theoretical issue involves not only problems of representation but of presentation: namely how diseases "communicate" between bodies, "become visible" as symptoms in the body, how diseases are distributed geographically, and how they affect specific members/groups of people, including children, the poor, the elderly, and those with disabilities.

Recent studies move away from the Foucauldian alignment of discourse and power to look at the way cultural responses to disease attempt to work out the relation of presentation to representation, communicability to communication. The historical compendium by Delaurenti and Le Roux applies the logic of pandemics to other cultural phenomena of dynamic spreading; these include examples as diverse as antisemitism, the waltz as maniacal mode of socializing in post-Napoleonic France, and the violence of Mao's red guards (Delaurenti/Le Roux 2021). Other scholars have leveraged notions of contagion to explore the dissemination of narratives, rumors, and conspiracy theories (Bar-On/Molas 2020, Castrillón/Marchevsky 2021). On the other hand, Magnusson and Zalloua have cautioned against using contagion as the "metaphor of choice" to describe other spreading threats to humanity from "global terrorism … to obesity" (Magnusson/Zalloua 2012, 4). Besides leading to questionable political consequences, metaphors of contagion can, when overused, simply lose their rhetorical force. Here it is also worth citing Thomas Piketty, who sees the global spread of Covid-19 as contagious in the way that ideas and practices of containment are contagious (mass lockdown, for instance, becoming a global trend). But Piketty also acknowledges that "the processes governing the spread of ideologies always entail a multiplicity of possible choices, sociopolitical trajectories, and opportunities" (Piketty 2021, 333–334).

Another emergent area of study focuses on specific genres and fields of cultural production such as the "viropolitics" of horror fiction (Becker/de Bruin-Molé/Polak 2021), the metaphorical application of the Corona virus in scientific communication (Charteris-Black 2021), and the role played by narratives in the reception of the 2009 swine flu epidemic (Davis/McGregor/Lohm 2020). In short, there is much pre- and early Covid-19 work in the humanities and social sciences that emphasizes the power of narrative as a tool of policy-making and sense-making in the face of natural disaster.

The still recent exposure to the deadly force of a viral agent – however strongly mediated by cultural practice – has heightened awareness of the dangers of a purely cultural or political reading of a pandemic. The question of the nature of the relation between the biological fact of the disease and the stories we tell about it still looms large. Add to this the complicating factor that not every pathogen is transmitted in the same way, at the same speed, under the same circumstances, or with the same physical consequences. It is important to remember this specificity, along with the difference between the transmission of pathogens and messages, when considering how narratives respond to and shape infection. Few works of research look beyond the discursive model in order to consider disease as a co-production of nature and culture – not necessarily in the literal sense of having originated in and spread from a lab, although this theory of the emergence of Covid-19 is gaining credibility, but in the sense that the agency of the disease becomes visible through techno-scientific and social processes (e.g., on yellow fever/malaria and empire, cf. McNeill 2010, Mitchell 2002). Bruno Latour, whose work is key here (1999), has chosen to give "the virus" a much more symbolic presence in his recent pandemic writing, namely as a harbinger of a future universal lockdown induced by the climate catastrophe – inflicted on humanity trapped on a planet with dwindling resources and shrinking habitability (Latour 2021). This is meant as a warning about the overconsumption of natural resources and should be contrasted with Giorgio Agamben's complaints about the state's biopolitical overreach against society (Agamben 2020). Agamben's interventions demonstrate, for some, the problems inherent to any approach that conflates discourse and power (cf. the critique by Ginzburg 2020 and, more generally, Latour 2004). We need a transdisciplinary approach to the stories we tell about disease in order to map the relations of culture to biology in a more complete picture of social reality.

Morality and Narration: From the Diagnostic and Systematic to the Communal and Personal

The contributions to this collection of essays consider the relation of contagion to narration not only in terms of justice but *injustice*, most notably Silke Schicktanz's concluding essay on the philosophical and ethical framing of pandemics. There is body of work in public health policy and the ethics of infection control on how viable concepts of justice need to balance public health with compassion and personal freedom (Arnold/Flügel-Martinsen/Mohammed/Vasilache 2020, Baron/Lenz/Hasenfratz 2021, Reis/Schmidhuber/Frewer 2021, Thießen 2021, Lupton/Willis 2021). In addition to injustice, related concepts of solidarity and vulnerability have gained much more relevance in the last decade due to an enlarged sensitivity to economic disparities and structural inequalities related to infection disease.

Why injustice? Various groups and individuals claimed that the official responses to the recent pandemic were unjust. To claim *injustice* is to express the value judgment that the suffering caused by the pandemic, and/or by responses to it, was not only unfortunate but wrong. While this can, when taken to the extreme, reflect conspiratorial or even magical thinking, mistakenly assigning blame where agency is dispersed or nonexistent, narratives of injustice also draw attention to inequalities in healthcare or education that only come to light in moments of crisis. The moral calculus involved does not have to be systematic, and that is the point. Claims of injustice do not presuppose a coherent theory of justice, nor do they depend for their moral force on the impersonality of science or law. The moral sentiment expressed by the claim of injustice reflects a particular point of view – that of the person or group that believes itself to be unfairly disadvantaged – even when it points to problems that can be measured statistically.

This particularity, in turn, reveals something essential about narrative and the way stories differ from, and respond to, the spread of disease. Particularity is a basic feature of narrative and one of the ways it differs from other modes of description. As David Herman puts it in *Basic Elements of Narrative*, "the degree to which represented events are particularized provides a parameter along which narratives can be distinguished from explanations" (Herman 2009, 92). Particularity, in storytelling, tends to express itself through characterization and point of view, but also through the vagaries of fate, revealed through a narrative arc, that distinguish the individual from the statistical average. The subjects of narrative are cast as protagonists and antagonists, not as examples or types. There can be average heroes – in the sense of Everyman – and parables tend to leave their protagonists unnamed. Nevertheless, the kind of universality achieved through such narratives is representative rather than statistical. Everyman acts for reasons that may be widely understandable; his actions, however, are not the predictable results of quantifiable causes (cf. Herman 2009, 97).

The particularity of narrative does not necessarily make it more biased than other modes of reasoning, but it does impact the way narrative produces knowledge. Using "system" in a looser sense than we mean it here, literary scholar Peter Brooks argues that "[n]arrative is one of the large categories or systems of understanding that we use in our negotiations with reality, specifically, in the case of narrative, with the problem of temporality: man's time-boundedness, his consciousness of existence within the limits of mortality" (Brooks 1984, xi). This is the second feature of storytelling that needs to be emphasized: narratives are particular; they also unfold over and are bound by time (Cohan and Shires 1991, 52–53; Hermann 2009, 90). The features are linked existentially: one event follows another in narrative in the way one experience follows another in life. The lifespan of narrative gives it a beginning, middle, and end – designations that go beyond mere sequentiality. The beginning and end of a story stand in a special relation Frank Kermode calls "consonance," which involves the end commenting on the beginning (Kermode 2000, 17). Consonance invests the middle of the story with a fullness that liberates it from "chronicity," the mechanical sequencing of one event after another, because elements *in medias res* recollect the beginning through analepsis, and anticipate the end through foreshadowing, in an order that is diegetic rather than strictly serial (Kermode 2000, 50). Kermode, like Brooks (1984), points out that narrative order is above all existential. He also stresses the religious dimensions of narrative, the way every beginning echoes Genesis, and every end anticipates the Apocalypse, so that the existential qualities of narrative draw their moral force from eschatology (Kermode 2000, 12–15).

It is not necessary to invoke the Final Judgment to note that narratives invite judgment. The patterns are also amenable to logics of secular morality. The beginning and end of narrative can be understood as terminal points of an arc spanning the is/ought gap. Conventions like the plot twist or the surprise ending, and even basic elements of storytelling like suspense, depend on the fact that even casual readers have strong feelings about how stories are supposed to develop, in part because we learn from common stories, such as fairy tales, from a very early age. Alasdair MacIntyre invokes this quality of narrative, its tendency to point towards a fitting ending, to explain how personal and collective stories intersect in ways that result in shared values. His teleological model of ethics is not consequentialist. He does not propose evaluating the results of actions in terms of a fully developed ethical system; rather, he is interested in how collective stories link up with the open-ended stories we tell about ourselves as we go along:

> We live out our lives, both individually and in our relationships with each other, in the light of certain conceptions of a possible shared future, a future in which certain possibilities beckon us forward and others repel us, some seem already foreclosed and others perhaps inevitable. There is no present which is not informed by some image of some future and an image of the future which always presents itself in the form of a *telos* – or of a variety of ends or goals – which we are either moving or failing to move in the present. Unpredictability and teleology therefore coexist as part of our lives; like characters in a fictional narrative we do not know what will happen next, but nonetheless our lives have a certain form which projects itself towards our future. Thus the narratives which we live out have both an unpredictable and a partially teleological character. If the narrative of our individual and social lives is to continue intelligibly – and either type of narrative may lapse into unintelligibility – it is always both the case that there are constraints on how the story can continue *and* that within those constraints there are indefinitely many ways that it can continue. (MacIntyre 2020, 250)

Narratives provide a heuristic basis for judgment because they are open-ended and end-directed at the same time, at least for the agents experiencing and shaping them as they unfold. We are actors in dramas we compose collectively, as we go along, with a number of possible ends in mind – not authors of stories whose end is already clear.

MacIntyre points to a third quality of narrative worth invoking here. Besides being particular and temporal, narratives can be personal and communal at the same time. This aspect of narrative goes by various names in literary criticism: tradition, archetype, paradigm, genre. MacIntyre's account of the confluence of personal and collective narratives is an attempt to theorize virtue. This is not the same as injustice. Nevertheless, he illuminates some of the ethical issues at stake when personal – or small group – and public accounts of behavior diverge.

Narratives of injustice derive their pathos, their emotional charge, from the claim that dominant stories, sometimes labeled in populist terms as the "system" or the "establishment," are indifferent to the particular. While the emergence of systematic thinking in science has its own history, as does the relation of narrative to system and method in scientific research, for our present purposes it suffices to say that public health measures, and a bureaucratic healthcare system, can seem indifferent to the individual. The significance of this indifference antedates the most recent pandemic. For several years, programs in narrative medicine have stressed the importance of listening to the stories patients tell about themselves inorder to resist "the individual's abstraction into the institutional space of diagnostic categories," as one of the contributions to the standard textbook in the field puts it (Charon et al. 2016, 72). The first page of the introduction to that textbook raises the relation of narratives to injustice: "Narrative medicine ... emerged to challenge a reductionist, fragmented medicine that holds little regard for the singular aspects of a patient's life and to protest the social injustice of a global healthcare system that countenances tremendous health disparities and discriminatory policies and practices" (Charon et al. 2016, 1). The goal of narrative medicine is to address injustice in healthcare by telling stories that put the particular back into focus.

Social Inequalities and Narration

It does not always make sense to rail against the injustice of infection per se. The narratives impugning biology are often misdirected, from an epidemiological point of view, because sickness as such cannot be put on trial. Nevertheless, the sick curse their fate, family members accuse those who infect their relatives (Battin 2009), protestors condemn governmental policies and the advice of experts, the vaccinated disparage the anti-vaxxers, citizens close ranks against foreigners (Bobba/Hube 2021). We could observe all of this in real time in 2021 and 2022. Now, after a pause, we can begin to reflect on what was at stake when narratives of injustice began to spread in newspapers, in social media, and the academic literature. The narratives often register a basic human sense of unfairness; they also testify to the inequities built into collective responses to contagion. A virus like Covid-19 does not respect borders, but richer nations did have better access to vaccines, as did wealthier individuals within their communities. Political power and economic interest limited access to vaccines for poorer countries by protecting some patents. This is unjust. The rich within one nation could better avoid exposure to pathogens than could the poor (Harsh 2021, Timmermann 2021, ten Have 2022). This is unjust. On a closer look, the social epidemiology of the Covid-19 pandemic offers a veritable pandemonium of very real inequalities with regard to exposure, mitigation, and recovery in health care, but also economically and for society as whole (Duncan/Kawachi/Morse 2024). Of course, this echoes pre-existing societal and global inequalities perceived during earlier epidemics (e.g., Farmer 1999). It is, however, not a given that narratives of injustices reflect social inequalities in a direct or impartial manner, or that they simply "give voice" to them. The hypothesis of this volume is that the relationship between narratology of pandemics and the social epidemiology of pandemics is complex but also productive (in a social and poetic sense) and therefore needs to be examined.

At first glance, it seems that viruses are great equalizers that infect the rich and the poor alike. If society were nothing but a densely packed biomass, a pandemic would unfold in a most democratic fashion. However, the structures that define social life by separating inside from outside, rich from poor, public from private, and various identity groups from one another impact infection patterns and rates in ways that are patently unfair. Stories address these inequalities, and they contribute to them as well, motivating actions that lead to more injustice, e.g., by scapegoating vulnerable groups as the spreaders of infection. Narratives of infection can stigmatize or voice injustice; they can also inspire compassion or solidarity, provide assurance by signaling organizational strength and scientific insight, mark crises and turning points, provide hope, voice despair, and highlight self-sacrifice or the sacrifices made by others.

Focus and Scope of this Collection

This volume contributes to the growing field of infection-related work in the humanities and social sciences by bringing a transdisciplinary perspective to narratives of pandemics. To this end, we employ a broad set of research perspectives integrating social sciences (sociology, social and cultural anthropology, STS), humanities (literary studies, history), and ethics. We engage with a variety of historical and contemporary settings as well as social contexts of narration (scientific, humanitarian, religious, popular, political). The common denominator is an emphasis on narration / narratology in the analysis of the "making sense of epidemics." Privileging narration as a bridging concept between various disciplines, this volume aims to provide a complementary approach to research that focuses on concepts such as "discourse" and the "imaginary" (Lynteris 2021), and also on the outbreak narrative (Wald 2008). The contributions attempt to link a cultural approach with perspectives that expose the material conditions and social inequalities that characterize pandemic events (e.g., Duncan/Kawachi/Morse 2024).

The interdisciplinary layout of this volume allows for a dialogue between various perspectives: historical, contemporary, sociological, organizational, narratives of everyday experiences, as well as movement-oriented, ethics-oriented, policy-oriented, and communication-oriented narratives. The authors engage with diverse social formations in Western, post-socialist, and colonial societies. The various contributions discuss issues of mediality as well as the ability of narratives to translate and transform the materialities ("the nature") of specific epidemic diseases.

The volume has a geographical focus on the German-speaking countries of central Europe (Germany, Austria, Switzerland), but also includes flanking studies of the United States and England. Various contributions draw attention to the international as well as colonial angles of Western narrations of pandemics. In this respect, the chapter complements a growing body of work that focuses mainly, and sometimes exclusively, on North America or colonial health regimes. A global approach would of course resonate metaphorically with the global nature of a pandemic such as Covid-19. However, regional studies, like those making up this collection, can also contribute to an understanding of particularities that more global perspectives sometimes miss.

The volume is structured by three sections devoted to, firstly, *Literary Narratives and Metaphors*; secondly, *Social and Historical Narratives*; and thirdly, to the relationship of *Narratives and Morality*.

Literary Narratives and Metaphors: Andrew S. Gross traces the development of the figure of the "lone survivor" in a genre he calls the pandemic pastoral. The post-apocalyptic literature that fits this definition presents the world (in which humanity has been nearly eradicated by a pandemic) as a garden on the far side of catastrophe. Only the "lone survivor," who remembers what life was like before, is able to make sense of the ruins preserved in the garden and explain what they mean for civilization, which has disappeared in the present tense of the narrative (the lone survivor has no neighbors) but is preserved in the readership. The difference between neighbors and readers, built into the language of the narratives, accounts for the survivor's loneliness, but it is also the novel's means of exploring the difference between communication and communicability. The essay offers readings of six novels and novellas: Mary Shelley's *The Last Man* (1826), Edgar Allan Poe's "King Pest: A Tale Containing an Allegory" (1835) and "The Masque of the Red Death" (1842), Jack London's *The Scarlet Plague* (1912), Katherine Anne Porter's *Pale Horse, Pale Rider* (1939), and Richard Matheson's *I Am Legend* (1954).

Franziska Meier traces how Western writers struggled to find an adequate form for pandemic fiction. She uncovers the intertextual relations of narratives through many centuries, from Thucydides' *The Peloponnesian War* to Giovanni Boccaccio's *The Decameron*, to more modern works by Daniel Defoe, Alessandro Manzoni, and Albert Camus. One feature these texts have in common is the centrality of eyewitness accounts. As Meier demonstrates, Thucydides discusses his own role as a contemporary witness of the plague, while Boccaccio has an eyewitness relate scenes of turmoil. The centrality of the eyewitness is emphasized by Defoe, who uses a first-person eyewitness as narrator in his account of the London plague of 1665, much as Camus does with his account of a fictitious plague in a fictional German-occupied Algeria set in 1940. Manzoni's early 19th-century novel, on the other hand, has a first-person narrator discuss the reliability of various eyewitness accounts of the Milan plague of 1629–30.

In his essay on the entanglement of medical and communication discourses, Pierre-Héli Monot approaches a key issue of this book: the morphology of the pandemic narrative as a form. Issuing an apt warning about the danger of metaphorical health communication, he contends that the public is misled when warned of the "viral" spread of misinformation, even when international organizations such as the WHO include this in their well-meant health messaging. Monot's argument is gathered from current observations and underpinned by several loosely connected cases of medico-literary history. The key figures here are Oliver Wendell Holmes, Ignaz Semmelweis, and Louis-Ferdinand Céline. Monot demonstrates how when medical discourse intersects with political pamphleteering, it can spiral out of control, most viciously in Céline's murderously antisemitic texts of the late 1930s and early 1940s.

Social and Historical Narratives: Yvonne Völkl takes a deep dive into recent examples of Corona writing, including diaries and self-narrations, which helped some people cope with the hardships of the pandemic lockdown. Analyzing two online journals – one in French and one in Spanish – Völkl explores what renders them effective and which narrative tools seem best adapted to therapeutic, commemorative, and testimonial goals.

Jan Hinrichsen shares his reflections on the changing nature of the modern experience of immunity, which can no longer be defined as a personal boundary created by the body's immune system. Both the contingency of the pandemic and the implications of new vaccines based on messenger-RNA technology, call for new narratives that stress multi-relational concepts rather than corporeal boundaries. In the course of his analysis, Hinrichsen revisits key theoretical works of cultural anthropology (and other related fields of study) by authors such as Barbara Duden, Emily Martin, Donna Haraway, Bruno Latour, and others.

How to educate the public about sexually transmitted diseases, such as syphilis, that come with moral and religious baggage as well as a stark class and gender bias? The question bothered European doctors around the time of the First World War. Their answer was to put a stop to the stigmatization of syphilis and to address the problem publicly, rationally, and scientifically. This was the proclamation of a professional group of doctors, but it did not necessarily correspond to public opinion. Victoria Morick examines the outcomes of this new, supposedly non-moralistic approach by focusing two photographic slide shows originating from the Dresden Hygiene Museum in the mid-1920s and intended for medical presentations all around

Germany. Based on a reading of the visual narratives implicit in the two series of photographic representations, Morick asks whether the moralizing/non-moralizing binary can capture what the images were doing in terms of medical communication. She concludes much more complicated "re-coding" of traditional syphilis narratives was really taking place.

In another historiographical inquiry, set in colonial health care systems of the 1920s to 1940s, Richard Hölzl traces the impact of African and European historical actors (doctors, nurses, missionaries, patients) on imperial narratives of "leprosy eradication." He argues that narrative plots and characters depended on the social contexts of empire, but also on the imaginary of therapeutic success and failure. A masculine, heroic, and curative paradigm could only govern leprosy narratives as long as success in the form of an effective drug therapy was deemed available. Once the success of the drug-based "leprosy eradication campaign" of the 1920s and 1930s was called into question, the highly symbolic, heroic tales of "curing empire" gave way to more care-focused stories, often highlighting the "selfless female care worker." The case study focuses leprosy work in Southern Tanzania, local agency, and missionary care workers, as well as on medical health campaigners of the British Empire Leprosy Relief Association and a Catholic mission society.

Cultural anthropologist Laura Bäumel turns to the contemporary scene to analyzing the meaning and reception of a common Covid-19 pandemic narrative ("We're all in this together") in an everyday work environment. Bäumel conducted qualitative interviews with working mothers, most of them in temporary employment, in Austrian factories. Situating their stories in the wider discourse on Covid-19 in Austria and the German speaking countries, the analysis uncovers connections between self-narration and the medico-political grand-narrative, especially in the way the mothers address issues of social cohesion rather than their own vulnerability and potential social injustices.

This representation of social respectability is contrasted in the following chapter by the "social figure of 'the jailbreaker.'" The sociologists Böhrer, Döbler, and Pfaller take a close look at the narratives surrounding an incident in the Bavarian small town Mitterteich. The town was locked down after a local beer festival developed into a potential "super-spreader" event in March 2020. The authors argue that social figures, such as "the jailbreaker," emerge in mass mediated societies as shorthand for complex social events; social figures personalize blame and simplify complex situations, but they also provide tools for individuals and groups to position themselves within society.

The essays in the third part *Narratives and Morality* explore the moral implications of pandemic narratives. The authors ask how pandemic narratives represent behavior and how they attempt to provide moral guidelines.

The cultural anthropologists Moritz Ege and Julian Schmitzberger trace a particular social phenomenon in relation to the increased concern with ethical communication during the Covid-19 pandemic: anti-judgmentalism. Employing a transdisciplinary lens, the authors follow a widespread resistance to judging (as in "don't judge me!") through various discourses and social environments. They note, for instance, that the English verb "to judge" has entered German youth culture with the negative connotation of judgmentalism ("judgen"). This observation sets the scene for the narrative analysis of interviews with activists from the Berlin hedonist youth culture and clubbing scene. The interviews were conducted during the Covid-19 pandemic.

Julia Brose examines narratives of injustice in conversations of German anti-vaccination groups on the social media platform Telegram. Asking how vaccination critics perceive their social positions and voice their claim of having experienced injustices during the Covid-19 pandemic – by others, by the state, by society – Brose addresses the larger question of how right-wing movements mobilize members and potential members by questioning resource distribution, access to social opportunities and mobility, as well as health policy decision-making. Brose notes the circularity of group discussions, the devaluation of opponent groups, and the utopian trajectory plotted by discourses of "systemic change."

Jennifer Reich's chapter takes a complementary look at groups opposed to vaccination in the United States. Reich highlights the extent to which anti-vaccination narratives reinforce inequalities within society by stressing personal responsibility over public health. Often vaccination opponents argue in highly individualistic terms, claiming responsibility for "one's own body" and portraying health and disease as matters of life choices and bodily practices. Brose's and Reich's findings highlight both important transnational similarities, but also marked differences in the way vaccination is opposed across the Atlantic.

Turning towards a line of argument that advocates societal protection of vulnerable social groups, Niklas Ellerich-Groppe and Mark Schweda highlight a variety of storylines that put forward the motif of intergenerational solidarity. Based on a narrative analysis of German newspaper commentaries, the authors differentiate the ethical potential of intergenerational stories of missing, required or even successful solidarity. Most of these emphasize already existing relations between age groups. However, the same stories can also result in a "blame game" by pointing the finger at an alleged lack of gratitude among the younger generation. In this sense, the various claims for more solidarity should also be understood as discursive attempts to frame structural injustices, marginalization or misrecognition of particular social groups.

These various forms of injustices are taken up in the concluding contribution to this volume by Silke Schicktanz. She provides a philosophical overview of different concepts of injustice, ranging from maldistribution, oppression, unfairness, epistemic, and everyday injustices. She argues for the analytical need to preserve multiple meanings relative to the scenarios in which they are deployed and suggests the importance of maintaining nuance in concepts of injustice, especially those involving concepts of social recognition. The point of this concluding chapter is to show how the theme of injustice, with its emphasis on the particular story rather than the systematic diagnosis, unites the various contributions to this volume.

Bibliography

Agamben, Giorgio. 2020. "Lo stato d'eccezione provocato da un'emergenza immotivata." *Il Manifesto*, February 20, 2020. https://ilmanifesto.it/lo-stato-deccezione-provocato-da-unemergenza-immotivata.

Amrith, Sunil S. 2012. "Eugenics in Postcolonial Southeast Asia." *The Oxford Handbook of the History of Eugenics*, edited by Alison Bashford and Philippa Levine, Oxford UP, 301–314.

Anderson, Warwick. 2006. *Colonial Pathologies: American Tropical Medicine, Race, and Hygiene in the Philippines*, Duke UP.

Arnold, Clara, Oliver Flügel-Martinsen, Samia Mohammed, and Andreas Vasilache, editors. 2020. *Kritik in der Krise. Perspektiven politischer Theorie auf die Corona-Pandemie*, Nomos.

Arnold, David. 1993. *Colonizing the Body. State Medicine and Epidemic Disease in Nineteenth-Century India*, U of California P.

Baron, Christian, Sarah Lenz, and Martina Hasenfratz, editors. 2021. *Gesellschaft als Risiko. Soziologische Situationsanalysen zur Coronapandemie*, Campus Verlag.

Bar-On, Tamir, and Bàrbara Molas, editors. 2020. *Responses to the COVID-19 Pandemic by the Radical Right: Scapegoating, Conspiracy Theories and New Narratives*, Ibidem Verlag.

Bashford, Alison, editor. 2016. *Quarantine. Local and Global Histories*, Palgrave Macmillan.

Bashford, Alison, and Claire Hooker, editors. 2001. *Contagion. Historical and Cultural Studies*, Routledge.

Battin, Margaret Pabst. 2009. *The Patient as Victim and Vector: Ethics and Infectious Disease*, Oxford UP.

Bauche, Manuela. 2017. *Medizin und Herrschaft. Malariabekämpfung in Kamerun, Ostafrika und Ostfriesland (1890–1919)*, Campus Verlag. Universität Leipzig, dissertation.

Becker, Sandra, Megen de Bruin-Molé, and Sara Polak, editors. 2021. *Embodying Contagion: The Viropolitics of Horror and Desire in Contemporary Discourse*, U of Wales P.

Bobba, Giuliano, and Nicolas Hube, editors. 2021. *Populism and the Politicization of the COVID-19 Crisis in Europe*, Palgrave Macmillan.

Brooks, Peter. 1984. *Reading for the Plot. Design and Intention in Narrative*, Harvard UP.

Castrillón, Fernando, and Thomas Marchevsky, editors. 2021. *Coronavirus, Psychoanalysis, and Philosophy: Conversations on Pandemics, Politics and Society*, Routledge.

Charon, Rita et al. 2016. *The Principles and Practice of Narrative Medicine*, Oxford UP.

Charteris-Black, Jonathan. 2021. *Metaphors of Coronavirus. Invisible Enemy or Zombie Apocalypse?*, Springer.

Cohan, Steven, and Linda M. Shires. 1991. *Telling Stories. A Theoretical Analysis of Narrative Fiction*, Routledge.

Daston, Lorraine. 1991. "The Ideal and Reality of the Republic of Letters in the Enlightenment." *Science in Context*, vol. 4, no. 2, 367–386.

Davis, Mark, David McGregor, and Davina Lohm. 2020. *Pandemics, Publics, and Narrative*, Oxford UP.

Delaurenti, Béatrice, and Thomas Le Roux, editors. 2021. *Cultures of Contagion*, MIT Press.

Duncan, Dustin T., Ichiro Kawachi, and Stephen S. Morse, editors. 2024. *The Social Epidemiology of the COVID-19 Pandemic*, Oxford UP.

Ernst, Waltraud, and Bernard Harris, editors. 1999. *Race, Science and Medicine, 1700–1960*, Routledge.

Farmer, Paul. 1999. *Infections and Inequalities*, U of California P.

Foucault, Michel. 1995. *Discipline and Punish. The Birth of the Prison*, Vintage Books.

Ginzburg, Carlo. 2020. "Une démocratie grégaire?" *En Attendant Nadeau*, July 12, 2020. https://www.en-attendant-nadeau.fr/2020/07/12/democratie-gregaire-ginzburg/.

Gross, Andrew. 2020. "Vaccination, Inoculation, and Franklin's Grief." *American Counter/Publics*, edited by Ulla Haselstein, Frank Kelleter, et al., Universitätsverlag Winter, 137–158.

Harsh, Mander. 2021. *Locking Down the Poor. The Pandemic and India's Moral Centre*, Speaking Tiger.

Herman, David. 2009. *Basic Elements of Narrative*, Wiley-Blackwell.

Kermode, Frank. 2000. *The Sense of an Ending*, Oxford UP.

Latour, Bruno. 1999. *Pandora's Hope. Essays on the Reality of Science Studies*, Harvard UP.

Latour, Bruno. 2004. "Why Has Critique Run out of Steam? From Matters of Fact to Matters of Concern." *Critical Inquiry*, vol. 30, no. 2, 225–248.

Latour, Bruno. 2021. *Wo bin ich? Lektionen aus dem Lockdown*, Suhrkamp. (French original: 2021. *Où suis-je?: Leçons du confinement à l'usage des terrestres*, Empêcheurs).

Lynteris, Christos, editor. 2021. *Plague Image and Imagination from Medieval to Modern Times*, Palgrave Macmillan.

Lupton, Deborah, and Karen Willis, editors. 2021. *The COVID-19 Crisis. Social Perspectives*, Routledge.

MacIntyre, Alasdair. 2020. *After Virtue*, Bloomsbury Academic.

Magnusson, Bruce A., and Zahi Anbra Zalloua, editors. 2012. *Contagion. Health, Fear, Sovereignty*, U of Washington P.

Marks, Lara, and Michael Worboys. 1997. *Migrants, Minorities and Health. Historical and Contemporary Studies*, Routledge.

McMillan, John. 2020. "COVID-19 and Justice." *Journal of Medical Ethics*, vol. 46, no. 10, 639–640.

Mitchell, Timothy. 2002. *Rule of Experts. Egypt, Techno-Politics, Modernity*, U of California P.

McNeill, John R. 2010. *Mosquito Empires: Ecology and War in the Greater Caribbean, 1620–1914*, Cambridge UP.

Piketty, Thomas. 2021. *Time for Socialism. Dispatches from a World on Fire, 2016–2021*, Yale UP.

Reis, Andreas, Martina Schmidhuber, and Andreas Frewer, editors. 2021. *Pandemien und Ethik. Entwicklung – Probleme – Lösungen*, Springer.

Sarasin, Paul. 2020. "Understanding the Pandemic with Foucault?" *Genealogy+Critique*, March 31, 2020. https://blog.genealogy-critique.net/essays/254/understanding-corona-with-foucault.

ten Have, Henk. 2020. *The Covid-19 Pandemic and Global Bioethics*, Springer.

Thießen, Malte. 2021. *Auf Abstand. Eine Gesellschaftsgeschichte der Coronapandemie*, Campus Verlag.

Tilley, Helen. 2011. *Africa as a Living Laboratory. Empire, Development, and the Problem of Scientific Knowledge, 1870–1950*, U of Chicago P.

Timmermann, Cristian. 2021. "Pandemic Preparedness and Cooperative Justice." *Developing World Bioethics*, vol. 21, no. 4, 201–210.

Wald, Priscilla. 2008. *Contagious: Cultures, Carriers, and the Outbreak Narrative*, Duke UP.

Literary Narratives and Metaphors

Pandemic Pastoralism

The Legend of the Lone Survivor in American Literature

Andrew S. Gross

The devastation wrought by pandemics has led writers to imagine a world devoid of humanity. Empty streets and deserted houses manifest the fear that when a disease is contagious enough to infect everyone, no one will be left alive. No one, that is, except the lone survivor. As the protagonist of Katherine Anne Porter's (1939) semi-autobiographical novella of the 1918 flu pandemic puts it, "[d]eath always leaves one singer to mourn" (240). The protagonist is referring to an (invented) spiritual that lends its title to the novella, "Pale Horse, Pale Rider"; and indeed, the legend of the lone survivor draws some of its authority from biblical archetypes. The allusion here is to the Book of Revelation and, to a lesser degree, The Book of Job, but it is important to note that the implications are secular rather than eschatological: there is no final judgment at the end of Porter's novella, just loneliness. Survival thus lends poignancy to the devastation; it also adds a plot, ensuring that the end of the pandemic is not the end of the story.

This paper argues, perhaps counterintuitively, that stories about the aftermath of pandemics are versions of the pastoral. Pandemic pastorals are (nearly) void of humanity because they imagine infection leading to the worst-possible conclusion in order to depict the end of civilization from the perspective of someone who knows what life was like before. Because the worst-case scenario is not the end of the story, it provides a contrast that allows the pandemic to operate as a symbol in two complementary ways:

First, the cityscape, denuded of its inhabitants, serves as a diagram of society at its final stage of development. That diagram is synchronic, or frozen in time, and it is read or interpreted by someone who is a product of civilization but who now lives in a post-civilized space. The view of civilization from an outside (but still sophisticated) perspective is central to pastoralism.

Second, the empty city serves as a cordon sanitaire between the vector of infection, which decimates civilization, and the trajectory of the narrative, which constitutes the survivor's tale. This separation is essential because infection, in these narratives, is both a means and a symbol of transmission. The premise here is that language is like a virus when it spreads uncontrollably; indeed, all sorts of social interaction can prove infectious and take on the natural inevitability of disease. Nature (in the form of disease) thus stands in contrast to civilization and emerges as a destructive force within it. The survivor, having passed through infection to the other side, speaks a language that has, in effect, been immunized. He or she stands on the other side of the cordon sanitaire. The pandemic pastoral thus offers a kind of a cure to social ills, but one that comes with a melancholy disclaimer: It is sometimes easier to contemplate the end of civilization than to reform it.

Three Historical Sources

Contemporary pandemic narratives build on biblical tropes and on two secular figures, one historical and the other fictional, who are Job-like in their suffering but not their faith. They also register a secular view of contagion put forth by an eighteenth-century philosophical treatise that helped establish the reformist agenda of pandemic pastoralism.

The historical lone survivor is Squanto, the last of the Patuxet, whom William Bradford mentions appreciatively in his journal of early American colonization, *Of Plymouth Plantation* ([1651] 1981). Squanto survived the decimation of his tribe and could help the Pilgrims colonize the "new world" because he had been kidnapped and transported to Europe before his tribe was infected by disease (probably smallpox transmitted by explorers) (Cook 1997, 255–257). Returning after years of captivity to find his people gone, he taught Bradford and company to live off a land that seemed promised to the Pilgrims because it had already been cultivated (Bradford 1981, 87–91, 98, 108–127). The first generation of colonists, already exposed to smallpox during their childhood, had an immunological advantage over the natives. They interpreted this advantage religiously, taking the landscape, conveniently cleared of its inhabitants, as a judgment from God. Their own offspring, however, were not exposed in childhood and therefore proved susceptible to periodic outbreaks when ships landed carrying the disease. Bradford complained that subsequent generations lacked the religious fervor of the original colonists. Perhaps this had to do with their lack of immunity. In any event, Squanto endures in literature not as a religious but as a secular figure, opening the gates to a pastoral landscape that is half paradise, half wilderness. Versions of this lone survivor would later turn up in Westerns in the figure of the sidekick (Chingachgook, Hiawatha, Tonto): the last member of a vanished race whose role is to introduce white pioneers to native ways (but not to induct them into a native community).

Squanto, like the sidekicks modeled after him, suggests two things about pandemic narratives: 1) that the lone survivor provides a communicative but not a communicable link from the time before the pandemic to the time after, and 2) that the survivor crosses a frontier in time (before and after the plague) that seems to be patterned on the pastoral's frontier in space (civilization and wilderness).

Pandemics create the conditions for the pastoral when empty streets and houses go back to nature and animals start to inhabit dwellings built for people. This was a common theme in landscape painting of the nineteenth century, and one that received renewed attention during the recent lockdowns (Torgovnick 2022). If the deserted landscape suggests a version of the pastoral, pastoralism also provides a useful model for stories in which the end of civilization, which is to say the end of history, does not coincide with the end of time. The pastoral is a setting, but it is also a structuring device, allowing authors to map the frontier in time onto a frontier in space, civilization and its *aftermath* (the empty cityscape) onto the coordinates of civilization and its *other* (the countryside, the wilderness). Another way to put this is that pandemic pastoralism spatializes the end of history as landscape (empty buildings) and personal itinerary (the survivor's path). The end of history is not an apocalypse – it is not the end of the story – but a threshold event that transforms a collective calamity into a symbolic journey. On one side is civilization in its death throes, on the other empty ruins. The lone survivor, in crossing that threshold, moves through and makes sense of the ruins, transposing their significance into a personal – and less complicated – register.

Frank Kermode's ([1967] 2000) observations in *The Sense of an Ending* can serve to sharpen the contrast between the apocalypse and pandemic pastoralism's version of the end of history. Kermode argues that literary narratives "escape from chronicity" by bringing the end of the story in relation to the beginning (50). This is a pattern he usefully characterizes as a weak or naïve apocalypse: narrative is a sequence that doubles back on itself, commenting on its own development (8–18). The end and the beginning stand in symbolic relation to each other in any narrative that is not a mere chronicle of events. Thus, Kermode argues that the apocalyptic structure of narrative is preoccupied with endings in a way that is "time-redeeming" (52). It is my claim that pandemic pastorals offer a partial exception to this rule because they do not redeem the past, which is to say civilization, rather spatialize it as empty landscape. This provides the setting for pastoral simplification.

The First Pandemic Novel

The link between traditional pastoralism and pandemic pastoralism is confirmed by the novel that gives the figure of the lone survivor another moniker – the "last man" – and develops him into a protagonist. Mary Shelley's *The Last Man* ([1826] 1994), the first pandemic novel, takes its title from its catastrophic ending, when a plague wipes out the entire human population with the exception of Verney, a former shepherd who has been civilized by a character (Adrian) modeled on Shelley's recently deceased husband, the poet Percy Bysshe Shelley: "I was an untaught shepherd-boy, when Adrian deigned to confer on me his friendship" (ix, 451). Mary Shelley could have given her hero any vocation. Why a shepherd? I would argue that Verney's idyllic background helps her plot the historical implications of a pandemic onto the spatial dimensions of the pastoral.

In *The Last Man*, time *after* the end of civilization resembles the space *beyond* the boundary of the city insofar as both constitute civilization's other. However, civilization's other is not civilization's opposite. This is evident in the irony that Shelley's child of nature has already been civilized, but only to see all of civilization, including his mentor, perish. He is accompanied by a dog, which will also establish itself as standard trope in post-pandemic literature. The dog's behavior is similarly ironic, which is to say civilized in ways that stand out against the backdrop of the catastrophe:

> My only companion was a dog, a shaggy fellow, half water and half shepherd's dog, whom I found tending sheep in the Campagna. His master was dead, but nevertheless he continued fulfilling his duties in expectation of his return….Riding in the Campagna I had come upon his sheep-walk, and for some time observed his repetition of lessons learned from man, now useless, though unforgotten. (467)

The sheepdog raises an addendum to the previous question about the shepherd: why does Shelly give her survivor a trained dog? The answer seems to lie in the cliché that owners resemble their pets. The last man, as a former shepherd, is like the sheepdog in his connection to rural life and in the persistence of his training. Neither one of them is wild, but both are connected to nature, and their fateful meeting reveals that both have been "civilized" in ways rendered obsolete by the pandemic (but indispensable to its narration). The pandemic puts a stop to history, understood as the story of civilization, but the survivor is a transition figure, bearing witness to the time *before* through his training. Because the narrative places the end of history in the timeline of the plot, it needs a protagonist who can record his memoir (the project is announced in an adjacent paragraph) in the same way the sheepdog herds sheep – performing "lessons learned from man, now useless, though unforgotten."

Here is how Verney describes his motivation to record his memories:

> I also will write a book, I cried – for whom to read? – to whom dedicated? And then with silly flourish (what so capricious and childish as despair?) I wrote,
> DEDICATION
> TO THE ILLUSTRIOUS DEAD.
> SHADOWS, ARISE, AND READ YOUR FALL!
> BEHOLD THE HISTORY OF THE
> LAST MAN. (466)

The irony here, implicit in the apostrophe "arise, and read your fall," is related to the other ironies structuring the narrative. The child of nature is civilized to witness the end of civilization in the same way the sheepdog is trained to herd sheep for no master and the dead are invoked to read of their own demise.

Verney pretends to address the dead here, but it is really Shelley addressing her readers. The "lessons learned from man" are not useless, but their currency must be denied (by the narrative) to transmit the emotional intensity of Verney's predicament. We apprehend the poignancy of survivor's emotions by pretending not to be his audience. This enables the pretense of a lyrical mode of communication that consists of the survivor talking to himself. This peculiar mode of address personalizes history by traversing the threshold of extinction, transforming the fate of civilization into a personal lament that, once again, cannot find a receptive public in the story world if it is to have any emotional impact on its actual readers.

Herein lies the difference between the time-redeeming function of the naïve apocalypse and the simplification strategy of the pastoral. The pandemic pastoral limits the communicability of disease by pushing it to the nth-degree, with one exception. Readers are not a part of the survivor's immediate community and therefore do not catch what he or she transmits; but we do learn from his knowledge (Squanto) or apprehend his emotions (Verney). The difference here is between contagion and communication. If, as I will argue in a moment, the pandemic represents a social ill, the "cure" involves a shift in register from the communal/communicative to the non-communicable and personal.

Pandemics and the Ruined Cityscape

As I already mentioned, pandemics create the conditions for pastoral when nature begins to push through cracks in the sidewalk and wear away the edges of the urban grid. The reverse is also the case. Empty ruins seem to evoke the specter of the plague, a mode of destruction that – unlike earthquakes or war – leaves infrastructure largely intact. A decisive text here is Constantin Volney's *Les Ruines, or Meditations on Revolutions and Empires* (1789), a philosophical treatise in which the author, contemplating the ruins of ancient civilization on the banks of the Euphrates, sinks into a pastoral reverie: "The shepherds had led the camels to their stalls," Volney remarks, before observing that deer now inhabit the former palaces of kings (2). The pastoral setting having been established, the narrator is visited by a "Phantom" or "Genius" who explains that human beings are responsible for the downfall of civilization. This sounds like divine judgment, but the Phantom emerges to explain that humans bring about their own demise. The plague is not a divine scourge but the symbol of a social ill. A standard translation provides this phrasing for Chapter 8, "The Sources of Evil in Society": "Thus that very principle of self-love, which, when restrained within the limits of prudence, was a source of improvement and felicity, became transformed...into a contagious poison....Yes, ignorance and the love of accumulation, these are the two sources of all the plagues that infest the life of man!" (20) Other translations substitute different words for "contagion" and "plague"; nevertheless, Volney seems to have played a role in forging the symbolic link between destructive human interaction and contagion. His book was extraordinarily influential – so much so that Thomas Jefferson translated all but four chapters before becoming President of the United States, then handed the rest of the job over to the poet and diplomat Joel Barlow. Significantly, Volney's *Ruins* is one of the books read by the Frankenstein monster in the novel Mary Shelley published before *The Last Man*. The monster is also a kind of lone survivor.

Volney's conceit reflects some basic assumptions of Enlightenment medical and political thinking. The countryside was safer than the city in plague times, and when the "state of nature," that common postulate of social contract theory, did not provide clear guidelines about how to improve society, it at least created an imaginary escape hatch and a conceptual baseline from which to contemplate social decay. Volney's treatise helped transform these principles into the formal conventions of pandemic pastoralism. In the story he tells of the rise and fall of civilizations, contagion serves as a metaphor of society gone awry but also as the threshold event producing the conditions necessary for a simpler life. There is thus a homeopathic element to pandemic pastoralism, with sickness representing the problem but also leading to a kind of a cure. That cure is conceptual: neither Volney, nor the other authors considered here seriously proposes depopulation as a corrective to social ills. They are not Malthusian. The empty landscape is a thought experiment whose point is not the end of civilization but a change in perspective from the historical to the personal. Volney's narrator is not infected by the self-love he ascribes to most of mankind; he is simply alone with his "Genius."

Pastoral Simplification

If sickness is a symbol of social ills, both isolation and spatialization are simplification strategies that limit its spread (compare Gessner 2013, 227–228; Kimpel 2013, 205). Simplification is a key element of the pastoral, which presents an alternative to the complexity of civilization, not because it is natural but because it is cultured in a straightforward way. As William Empson ([1935] 1974) puts it in his classic study, "The essential trick of the old pastoral...was to make simple people express strong feelings (felt as the most universal subject, something fundamentally true about everybody) in learned and fashionable language (so that you wrote about the best subject in the best way)" (11). He summarizes this as "the pastoral process of putting the complex into the simple" – a formula adapted by Leo Marx in his classic study of

American pastorals, *The Machine in the Garden* (Empson 1974, 22; Marx, 1967, 4–11). The shepherds living an idealized rural life are simple but not primitive; they speak the sophisticated language of the court (or in Marx are cognizant of the latest technological developments) for a cultivated audience. Empson terms this "the use of heroic language about the pastoral swain" (69). If Leo Marx is right in claiming that nature has always served as an American cultural ideal, then the city decimated by a pandemic (for instance in Charles Brockden Brown's *Arthur Mervyn*) is its recurring nightmare (Marx 1967, 4). The lone survivor, because of his isolation, is the swain of the secular apocalypse. His language is sophisticated, as is his knowledge, but the setting he inhabits has been simplified through depopulation.

There is a moralistic side to pandemic pastoralism. Susan Sontag famously cautions against treating illness as a metaphor *because* it leads to moralizing: "So indispensable has been the plague metaphor in bringing summary judgments about social crisis that its use hardly abated during the era when collective diseases were no longer treated so moralistically…." (Sontag 1991, 142). The point is well taken: from a medical perspective, disease is not a symbol but a pathology; it does not call for allegory but for diagnosis and treatment. Nevertheless, the *communicability* of disease seems to evoke some of the dangers inherent in *community* and *communication*. Sontag draws attention to this with the phrase "language is a virus" (153). Today we speak in a similar way of messages or videos "going viral."

In approaching illness as a metaphor for communication spreading out of control, it is important to recall that *communicable* diseases and *communicative* symbols circulate in different ways. Diseases thrive in tightly packed populations and tend to collapse society into a biomass; communication is structured and mediated in ways that facilitate the transmission of messages over distance. That we can read about diseases without catching them is one obvious result of this difference. The pastoral setting in which a survivor is no longer contagious because he or she is alone, is the fictional expression of the basic fact of publication and the media: communication is not the same as physical contact.

Two Limit Cases

Even a brief literary history of American contagion has to include Poe, but his stories are the exceptions that prove the rule. Poe denies any distance between contagion and communication, symptom and symbol, and hence closes off the space of the pastoral. The pandemic tales "King Pest: A Tale Containing an Allegory" ([1835] 1990a) and "The Masque of the Red Death" ([1842] 1990b) establish some of the conventions of pandemic narratives, but they either feature no survivor or a survivor who is not alone. They refuse to treat the pandemic as a threshold event, instead representing sickness as an allegory of social control or its opposite, anarchy.

"King Pest" is a story about escaping sickness by disobeying authority. "The Masque of the Red Death" sees in authority a cure that is that is just as bad as the disease. In the first tale, symptoms are mere symbols to be ignored in the spirit of anarchy; in the second, symbols are symptoms that, through a kind of sympathetic magic, produce the disease they are supposed to prevent. Like the authors who will follow, Poe uses the pandemic to project a simplified version of society, but he does not posit anything beyond or after civilization. The end of history is the end of time, not because of some final judgment – there is simply no difference between contagion and communication in Poe, no way to transform the end of history into the beginning of a story.

In "King Pest" two drunken sailors on shore leave in fourteenth-century London duck into the quarantined section of a city (these are the plague years) to avoid paying their bar tab, thus shirking their debt and disobeying the edict of the king – an act of insubordination that is punishable by death (Poe 1990a, 297). The irony is that one kind of death (sickness) seems to be the only alternative to the other (execution). The power of the king is not so different from the power of disease.

After making their way through a nightmare landscape of the dead and dying, the sailors encounter another ruler – the eponymous King Pest – who seems to be a nightmare version of the actual sovereign. He welcomes them to his drinking party on the condition that they consume a gallon of liquor "on bended knees" while toasting "to the prosperity of our kingdom" (301). True to their roguish nature, the sailors refuse to pay deference to any form of authority, defeating King Pest and his ghoulish court after refusing to "drin[k] the health of the Devil" and asking God to "assoilzie" or forgive their debts (302). The archaic word links injustice to infection and both to all forms of control. King Pest is the doppelgänger of the king who quarantines an entire section of the city and punishes disobedience with death. He is also a version of the devil or the grim reaper. This doubling, which suggests all power is satanic, is the story's major structuring device and what distinguishes it from the pandemic pastoral. There is no space *beyond* the frontier – the quarantined section of the city is the mirror image of the social world – and no time *after*. The contagion does not produce an alternate vision of a simpler life; it simply reveals power structures for what they are: a form of disease.

All of King Pest's ghoulish companions, who bear the word "pest" in their names, have deformed limbs or exaggerated physical characteristics, symbolizing the symptoms of various ailments. Ana-Pest, a woman whose beauty is marred by a syphilitic nose, is the king's consort. After defeating King Pest, the sailors kidnap her and escape back to the non-quarantined side of the city, acquiring a principle of aesthetic composition (anapest is the name of a poetic meter) and, one suspects, spreading the disease. The sailors, however, seem to be immune, and the characteristics of the lone survivor are distributed between the comic duo, who are like the comedians Laurel and Hardy in their complementary physical characteristics and temperaments (one fat and short, the other skinny and tall; one phlegmatic, the other hectic [296]). This is another form of doubling – one that prevents any kind of sympathy or identification with a main character and hence blocks the personal register that is built into pandemic pastoralism. The point of Poe's story is not to translate contagion into an emotion that the readers can apprehend. On the contrary, the antics of the sailors suggest that symptoms, properly regarded, are merely symbols without the power to do "real" harm. They can be ignored in the same way the sailors ignore their debt, the King of England, his quarantine, and King Pest, whom they accuse of being nothing but a ham actor (302).

If symptoms are merely symbols, and authority is just a performance, then health and justice lie in anarchy. The roguish sailors thus personify a libertarian rejection of public health measures: language is not a virus, but virus is merely language, or in today's parlance, fake news. Again, Poe's short story deploys most of the elements of a pastoral without qualifying as such because there is no *after* the pandemic, no other side of the frontier (here the *cordon sanitaire*) – both are just "allegorical" (to use Poe's term in the title) extensions of life under a sovereign monarch who views all disobedience as "treason" (302).

"The Masque of the Red Death" constitutes a volte-face in Poe's assessment of the relation of symbols to symptoms, but one confirming his distrust of authority. The source seems to be a Heinrich Heine story about a super-spreader event in Paris in the early nineteenth century. Perhaps the death toll made Poe reconsider his earlier fantasy about simply ignoring a pandemic. It is also worth noting that Poe wrote this story at a time when his wife was sick and he was financially strapped (O'Grady 2020).

In this short story, symbols *are* symptoms, and the attempt to totally exclude disease – in art and by decree – merely reproduces it as a social ill. The ruler is named Prospero, after the magician-duke from Shakespeare's *Tempest*, and when the plague strikes his dominion, he retreats into a sealed fortress with his court. Like his namesake, Prospero uses art to magically create a world apart. He exercises absolute political and cultural control, and his zero-plague policy seems at first to be effective. He throws a costume ball to celebrate his victory over the disease – prematurely it turns out (Poe 1990b, 461). The color-coded rooms in his palace follow an elaborate design that turns red and black in the final chamber – the very colors that the "red death" inflicts upon its victims. Prospero's taste is decadent, but it also suggests a link between art and magic (the black art). The authoritarian ruler is thus a figure of the author who seeks to ward off sickness through symbolic means: the "anapest" of the sailors has become the art-for-art's-sake style Poe called "arabesque" ("King Pest" appeared in the collection *Tales of the Grotesque and Arabesque* [1840]). When an uninvited guest dressed as a plague victim makes his way to the final chamber, it is difficult to distinguish his hue from the effects of Prospero's décor (462). Prospero is outraged at the hint of actual disease at his costume party. He unmasks the intruder in front of his shocked guests, only to find no face, no body beneath the bloody shroud.

This is the moment the contagion spreads, wiping out everyone in the fortress. The climax evokes a pre-epidemiological understanding of disease, where the pathogen is indistinguishable from its symptoms. (The masque or ball is not a virus, but a virus, insofar as it manifests itself through symptoms, always wears a mask [461].) It also suggests that symbolic attempts to control symptoms, here evoking the colors of the disease to magically ward off its ill effects, are futile. There is no escape, which means there is no survivor – the "mask" conceals nobody and nobody survives to tell this tale (unless the narrator is Death itself [464]). This story subverts pastoralism, canceling the temporal and spatial distinction between civilization and its other (civilization is just another name for sovereign power, and Death is the ultimate ruler). There is no *outside* or *after*: "And Darkness and Decay and the Red Death held illimitable dominion over all" (464).

These two stories are not pastorals but they stake out the generic limits of pandemic pastoralism. Their fairy tale-style effects a related symbolic strategy – one patterned on the schematic description of culture rather than an escape, over the threshold of disease, to a simplified cultural landscape. Poe's decidedly non-idyllic approach to disease helps establish the personal attributes of the lone survivor, whose character establishes a relation of communication to communicability. When symptoms turn out to be mere symbols, survivors triumph heroically over disease by simply ignoring it. When symbols are symptoms, which is to say when culture is sick, there is no aesthetic space of resistance and characterization approaches the point where the face disappears behind the mask. Both tales are skeptical of social and cultural attempts to control disease, and both caution against decadence, i.e., escaping the ills of civilization through art, which is presented as the pendant to despotism. The fairy tale quality of the stories, set in antique times and places, distinguishes them from the other narratives in this study, which employ the techniques of the pastoral to simplify and draw attention to particular features of actually existing society.

Three Case Studies: London, Porter, Matheson

By collapsing the distance between symbol and symptom, and closing off the possibility that the world *after* is different from that of the plague, Poe closes off the space of the pastoral. His stories are allegories of control, not narratives of threshold events. The other authors in this study use the threshold event of the pandemic to shift the register from social problems to personal journeys through simplified space. The problems symbolized by imaginary pandemics include the savagery of civilization in Jack London ([1912] 2018); wartime propaganda and groupthink in

Katherine Anne Porter (1939); and racism in Richard Matheson (1954). It is my argument that while the problems depicted in pandemic pastorals change over time, the formal characteristics remain consistent.

Jack London: "The Scarlet Plague"

Jack London's "The Scarlet Plague" ([1912] 2018), which alludes to Poe's "Red Death" in the title, is set in 2073, about half a century after a pandemic decimates the planet. Narrated by a former Berkeley English professor once known as James Smith but now called Granser, it traces the collapse of civilization into a few remaining hunter-gatherer tribes whose members are ignorant of their history (London 2018, 27, 34). This reversion-to-the-primitive is a common theme in London, who is best known for stories about dogs who turn out to be wolves beneath the skin. In this novella it is not the cultivated who survive, with the lone exception of Granser, but those who can thrive in a world where life is nasty, brutish, and short. The lesson of the pandemic is that men are wolves to men; its corollary is that civilization makes them so:

> And I knew, now, why it was that the fleeing persons I encountered slipped along so furtively and with such white faces. In the midst of our civilization, down in our slums and labor-ghettos, we had bred a race of barbarians, of savages; and now, in the time of our calamity, they turned upon us like the wild beasts they were and destroyed us. And they destroyed themselves as well. (85)

Though the "whiteness" of these faces will turn out to be significant, Granser is partially exaggerating for dramatic effect. Civilization produces savagery, but the savages do not destroy themselves. His own grandsons are primitive, and gleefully so: "the boys were true savages" (15). This is one of many hints that the relation between civilization and savagery is more complex than meets the eye. Indeed, invisibility turns out to be the key issue distinguishing civilization from savagery, and later good savagery from bad savagery. Civilization is complex because it masks power. In the savage state, on the other side of the pandemic, power is obvious and what is invisible does not exist. At least that is what the savages think.

Granser, who has witnessed the fall of civilization, is more knowledgeable than the primitives who are his immediate and unreceptive audience. When his grandsons unearth an old coin, he tries to help them understand money, numbers, and letters, but the young savages complain he is "always making believe them little marks mean something" (9). The irony of course is that these are the same little marks that must be decoded by the reader if the story is to make any sense (and by the author if he is to profit from his writing). We have already seen a similar kind of irony in "the last man's" invocation of his presumably dead audience.

Granser, as storyteller, finds himself in the thankless position of trying to make the savages believe what they cannot see; besides the value of the coin, this includes "wireless dispatches" (55), flying machines, and the germs that destroyed civilization and rendered technological innovation immaterial (42). His grandsons categorically refuse to believe in the meaning behind writing, the germs behind disease, or the history behind the present moment (43). Their serial refusals, like Granser's repeated frustrations, suggests that invisible forces – the forced concealed by civilization and those responsible for its destruction – are London's point. These are the forces of communication and contagion, both of which are noticeable primarily in their effects. Germs circulate in densely populated regions and communication over great distances, but they are both linked to the growth of civilization. Granser puts it like this: "The easier it was to get food, the more men there were; the more men there were, the more thickly were they packed together on the earth; and the more thickly they were packed, the more new kinds of germs became disease" (50). He goes on to link population density with communication, for instance in this passage that recalls speaking on the "wireless": "We talked through the air in those days, thousands and thousands of miles" (55).

The link between communication and contagion turns out to be the key problem in the time preceding the pandemic. Communicating over distance depends on the technological advancements that make increases in population density – and disease susceptibility – inevitable. How to separate the two in a way that retains the value of coins – and literature – without leading to their bankruptcy? This is where the pandemic comes in as a threshold event. The pastoral state following the collapse of civilization allows London to experiment with a kind of communication that is immediate in its oral register but ironic for his readers. The experiment leads to mixed results. By the end of the novella Granser is predicting the emergence of a society (like ours, only different) that does not contain the seeds of its own dissolution. However, he is frustrated by his audience's inability to follow his train of thought, and this begs the question of how the savages, his grandsons, will ever advance from their primitive state.

To see how London uses the pandemic to separate communication from contagion, it is important to recognize how irony works in the novella. London depends on irony to convey both the accuracy of Granser's knowledge and its irrelevance in his immediate context. The author is clearly on the side of the English professor when he laments the limited vocabulary (and knowledge) of his degenerate grandsons. The title of the novella and its main character both call the plague "scarlet," though the boys make a point of adopting the more straightforward "red." The simpler word is favored by the chief of the tribe, a former chauffeur who establishes his power by taking the daughter of his former boss as his wife and later murdering her – an injustice Granser never stops lamenting (23–24). The boys may be right to adapt their vocabularies to their context, but they are right in a way that reveals Granser also has a point – a point they cannot see because the significance of his tale, like the other invisibilities, is hidden.

The chauffeurs of the post-pandemic world are literally in the driver's seat, but if they present a savage alternative to a world governed by the wealthy and the cultured, they also embody its hidden principle. London has Granser explain that the last American president, Morgan the Fifth, was appointed by a Board of Magnates (10). This anti-democratic "election" reflects the author's conviction – one shared by many Social Darwinists of his generation – that the strongest members of society always prevail. When a plague wipes out civilization, the strongest are no longer the richest but those with the biggest muscles and the fewest scruples about using them. Is the post-pandemic world less unjust? It is certainly less cultivated, which is to say more straightforward in its privileging of naked power. Granser is unhappy in this world, but it is London's customary literary terrain. The author, who was a bestseller, is like Granser in his interest in symbols and money, but he is known for stories that predict the end of civilization and "call" domesticated creatures back to the "wild." He is the swain of the secular apocalypse, the sophisticate hiding behind pastoral simplicity.

London is aware of this second-order irony. He inserts his name into the novel as a plot device, for instance when the major cities cut off communication rather than broadcast their collapse, "not permitting the word to go forth to the rest of the world that London had the plague" (56). In what sense might *Jack* London be said to have the plague? Perhaps his stories about the end of civilization do more than diagnose a problem. Perhaps they also spread the disease. London serialized his novella in *London Magazine* at a time when his career seemed to be waning. The location named in the title is more than a setting, it is also an admission, on the part of the author, that – like a modern-day prepper – he may be trafficking in the collapse of the civilization on which he depends for his audience. Granser laments a civilization that breeds its own destroyers; London made his living by popularizing the barbarian creed.

Predicting the victory of savages in a language and through a medium they cannot read, London aligns himself with Granser, but also with a group of deceivers who make a surprise appearance at the end: the medicine men. Just as London distinguishes between contagion and communication, he distinguishes between those who diagnose disease and those who try to explain it away. The ultimate irony of the novella is when Granser calls for the death of doctors: "The doctors must be destroyed," he says in an uncharacteristic call for violence, "and all that was lost must be discovered over again" (144). Here he does not mean the scientists who discovered germs before the pandemic but the medicine men who call themselves doctors afterward. They sell spells and fetish objects that cannot cure anything. Is an author closer to a doctor or a witch doctor? Does he traffic in mere symbols or in actual cures? London diagnoses the sickness, but he does not want to be understood as deceiving the readers (or customers) who buy his symbolic objects/tales.

It is difficult for him to defend himself against an accusation that he raises. He does so by placing himself on the side of a simplified civilization that has purged itself of bad savagery and deception while retaining the good, simple life. This depends on distinguishing identification (the personal, which in this case will turn out to be the racial) from contagion (the cultural or communal). Near the end of the novel, Granser makes another surprise announcement, predicting (out of the blue) that "Aryans" will someday dominate the world again: "In time, pressure of population will compel us to spread out, and a hundred generations from now we may expect our descendants…[to engage in] colonization of the East – a new Aryan drift around the world" (142). This racist endorsement of white supremacy is hidden until the end, but it is the simplification London turns to in order to straighten out all the ironies that have been deviling both author and narrator since the announcement that civilization breeds its own destruction. While it is unclear how the "Aryan drift" would avoid problems like overcrowding, deception, and manipulation, in London the civilization to come will be superior to the one that has perished. Granser's immediate audience does not believe what he says about invisible things, but they will nevertheless inherit something else that is invisible (in the sense of merely unstated or presumed) in this story: namely, the race of the author and his narrator. The ultimate irony here is that the *whiteness* that is supposed to rise victorious over the plague is what "spreads out" like a virus. The pastoral space between contagion and communication is contaminated by racism. Put otherwise, the plague provides a structure of transmission that allows London to imagine a purified, pastoral society – a society that blames its savagery on the "races" that do not manage cross the frontier of the pandemic, which in this case is identical with the color line. Identification in this novella is not just personal, in the way the readers (like London) are encouraged to identify with the narrator; it is a matter of group identity.

The novella remains true to the paradox, common in the pastoral, of a sophisticated author calling for the simple life, but with a violent twist: "Ten thousand years of culture and civilization passed in the twinkling of an eye, 'lapsed like foam'" (71). The apocalyptic quality of "The Scarlet Plague" may have contributed to the legend – false as it turns out – that when London died a couple of years later, suicide was the cause (the actual cause was kidney failure). The despair evident in Granser's lament might be interpreted as personal resignation writ large. However, it is also a survival-of-the-fittest parable that works to distinguish good authorship from bad medicine men and good savages from, alas, "inferior" races. Blackness is ultimately what is invisible here, concealed behind the red faces of those who perish by the plague and the pale faces of those who flee a savagery they have created – and then go on to conquer the world.

Katherine Anne Porter: "Pale Horse, Pale Rider"

Katherine Anne Porter's "Pale Horse, Pale Rider" (1939) is a partially autobiographical tale that provides one of the few fictional accounts of the influenza epidemic of 1918 (it also uses the symptom of paleness to symbolize race – something I will return to in a moment). Porter takes advantage of the conjunction of the epidemic and the war to treat contagion as a symbol of patriotism and pro-war propaganda. The main character Miranda, who is a stand-in for the author, begins to experience flu symptoms when the audience at a concert is encouraged to stand up and sing a patriotic song (Porter 1939, 188). The germs prove to be catchier than the tune. At first, she thinks her headache is the result of exasperation. She is tired of being plagued by patriots, such as the men at work (a local Denver newspaper) pressing her to buy Liberty Bonds, even though her salary has been cut (189). The Liberty Bond salesmen are described as having connections to the Lusk Committee (183, 207). Charged with investigating seditious (meaning communist or anarchist) activities, the committee was formed on the heels of WWI (in 1919) – and in New York, not Denver. This anachronistic detail serves to expand the symbolic resonance of the plot. Porter seems to be recounting her experiences during WWI (she worked at a Denver newspaper and almost died from influenza) to reflect her discomfort with the resurgence of patriotism right before WWII (the story was published in 1939). She would later write patriotic, or at least anti-German stories such as *The Leaning Tower*. But this particular novella echoes the sentiments of the character who asks, "Suppose I said to hell with this filthy war?" (186)

The question is rhetorical, but it is voiced for the benefit of Adam, the soldier who is Miranda's love interest. Adam is loyal and willing to serve his country but hardly more patriotic than his beloved. His ironic rejoinder, that there won't be any more wars after this one, echoes her skepticism while undermining Woodrow Wilson's rationale for sending troops to the war that was supposed to end all wars (201, 222–223). The private affinity between these two characters stands in stark contrast to the public sentiment of patriotism. At one level the story offers a clear endorsement of love over war. There are even asides, such as a rumor that a German submarine is spreading influenza germs on the coast, intended to show how the paranoia caused by warfare turns all public discourse infectious (206).

However, contagion is an ambiguous metaphor, describing how feelings circulate (for instance through patriotism) in the public sphere but also how they pass from one lover to another in private. Porter underscores the ambiguity by strategically invoking made-up blues songs and spirituals, which bring a seemingly gratuitous racial dimension to the narrative. There is the title of the story, supposedly derived from a spiritual that does not exist, and then a refrain, invoked by Miranda, which also has a false derivation: "The blues aint nothin' but an easy-goin' heart disease" (218). Porter seems to be invoking blackness as a symbol for love and death, in short, for moments of passion in the affective but also existential sense, that threaten to subsume the individual into the beloved, the collective, or (as I will argue in a moment) the land of the dead. Porter's main point, however, is not about race, which is here fetishized as a cultural artifact and appropriated as a symbol of personal (and white) precarity. It is that patriotism and passion are both catching, so that turning to love as a refuge from war merely leads to bereavement. This is foreshadowed in the opening dream-sequence when Miranda imagines death as a pale suitor on a pale horse: "Ah, I have seen this fellow before. I know this man if I could place him. He is no stranger to me" (181).

Miranda demurs the date with the pale rider, but she goes out with Adam. The two male figures seem to become interchangeable at the end. When Miranda comes down with the flu at the concert they both attend, Adam nurses her until she is taken to an infirmary. Waking up after a close brush with death, she finds out that he has died of the flu after having been shipped overseas. The flu she catches at a patriotic event infects the lover who saves her from sickness and groupthink. Porter underscores the horrible irony with another dream sequence that shows Adam to be a "sacrificial lamb," as Miranda calls him (224). A conversation about protestant and Catholic prayer culminates in Miranda's incongruous pagan offering to "O Apollo" (239). Then, right after a discussion of the fake eponymous spiritual, which Adam claims to have "heard Negroes in Texas sing" (240), the two characters declare their love for one another, and Miranda falls into a troubled sleep:

> Almost with no warning at all, she floated into the darkness, holding his hand, in sleep that was not sleep but clear evening light...arrows from the invisible bow struck him again and he fell, and yet he was there before her untouched in a perpetual death and resurrection. She threw herself before him...and the arrows struck her cleanly through the heart and through his body and he lay dead, and she still lived. (243)

When she wakes up, she describes this dream as "something about an old-fashioned valentine. There were two hearts carved on a tree, pierced by the same arrow – you know, Adam –" (243). This is cupid's arrow but also Apollo's arrow – the god she invoked before. Apollo is the god of healing, but Greek mythology tells that his arrows also transmit the plague. (It is in this sense that Nicholas Christakis borrows the metaphor *Apollo's Arrow* for his 2020 book on the Corona pandemic). The arrows pass through Miranda, who lives, but Adam catches the disease and dies. What is noteworthy is that the arrows only kill him after passing through her, and after the two characters have declared their love. She makes him vulnerable. When Miranda wakes up, she feels alone, in a deep, existential way, with no connection to other people, excepting the notes Adam has left (246). Here Porter opens the space between symbols and symptoms, contagion and communication, in a way typical of pandemic pastoralism and in this case serving to underscore how writing takes the place of actual human connections, both in her own life (she was an avid letter-writer who had trouble maintaining relationships) and in her stories.

Writing and dreams, or writing *as* a dream: there is a sense in which this tale of a lone survivor is also a *Künstlerroman*. Another long dream sequence makes up the end of the novella. It contains Miranda's visit to the land of the dead, which ironically constitutes this novella's pastoral landscape. She knows the inhabitants, just like she recognizes death when he comes calling in the first paragraphs: "They were pure identities....each figure alone but not solitary...[but] something, somebody, was missing, she had lost something...left something unfinished" (254). Though Adam is probably the one who is missing – she has not yet recovered to read the final note and hence does not know that he is dead – the land beyond is a peaceful place where everyone is a lone survivor. This is a kind of a collective but it is not a community or a public – there is no danger of public passion (patriotism) or of private passion (love) because there are no groups or pairs, only "pure identities."

This land of pure, separate identities is preferable to the Armistice, a time of overriding national identity. Miranda experiences a sharp contrast between the two when she awakens from her sickness: "There was no light, there might never be light again, compared as it must always be with the light she had seen beside the blue sea that lay so tranquilly along the shore of her paradise" (259). Next time death comes for her it will be in the avatar of Adam, the stranger whom she recognizes at the beginning but who is still missing in her dream (263–264). Miranda thinks to herself, dreaming of a place that is the next best thing to isolation, "soon I shall cross back and be at home again" (263). Bereaved, she is actually already home, as the last line of the novella suggests: "Now there would be time for everything" (264). Eternity is now, though it is also predicated on a kind of distance or deferral. The pandemic pastoral of isolated "identities" living next to each other, but not with each other, has shown her a model of coexistence that is the opposite of contagion: it is the coexistence of pure communication, which is always predicated on a lack or distance between the word and its object or the word and its audience. The plot confirms her premonition that the joy she experiences with Adam has no future, but that is because it already exists, in a writerly form, in the present; her feelings are "pure poetry" but also "apocryphal" (207). Miranda, a young reporter modeled on her author, is the author of such poetry – poetry that identifies with the outsider status of (fake) spirituals – while keeping her distance from other people. The identity that is racialized in London is individualized in Porter, but in both cases, identification is the antidote to infection and the communal problems represented by race.

Richard Matheson: *I Am Legend*

Richard Matheson's *I Am Legend* (1954) is perhaps the most well-known example of the last survivor legend. There are three filmic adaptations of the science fiction novel, with a sequel reportedly in the works. The first is an Italian production (*The Last Man on Earth* [1964]) starring Vincent Price and partly written by Matheson, who withheld his name from credits because he was dissatisfied with the final product. *Omega Man* (1971), directed by Boris Sagal, is the second adaptation. Starring Charlton Heston and Rosalind Cash and featuring what is reported to be the first interracial Hollywood kiss, it uses depopulation – as W.E.B. Du Bois did in his short story "The Comet" (1920) – as a pretext for interracial romance. The latest version is a film bearing the same name as the novel (2007). Starring African American actor Will Smith, it builds on the racial politics of its predecessor at the level of casting rather than theme.

Racism is the problem evoked by a pandemic that destroys most of the earth's population. As the previous examples suggest, race almost always plays a role in US-American pandemic fiction because the conflict between the promise of equality and the fact of discrimination is simply too egregious to ignore. Before discussing the link between contagion and racism, I want to point out that Matheson borrows other elements from his predecessors such as the pet dog (from Shelley) and a fake musical allusion (as in Porter). The death of the dog – also a key element in the filmic versions – leaves the main character, Robert Neville, feeling lonesome and receptive to the advances of a woman who is infected in the novel and the first film, and who is Black in *Omega Man*. The implication seems to be that vectors of emotion, like vectors of infection, cross all sorts of boundaries: those between species, social groups, and of course between the infected and the healthy. The fake symphony, attributed to the fictional Roger Leie, is called *The Year of the Plague* (Matheson 1954, 8). The shift in medium involved in ekphrasis involves another form of boundary crossing or contagion.

In composing *his* account of the plague years, Matheson clearly taps into an established set of pandemic conventions; what he adds to them is the gothic convention of the undead. In *I Am Legend*, infection turns its victims into vampires. Some of them are reduced to biological shells – more like zombies or automatons, really – who are driven to behave in predictable ways by the virus that takes over their bodies; others develop into a new "race" who learn to manage symptoms, such as sensitivity to the light and an intolerance for garlic, through adaptation and treatment. Neville does not grasp the difference between the two types of vampires until the end of the novel. For the bulk of the narrative, he spends his days killing the infected and looking for a cure that might bring some of them back to the land of the living.

When Neville hides at night the less sophisticated vampires turn the tables, mindlessly attacking his fortified house (always in the same way) and trying to lure him outside. For automatons they are good at triggering his emotions. One of the attackers is his former friend, Ben Cortman, who seems to be happier now that he is dead (108). Neville, however, is especially susceptible to the women because "[a]ll the knowledge in those books [he spends a lot of time reading] couldn't put out the fires in him; all the words of centuries couldn't end the wordless, mindless craving of his flesh" (7). As the remark about "mindless, craving...flesh" suggests, Neville's sexual desire turns him into a kind of a zombie as well.

The reading helps Neville maintain self-control, but it is also part of his effort to solve, through research, the problem of vampirism. When not fighting, drinking whisky, listening to his hi-fi system, or fantasizing about vampire women, Neville attempts to separate legend from science in order to rationally explain the vampires' behavior (106). Here he is fighting centuries of superstition: "According to legend, they were invisible in mirrors, but he knew that was untrue" (16; 17). He also has to resist the religious hysteria that reaches its peak at the height of the pandemic (103), and the "yellow journalism [that] had spread a cancerous dread of vampires to all corners of the nation" in "pseudo-scientific articles" (105). Matheson is about as convincing at distinguishing Neville's findings from pseudo-science as London is at distinguishing Granser from the witch doctors. Neville "discovers" that while the vampire germ makes its victims sensitive to sunlight and garlic (two elements of the Dracula legend), their fear of the cross is just a bit of residual psychology left over from the legends the victims were familiar with when they were alive. Ben Cortman, raised Jewish, is sensitive to the Torah instead of the cross, as Neville tells Ruth, the woman he meets about halfway through the narrative: "A torah. Tablet of law, I believe it is....By using the torah, I backed him to the door and got rid of him" (129).

In his absurd struggle to uphold rationalism in the face of a vampire infestation, Neville shows himself to be deeply irrational: not only because some of the plot details could have been borrowed from Polanski's *Fearless Vampire Killers* (a Jewish vampire afraid of the Torah!), but because he has been deeply traumatized by his experiences. After he burns the body of his dead daughter in a firepit meant to limit the spread of contagion, all the infected children look like Kathy to him (15). He buries his wife Virginia, who then came back from the grave and has to be killed again – this time with a wooden stake (66, 138). The double murder/death of wife and daughter traps him in a chaos that he describes in terms of another pit, a pit of dualisms: "everything in the world seemed suddenly to have dropped into a pit of duality, victim to a system of twos" (65). The pit of duality also applies to the vampires, who are themselves split into two types, visible in mirrors, and mirroring Neville in their behavior. His speculations about traumatic "shocks" suffered by vampires might be justly applied to his own psychological state: "It could make them lonely, soul-lost slaves of the night, afraid to approach anyone, living a solitary existence, often seeking from the soil of their native land, struggling to gain a sense of communion with something, with anything" (105, 106; cf. 107).

For Neville the communion (holy or unholy) comes when a ghost seems to rise from Virginia's grave. It is Ruth, who later turns out to be a vampire, though she has hidden her ghostly pallor under dark make-up that is in effect a form of blackface (110, 125). When Ruth's identity becomes clear, she will warn Neville to abandon his home to avoid an organized attack from her compatriot members of the "new" race, but he remains stubbornly rooted – like the undead surrounding his house and with fatal consequences. The irrational attachment to place is underscored by an irrational attachment to the past that becomes clear when, prior to Ruth's revelation, Neville briefly considers marrying her and having children (128) and then calls her by his dead wife's name: "And he'd thought the past was dead. How long did it take for a past to die?" (137).

The past does not die in a novel about the undead. That is the point of the gothic convention. Neville's past haunts him, despite his efforts to remain rational, in the form of the revenant Ruth. The protagonist feels guilty for killing his own wife and child. Ruth makes him question his murderous rage and his so-called rationality, particularly when she reveals that the infected are still cognizant and that he has killed her husband and children in one of his rampages (135). The pandemic in this novel is a symbol of social conflict, as in London and Porter, but the conflict bears the stamp of its historical moment. The infected are racialized, though Ruth's blackface suggests this is a bit of a disguise, and Neville, whom Ruth later dubs "the last of the old race," is the quintessential angry white man, heavily armed, drunk on whisky, and driving around town in the precursor to an SUV (157).

I Am Legend was published the same year the Supreme Court handed down its ruling on *Brown vs. Board of Education* (a case that started making its way through the courts in 1951), at a time when interracial relationships were still illegal in some states. Neville picks up on the racialized language of the period when he describes the vampire question in the opening pages of the novel: "Friends, I come before you to discuss the vampire; a minority element if there ever was one, and there was one...Vampires are prejudiced against. The keynote of minority prejudice is this: They are loathed because they are feared...but, would you let your sister marry one?" (20–21). In considering the marriage question, which takes on a literal if short-lived significance in his relationship with Ruth, Neville confronts his own ghosts but also the ghost of racism, which despite the Supreme Court ruling, remained (and remains) undead.

If the gothic conventions evoke a chaos of dual (really multiple) hauntings, the pandemic works to simplify social conflict in ways typical of the pastoral. Because the vampire-hunting plot is in some ways more violent than death by contagion (though London may be an exception here), this pastoral is not only about inhabiting an empty cityscape but about emptying it – by killing the undead and disposing of their remains. While this might seem to stretch the meaning of pastoralism beyond the point of usefulness, the narrative does register the need to open a space between contagion and communication in the way we have seen in London and Porter. In Matheson, it is the firepit that offers an official antidote to the metaphorical "pit of duality": "Everyone without exception had to be transported to the fires immediately upon death. It was the only way they knew now to prevent communication. Only flames could destroy the bacteria that caused the plague" (62). Burning the bodies, thus, is not a form of pastoralism, but it is supposed to lead to the time *after*, where the infection has marked the landscape but is no longer raging. Two forms of communication come into play in this passage: the communication or contagion of the disease, and the communication of the official decree (Neville's own narrative, of course, is another form of communication). As official policy, the communication fails, as do Neville's efforts to uphold reason and restore the old order. He throws his daughter into the burning pit but not his wife, but it does not make any difference either way. The plague spreads, pseudo-science contaminates rationalism, mercy killing mutates into murder, and Neville's longing for his wife crosses the *cordon sanitaire* into necrophilia, or desire for the undead, which is troped as interracial desire. In short, communication collapses into contagion, which is why the lone survivor has to die, in spite of his bacteriological immunity.

But in dying Neville turns into a *legend* – and not only because he is more susceptible to legends and superstitions than he wants to be. The title *I Am Legend*, almost a posthumous utterance, is voiced by the protagonist as he lays dying in a jail cell – they are the final words of the novel. He has been captured by Ruth's compatriots – those who have been infected but have learned to live with the disease. She gives him a suicide pill so he can avoid execution which they see as justice but he understands to be a superstitious act of violence. ("My executioner, he thought, the justice of this new society" [154]). The new society is not more just than its predecessor, but it does need to sacrifice its monsters. Ruth puts it this way in her final words to the man she could have loved, had he not killed her family: "In a way we're like a revolutionary group – repossessing society by violence. It's inevitable. Violence is no stranger to you. You've killed. Many times" (156). Neville hopes the "new people of the earth" will be better, but he knows that is not the case: "Full circle, he thought while the final lethargy crept into his limbs. Full Circle. A new terror born in death, a new superstition entering the unassailable fortress forever" (160).

Sacrificing Neville does not purge the new society of the need for violence. On the contrary, the new people can kill monsters (Neville) and oppress others (their victims are the zombie-like vampires) in the same way Neville's world could believe in vampires and repress racial minorities. The novel devotes nearly three pages to the new people's prolonged murder of his friend Ben Cortman, a gratuitous act of violence prior to their raiding of Neville's house. He resents seeing his friend killed by strangers, and "he felt more deeply toward the vampires than he did toward their executioners" (148–149). That Cortman is Jewish suggests that anti-Semitism sets the social coordinates for other forms of racism in this decade after the Holocaust.

Neville, in seeing his friend killed, finally identifies with the vampires who are his doubles, and we identify with him in his sympathy – especially now that he is a legend, and therefore undead in a different way. At the eponymous and nearly posthumous moment, this novel does follow the conventions of pandemic pastoralism: translating a social problem into the first-person sentiments of "I am" and the city into a diagram of race relations. Identification, at the personal and racial levels, is the alleged antidote to contagion.

Conclusion

I Am Legend brings up an issue that is central to this volume but was only raised intermittently in connection with the narratives analyzed in this essay. That is the issue of injustice. When injustice is systemic in the way that racism is systemic, it spreads beyond individual cases of prejudice and discrimination to infect an entire society.

The narratives explored in this essay represent this kind of systemic injustice as contagion. Poe's stories demonstrate the possible range of symbolic responses to contagion: either the collapse of the entire system into despotism and disease ("The Masque of the Red Death") or denial of the validity of authority ("King Pest"). Neither response offers a solution to the social problem, however, and neither is a pastoral. Pastorals mobilize contagion as a metaphor for social problems, but they push the spread of disease to the point where it becomes a threshold event. The lone survivor crosses the threshold from the time of social contagion to the time after, a time of depopulation, thereby shifting the symbolic register from the communal to the personal. Readers, cut off from the symbolic world of the fiction by a pandemic apocalypse that theoretically would have killed them as well, are asked to identify with the survivor – they do not catch the disease. This shift from the communal/contagious to the personal, usually in the emptied and schematized space of the city, is the essential feature of the pandemic pastoral.

This essay establishes the historical genesis of this feature of pandemic pastoralism, drawing on the writing of early colonists and the work of Mary Shelley and Volney. It then traces the conceptual boundaries of pastoralism through Poe, before providing close readings of three examples from the first half of the twentieth century. Further research would push this genealogy into the second half of the twentieth century. Particularly interesting here is Colson Whitehead's *Zone One* (2011), which uses the zombie-pandemic metaphor to respond Matheson in a way that complicates the connection between race, as a marker of group identity, and the radical individuation – perhaps *atomization* is the better word – characteristic of neoliberal employment practices.

Whitehead's African American protagonist Mark Spitz – mockingly named after the Olympic gold medalist because he cannot swim – escapes numerous encounters with the infected (their bite spreads infection) because when push comes to shove, he is willing to abandon all compatriots and go it alone. This anti-group aversion may be (ironically) post-racial, as the name of the white swimmer suggests. It is also the ultimate expression of pandemic pastoralism. The city is not the space of community for the lone survivor; it is like a diagram frozen in time. Mark Spitz, who often recalls the view of Manhattan from a relative's skyscraper apartment, grasps communicability for what it is: the danger of proximity in any community. The antidote, if that is the right word, is communication purged of all bodily contact; thus, one of Mark Spitz's fellow survivors arranges abandoned cars on the road into patterns she hopes will one day be deciphered from outer space. Pandemic pastorals provide that antidote, but only for readers who agree to engage in a collective fantasy of isolation.

Bibliography

Bradford, William. 1981. *Of Plymouth Plantation*, Random House/Modern Library.

Cook, Sherburne F. 1997. "The Significance of Disease in the Extinction of the New England Indians." *An Expanding World, Vol 26. Biological Consequences of the European Expansion, 1450–1800*, edited by Kenneth F. Kiple and Stephen V. Beck, Ashgate/Variorum, 251–274.

Empson, William. 1974. *Some Versions of Pastoral*, New Directions.

Gessner, Ingrid. 2013. "Contagion, Crisis, and Control: Tracing Yellow Fever in Nineteenth-Century American Literature and Culture." *Communicating Disease: Cultural Representations of American Medicine*, edited by Carmen Birkle and Johanna Heil, Universitätsverlag Winter, 219–242.

Gross, Andrew. 2022. "American Crisis: An Introduction." *New American Studies Journal: A Forum*, vol. 72 (April). http://doi:10.18422/72-01.

Kermode, Frank. 2000. *The Sense of an Ending*, Oxford UP.

Kimpel, Imke. 2013. "'Like Hermits in Holes and Caves.' Isolation as a Narrative Mode for Writing the Plague in Daniel Defoe's *A Journal of the Plague Year 1665*." *Communicating Disease: Cultural Representations of American Medicine*, edited by Carmen Birkle and Johanna Heil, Universitätsverlag Winter, 199–218.

London, Jack. 2018. *The Scarlet Plague*, Seawolf Press.

Marx, Leo. 1967. *The Machine in the Garden: Technology and the Pastoral Ideal in America*, Oxford UP.

Matheson, Richard. 2010. *I Am Legend*, S.F. Masterworks.

O'Grady, Megan. 2020. "What Can We Learn from the Art of Pandemics Past?" *NYT Magazine*, April 8, 2020. https://www.nytimes.com/2020/04/08/t-magazine/art-coronavirus.html.

Poe, Edgar Allan. 1990a. "King Pest." *The Short Fiction of Edgar Allan Poe*, edited by Stuart Levine and Susan Levine, U of Illinois P, 296–303.

Poe, Edgar Allan. 1990b. "The Masque of the Red Death." *The Short Fiction of Edgar Allan Poe*, edited by Stuart Levine and Susan Levine, U of Illinois P, 461–464.
Porter, Katherine Anne. 1939. *Pale Horse, Pale Rider: Three Short Novels*, The Modern Library, 179–264.
Shelley, Mary. 1994. *The Last Man*, edited by Morton D. Paley, Oxford UP.
Sontag, Susan. 1991. *Illness as Metaphor & Aids and its Metaphors*, Penguin.
Torgovnick, Marianna. 2022. "Bomb and Climate Change in Fact and Fiction." *New American Studies Journal: A Forum*, vol. 73 (December). http://doi:10.18422/73-14
Volney, Constantin-François. 1789. *Volney's Ruins, or, A Survey of the Revolutions of Empires*, 3rd edition, J. Johnson, St. Paul's Church-Yard. https://oll.libertyfund.org/title/volney-the-ruins-or-a-survery-of-the-revolutions-of-empires.
Whitehead, Colson. 2011. *Zone One*, Doubleday.

Intertextuality and the Role of the Eyewitness in Plague Descriptions

Giovanni Boccaccio, Daniel Defoe, and Albert Camus

Franziska Meier

Besides wars, natural disasters and famines, epidemics figure most prominently among the disasters that occasionally strike humankind and have therefore become an integral part of our apocalyptic visions. As far as the literary representation of these disasters is concerned, it is hardly surprising that, much more than epidemics or famines war holds an enduring interest for authors whether they describe it in a celebratory or a highly critical way. To some extent, this is due to the simple fact that epidemics do not occur as often as military battles. Moreover, there are special challenges that their description posed to writers throughout the ages. For instance, pandemic situations do not offer many opportunities to praise outstanding heroic individual or group performances – a convention of narrative genres in ancient times; diseases rather seem to beset cities and countries suddenly, striking in an uncontrollable as well as, for a long time, incomprehensible way. It was not until the end of the 19th century that they could finally be somewhat mitigated and contained. Beyond that, epidemic outbreaks attacked and annihilated what is considered to be essential to humankind, in particular the notion of the individual's dignity, the evidence of natural bounds between kins and friends, and the most elementary achievements of civilization: the basic social order and the burial rites an individual was entitled to enjoy.

Beyond the lethal threat, once an epidemic had gained momentum, those who survived and, in the aftermath, took to writing about the events had to face several issues. First, which genre should they select? Epidemics could hardly fit into the traditional narrative genres that usually plotted the adventures of individuals or groups of more or less heroic characters. Unsurprisingly, in the ancient and medieval era, authors fell back on the chronicle style. It took a very long time until epidemics and their outcomes would appear in fictional or novelistic writing.[1] This long-lasting un-

1 This is a question that in my view still awaits to be explored. In a very cautious manner, I would state that whereas Defoe's *Journal of Plague* and Manzoni's *Promessi Sposi* are rightly qualified as "boundary-texts," for different reasons though, Albert Camus is likely to be one of the first

certainty about the adequate genre contributed to the formation of a tradition of its own, a legacy of Western plague writing that stretches from Thucydides' famous depiction in the *History of the Peloponnesian War* to his much later heir, Giovanni Boccaccio, as well as to their modern successors Daniel Defoe, Alessandro Manzoni, and Albert Camus not to name but the most important who figure among the top ten on Western reading lists during the first year of COVID-19. This legacy can be immediately grasped in the high degree of intertextuality that becomes visible in these otherwise very different depictions.[2]

Secondly, how could writers give structure and coherence to what, by its very nature, defied any order? Should they transmit the spreading of the disease to readers from the limited perspective of an individual or rather from the perspective of a detached observer?

Scholars have already acknowledged the use of a first-person narrator or eyewitness in plague depiction, mostly however, without giving further attention to it. The only exception is Jennifer Cooke's book *Legacies of Plague in Literature, Theory and Film*, according to which the first-person narrator is "clearly a fictional device" (Healy, 25–44; Cooke, 31) – an insight she drew from her readings of Daniel Defoe's *Journal of a Plague Year* and, to a lesser extent, from Albert Camus's novel *La Peste*. The device allowed literature to step into the gap that divided the "official account" of history and the personal points of view on what had happened (Cooke, 42). However, even a superficial look at the two major depictions written long before Daniel Defoe's *Journal of a Plague Year* makes us aware of the fact that the figure of an eyewitness can also serve other purposes and is not simply a fictional device to bridge the gap between official historiography and personal histories. Thucydides, for instance, includes a non-fictional eye-witness-passage in his depiction. Therefore, despite many obvious differences between the five major plague narratives discussed here, a comparison may well provide deeper insights into how writers dealt with the issue of being a witness in and of an epidemic.

---

who achieved a novel about a fictitious epidemic. I presume that the modern dystopian novels, probably starting with Mary Shelley's *The Last Man*, lent themselves best to incorporate a plague within a fictional text.

2 The fact that plague depictions highly depend on their predecessors has already been acknowledged; cf. David Steel. 1981. *Plague Writing: From Boccaccio to Camus. Journal of European Studies*, vol. II, 88–110. Jennifer Cooke's monograph *Legacies of Plague* offers a very extreme take on this phenomenon: "There is a logic of contamination at work between plague and the narratives that tell of it. For instance, the role of the parasitic flea in plague outbreaks has as its textual corollary a tendency among plague writers to parasitise (sic!) one another," Jennifer Cook. 2019. *Legacies of Plague in Literature, Theory and Film*, Palgrave Macmillan, 18.

Thucydides and the Body of the Historian

The Greek historian Thucydides includes the description of a plague in Athens in his *History of the Peloponnesian War*, although, as he tells his readers, this horrible event was not really part of this long war. The historian decided to place a summary of the three-year-long plague in the second chapter of the second book, at the moment of its outbreak. More precisely, he positioned his account at a significant point in the *History of the Peloponnesian War*, between the brilliant funeral speech in which Pericles praised the greatness of the Athenian polis in the previous chapter and the death of the same statesman that is mentioned shortly after the plague description.[3]

The admiration which Thucydides's depiction enjoys, conveys an idea of how skillfully the extremely chaotic sequences of the epidemic are brought into a perfectly ordered and highly balanced picture. In the voice of a detached historian, the depiction starts with some chronological and geographical details about the disease's origins and its arrival in Attica. It then focuses on the symptoms and the progression of the disease and, subsequently, to its disastrous impact on social order, laws, and on the achievements of human civilization. Thucydides carefully highlights the extent to which the doctors as well as the city's government had been overpowered by the sudden outbreak of an entirely unknown disease and therefore did not know how to prevent the total breakdown of order and customs.

At the beginning of the *History,* the author had already identified himself as a contemporary of the Peloponnesian war who had immediately assessed its importance. Consequentially, there would be no need to repeat it in this chapter. Interestingly, he nevertheless mentions his personal involvement – in a rather cursory manner – within the highly elaborated, well-structured description of the epidemic's many disturbing aspects and effects on the population. In the second paragraph, he says:

> All speculation as to its origin and its causes, if causes can be found adequate to produce so great a disturbance, I leave to other writers, whether lay or professional; for myself, I shall simply set down its nature, and explain the symptoms by which perhaps it may be recognized by the student, if it should ever break out again. This I can the better do, as I had the disease myself, and watched its operation in the case of others. (Thucydides)[4]

3 According to Karl Reinhardt, by placing the plague between the two scenes Thucydides may have made a tacit critical comment on Pericles' funeral speech. "Thukydides und Machiavelli," Karl Reinhardt. 1966. *Vermächtnis der Antike. Gesammelte Essays zur Philosophie und Geschichtsschreibung*, Vandenhoeck & Ruprecht, 184–218.

4 The English translation by Richard Crawley can be found on http://www.gutenberg.org/files/7142/7142-h/7142-h.htm#link2HCH0007.

In this passage, the first-person singular first refers to the self-understanding of a historian whose principle is not to yield to speculations that cannot be proven by rational arguments. Instead, he claims to stick only to what had actually happened, which in this context means the symptoms of the disease. His aim is not to understand why the disaster had struck the city, but to collect and record as many details of the novel medical signs as possible since nobody had ever heard of them beforehand. His ambition is to alert future generations so that they may be better prepared to fight a similar outbreak. It is only in the last sentence of the passage that the historian turns to his being an eyewitness, or more precisely, a lucky survivor who can testify about the atrocities. Here, the historian who is proudly displaying his objectivity and inner detachment brings into play his body. The emphasis is not so much put on his point of view as on his physical body that suffered from and witnessed the infection and thereby proved the pertinence of the indications. In other words: it is the memory of the sick body which gives major credibility to the account.

Although the historian does not give information about his own recovery from the plague, it is interesting to read what he later states about a behavior specific to all those who were lucky to survive.[5] After having depicted the dehumanizing effects of the plague on the citizens, Thucydides adds:

> Yet it was with those who had recovered from the disease that the sick and the dying found most compassion. These knew what it was from experience, and had now no fear for themselves; for the same man was never attacked twice – never at least fatally. And such persons not only received the congratulations of others, but themselves also, in the elation of the moment, half entertained the vain hope that they were for the future safe from any disease whatsoever. (Thucydides)

Apparently, those who recovered from the infection had not been oppressed by the trauma of having survived. On the contrary, they stood out among their compatriots for their enhanced moral fortitude in the face of the plague's dehumanizing effect. I'm wondering whether this remark can also be referred to the historian in general, or, specifically, to the way in which he depicts the plague. Since we do not have other contemporary sources, it is impossible to say if his account proves to be more lenient in relation to the saddest and most horrible effects of the plague. It is obvious that Thucydides shies away from criticizing the doctors or the government for any shortcomings in their response to the plague. The only benefit that can be drawn from the survival seems to consist in processing what had happened and in giving to future generations the most accurate account of it.

---

5 Interestingly, this second hint is not taken into account by recent researchers, such as Elena Gome. 2000. "The Plague of Utopias: Pestilence and the Apocalyptic Body." *Twentieth Century Literature*, vol. 46, no. 4, 405–433 (in particular 410).

It is yet intriguing that Thucydides assigns a state of hubris to those who survived. Of course, it mainly pertains to their confidence in being immune to any disease or, to be blunt, in being granted a longer life. Amid countless dead, they felt almost like being immortal and, thereby, somehow detached from the earthly world. It is noteworthy that Thucydides inserted these two hints regarding his personal and subjective experience with the disease in a depiction that is otherwise marked by its objectivity and detachment. On a literal level, the figure of the witness is deployed to authenticate the specifically medical aspects of the depiction of the disease. On a metaliterary level, it may have exempted the author from the dehumanizing effect of the plague and, thereby, conferred authority onto him.

Giovanni Boccaccio or Eye-witnessing the Marvelous

Like Thucydides, Boccaccio incorporates his description of the Black Death that had struck the city of Florence in 1348 and wiped out more than half of the population, into a much longer text. His chronicle of the outbreak that opens the *Decameron* had been promptly admired as a rhetorical and stylistic masterpiece that soon circulated on its own. In the vernacular, Boccaccio had achieved an elegant prose style modeled on the sophisticated Latin syntax which could compete with the best ancient prose writings. He took inspiration from a Latin model, the *Historia Langobadorum* in which Paulus Diaconus, treading in the footsteps of Thucydides, depicted the Justinian plague that had devastated the countryside of Milan in the 6th century. Ironically, the more Boccaccio adapted his medieval model to the reality of the Black Death in the city of Florence, the closer he came to the Greek antecedent to which he did not have access.

Following this ancient model, Boccaccio gives an astoundingly balanced and thematically well-ordered account of the chaotic confusion brought upon Florence by the Black Death. His representation of the epidemic stretches from initial chronological and geographical considerations to the symptoms and progression of the disease and, finally, to the social and political breakdown of the city that fell into anarchy once the prevailing natural, moral, and social bonds completely deteriorated. Like Thucydides, Boccaccio takes on the role of a detached chronicler who retrospectively draws an insightful picture of the frightful months. Contrary to Thucydides, however, he does not bother to point out that he is a citizen of Florence, and, therefore, a contemporary of the plague. It is hard to tell whether this omission is due to the convention of medieval literature or to the personal circumstances in the author's life about which we don't know much or if his presence was simply taken for granted.

Boccaccio only briefly adopts a first-person perspective. Contrary to Thucydides, he does not mention that he survived the disease, nor that he had lost friends and members of his family. As a result, this first-person perspective is comparatively impersonal. He places the passage at a significant juncture in the well-planned description, that is at the very end of the medical report and immediately before the chronicler turns to the epidemic's horrendous impact on the social and anthropological order. More precisely, the first-person perspective occurs when the incredibly high risk of infection is addressed. Like Thucydides, Boccaccio switches from the I of the detached author to the subjective I of a witness. He accurately introduces and emphasizes the reason why he had to revert to his personal testimony:

> So marvelous sounds that which I have now to relate, that, had not many, and I among them, observed it with their own eyes, I had hardly dared to credit it, much less to set it down in writing, though I had had it from the lips of a credible witness. (Boccaccio 0.17-0.18)[6]

The first-person perspective is employed to give credibility to something "miracoloso" that contradicts the common rules of reality. Strikingly, the chronicler is not the only witness to what happened. He stresses that he would not have dared to write down the scene if he had not seen it himself. He does not so much insist on his personal involvement and intimate exposure to the historical event of the Black Death, he rather highlights that he is about to recount something unlikely to be believed. This insistence is astonishing in the context of a chronicle, it is much more familiar in poetry. It regularly occurs when poets are forced to break a rule established by Horace in his *Ars poetica* according to which poetry should always stick to what is probable.

Apart from being a rhetorical device employed in poetry, the figure of an eyewitness may also relate to a more recent use of this testimonial mode that had gained momentum during the 13th century. Boccaccio, who was trained in canon law, was aware of the essential role that the eyewitness had begun to play in lawsuits as well as in procedures of canonization. Whenever a dead contemporary who had been already venerated as a saint was proposed to be canonized, the committee asked for proof of a miracle. The evidence, in turn, requested an eyewitness.[7] Boccaccio may have been inspired by this juridical procedure when he refers to his having been an eyewitness to a marvelous event that heavily contested the well-established hierarchical divisions of God's creation. He may even have had in mind to parody the procedure, as is often the case in the novellas of the *Decameron*.

---

6 Translation by J. M. Rigg. https://www.brown.edu/Departments/Italian_Studies/dweb/texts/DecShowText.php?myID=d01intro&lang=eng.

7 Cf. Roberto Righi. 2019. *Mediante specie: note a Francesco stimmatizzato*, 71–87; Franziska Meier. *Poesia e diritto nel Due – e Trecento italiano*, Longo.

Boccaccio's direct testimony concerns a scene that at first sight is only supposed to give an idea of how infectious the plague had been:

> I say, then, that such was the energy of the contagion of the said pestilence, that it was not merely propagated from man to man, but, what is much more startling, it was frequently observed, that things which had belonged to one sick or dead of the disease, if touched by some other living creature, not of the human species, were the occasion, not merely of sickening, but of an almost instantaneous death. Whereof my own eyes (as I said a little before) had cognizance, one day among others, by the following experience. The rags of a poor man who had died of the disease being strewn about the open street, two hogs came thither, and after, as is their wont, no little trifling with their snouts, took the rags between their teeth and tossed them to and fro about their chaps; whereupon, almost immediately, they gave a few turns, and fell down dead, as if by poison, upon the rags which in an evil hour they had disturbed. (Boccaccio 0.18)

The epidemic questions the clear-cut distinction between animals and human beings. In Boccaccio's Christian humanistic worldview, the human species is considered to be superior to animals. The Black Death, however, challenges this view. Contrary to the context of religious canon law in which the eyewitness serves to prove that someone had risen beyond the limits imposed on human beings, Boccaccio employs it to debunk the supposedly self-evident superiority of humankind – incidentally, this procedure is consistent with the satirical and parodistic style in some novellas. From here, it does not come as a surprise that Boccaccio placed the passage just before addressing the deterioration of the social and moral order. While Thucydides referred to his first hand-knowledge in a medical context, Boccaccio deploys the first-personperspective in a medical context as well, but at the very point of the text where the topic of the medical peculiarities yields to the epidemic's anguishing impact on civilization. The brief eye-witness passage, therefore, serves as an eye-opener to what remains at the core of Boccaccio's plague description, i.e., the very questioning of the widespread belief in human achievements and superiority. The scene of the sudden infection followed by the death of two hogs brings a more general anthropological dimension to the fore: the abyss of human behavior, the bestiality inherent to mankind[8] – an aspect that will be reflected in manifold ways by the ten young people who escape from the plagued Florence to build a harmonious alternative world.

---

8 According to David Steel, in the *Decameron* "the age of modern fiction was ushered in by a virus" because the plague directly caused the gathering of the young people. Seemingly, Steel does not acknowledge how neatly Boccaccio separates the historical part from what is called "novella portante," the story of the ten young people flying from Florence. Nonetheless, Steel's assessment was resumed by Jennifer Cooper, op. cit. on p. 17.

The First Eye-Witness Narration: Daniel Defoe's *Journal of a Plague Year*

Daniel Defoe's depiction of the "Great Visitation" of the plague in London differs from the two predecessors in many ways. The author was only five years old when the plague came to London in 1665.What is more, he did not only dedicate an entire book to the topic but described the spread of the epidemic from the perspective of an eyewitness. Interestingly, the literary depiction in *Journal of a Plague Year* published in March 1722 had been preceded and accompanied by a prolific journalistic activity starting in 1709.[9] In fact, as a journalist and novelist, Defoe had been obsessed with the idea that another plague might spread from the continent to the island.[10] Around 1720, at the time when a plague broke out in Marseille, the journalist Defoe seemed to have supported the preventive measures taken by the Walpole government.[11] Two years later, when the plague had reached the English shores, he published the pamphlet *Due Preparations for the Plague, as well for Soul as Body*, a kind of guidebook on survival techniques. Roughly a month later, the *Journal* came out, in which the novelist tried to take advantage of the current anguish.[12]

A Journal of the Plague Year is the first literary "plague text" of the Western canon written in a first-person perspective. However, the subjective point of view as well as the stance of the self as a witness is far from being firmly established. This is already reflected in the graphical arrangement of the front page of the first edition. Contrary to *Robinson Crusoe* or *Moll Flanders*, it is not the name of the first-person narrator but the plague that is put center stage. This may be due to the marketing of a book that responded to and played with the fears of contemporaries who were anxious to get information about how to protect themselves. Incidentally, even the historical dating of the plague – the "Great Visitation" took place fifty years ago – is printed in smaller letters. Finally, it is only in the lower half of the front page and in still smaller letters separated by two lines that the author of the *Journal* is mentioned. According

9 It would be interesting to know more about the reason why in the centuries after the *Decameron*, poets seem to have almost lost interest in the description of plagues. The many plagues that continued to devastate Europe, instead, left their mark on written documents such as chronicles or ego-documents and on scientific, most of all medical treatises. In Defoe, the two lines merge again.

10 Cf. David Roberts's introduction to Daniel Defoe. 2010. "*A Journal of the Plague Year*," Oxford UP, x.

11 Patrick Reilly. 2015. *Bills of mortality. Disease and Destiny in Plague Literature from Early Modern to Postmodern Times*, Peter Lang.

12 The editor of *A Journal of the Plague Year*, Louis Landa, recommends that readers "do better to consider the Journal not as an isolated work: it is, in fact, the culmination of a persistent interest in plague expressed in Defoe's writing for at least a decade before he wrote the Journal. The very idea of plague seems to have been an abiding fact in his consciousness." Quoted by Cooke, 25.

to the front page, the account is "written by a Citizen who continued all the while in London" and has never been published before. Thus, the only aspects that seem to matter are that the author is a Londoner and an eyewitness.

The citizen does not have a name nor is there any hint at his editor, Daniel Defoe. It will be only at the very end of the account that the reader learns the initials of the narrator. As scholars already pointed out, H.F. matches those of Defoe's uncle, Henry Foe. Be that as it may, Defoe does not seem to be interested in a more individualistic self-portrait of the narrator. The use of initials may simply be due to a juridical convention according to which the account of a witness had to be signed and, thereby, authenticated.

The omission of the name indicates a revealing uneasiness about the first-person perspective that pervades the entire account. Admittedly, the narrator speaks about his whereabouts, his family, his profession, and his living in London during the plague, but his account does not reach a level of completeness as to how an individual may intellectually, practically, and emotionally have coped with the plague. It has already been pointed out that the account starts with an "I" in the first sentence and, famously, ends with an "I" in the fourth line of the concluding stanza: "Yet I alive."[13] However, from the very first sentence the "I" is eager to be part of a collective experience and to identify with others. In fact, the account is not limited to his first-hand experiences. The self rather transforms itself into a representative of his fellow citizen who collected numerous second-hand experiences. By doing so, his account meshes a polyphony of small stories and anecdotes which H.F. had observed or heard about. Moreover, the multitude of second-hand experiences does not show different or contrasting individual points of view against which the writer sets his own. In case he takes sides between diverging opinions, he significantly prefers a standpoint that holds the golden middle.[14] His purpose rather is to filter or, better, to generalize them. He deals with the others' experiences as if they were *exempla*: "cases" (Defoe 2010, 50) in the ancient and medieval sense of the term.

Although the *Journal* is written in a first-person perspective, the narrator does not conceive of his account as "a History of my actings," but as a "Direction" "to act by" (Defoe 2010, 9). From the start, however, his acting is far from being sensible or an example to be followed. Whereas his brother, for instance, brings forward many rational arguments in favor of leaving the city, the self yields to what he calls signs

13 Jennifer Cooper, for instance, insisted on this continuous presence, 38–39.

14 Telling in this regard is the first paragraph. The opening sentence introduces the first-person pronoun; the I, however, immediately adheres to a group of neighbors who face diverging opinions and rumors. Eventually, the narrator settles on the "all-agreed" consensual assessment of the last "transmitter" that matters only.

"from Heaven" (Defoe 2010, 10).[15] Even though the narrator interprets a series of hazards, such as a sudden illness, as heavenly signs, he does not go on to understand all his following actions or his writing as stemming from a religious calling. On the contrary, he tries to fashion himself as a craftsman who applies the rules of reason and common sense.[16]

A similar uneasiness can be sensed when the narrator justifies his walking across the city, the foundation on which the account is built. He admits that he transgressed the very measures that had been taken to prevent the spreading of the plague. Moreover, he acknowledges that the search for news and particularities was none of his business. However, he could not help that "my Curiosity led, or rather drove me to go and see this Pit again" (Defoe 2010, 53). He does not condemn his curiosity, but neither does he feel entitled to observe or collect all the information and experiences regarding the plague; nor does he think to have the right to evaluate the success of the government's many policies, though he does so throughout the book. In short, in the *Journal* the role of the self in the plague and in its representation is far from being self-evident. It is aware of violating a taboo.

The witness seems to have struggled also with staying at home, with isolating in accordance with the severe quarantine rules imposed by the government and praised by the journalist Defoe. Interestingly, it is during these days in which he had to stay in place that he took to writing to fill the void:

> Terrified by those frightful Objects, I would retire Home sometimes, and resolve to go out no more; [...] Such intervals as I had, I employed in reading Books and in writing down my Memorandums of what occurred to me every Day, and out of which, afterwards, I [took] most of this Work as it relates to my Observations without Doors. What I wrote of my private Meditations I reserve for private Use, and desire it may not be made publick on any Account whatever. (Defoe 2010, 67)

It seems that every time he observes the imposed quarantine, he felt compelled to write. Among his several notebooks, he mentions a "Memorandum" that contains a kind of day-to-day writing log. The account we read, however, is not a simple copy of this diary. It is based on a rigid selection and redrafting of selected passages by the first-person narrator. Only the passages which deal with what was happening outside of his home were included in the draft. It is hard to say what he means by "private Meditations," for the account itself does contain judgments and musings

15 Following a chance reading of the "91st Psalm" (13), in particular, a verse that promises God's protection and shelter, he decides to stay. According to Patrick Reilly, H.F. follows a "puritan practice of *sortes Biblicae*," 29.

16 Cf. Patrick Reilly, according to whom the narrator prefers "the measure of reason and the voice of sanity," 31.

on what he saw or heard. Anyhow, the first-person account is preceded by an intentional omission of anything private. Moreover, the selected diary entries are clearly remodeled by a first-person narrator in the aftermath of the plague. This can be deduced from his hinting at the first and second part of the plague year which implies that he narrated the entire development of the epidemic from hindsight, or from his comment that the same emotions welled up in him again while writing. (Defoe 2010, 16, 49) Thus, on the one hand, the narrator is eager to emphasize that many highly emotional aspects of the plague are still present in his mind and, consequentially, in his writings, and, on the other hand, that he takes control of what he had lived on the spot in a probably very confusing way.

This thematic order in which the narrator organizes the sequence of the plague and its representation, strongly marks the account. Although the title of the book promises a "journal" – a term that in the Eighteenth century meant both "[a] diary; an account kept of daily transactions" and "any paper published daily" (*Johnson's Dictionary*) –, the book is neither a personal diary nor a newspaper. It is not even arranged along a chronological structure since the timeline is not put into evidence. Although the inserted weekly statistics or orders do suggest a chronology, it becomes clear on closer inspection that the narrator implements a structure that is largely based on thematic headings under which he unrolls over many pages his observations and experiences. He pieces together those which refer to the symptoms of the disease, those that feature the measures taken by the government adding to them the people's various reactions, including his observations about the range of behaviors of the afflicted as well as the not-yet infected Londoners. He completes his account with descriptions of the mass burials. The weekly statistics are placed when the author addresses the speedy spreading of the plague or the astronomically high number of buried dead. In contrast with the title "journal of a plague year"[17], the writer transfers the traumatizing months into a tableau of themes, of specific aspects respectively illustrated by individual cases. It is possible that it was this attempt to bring order into the confusing memories of the plague that undermined a full-blown articulation of the first-person narrative.

It is remarkable that the retrospective account does not stage the interplay between the former witnessing and the later writing self. The first-person is the agent who moves within the epidemic situation, but not the protagonist who confesses and tries to process the many traumatizing experiences that marked him. He does not mention how he integrated them into his biography. In his view, the first- as well as second-hand experiences seem to be valuable only inasmuch as they may improve governmental policies against the plague and, thereby, enhance the welfare of the community. The narrator cannot connect his personal experiences to a religious or

17 In his introduction, David Roberts calls the *Journal* a "boundary text" (XVI) and then a historical novel (XIX).

moral framework even though the idea intermittently emerges. In fact, the narrator does not conceal his utter disappointment that the plague – sometimes qualified as a divine punishment – had not morally improved the Londoners (cf. Defoe 2010, 212). In hindsight, the plague seems to have only caused senseless suffering.

It seems to have been this profound disillusion that compelled the narrator to conclude his account of the *Plague Year*:

> I can go no farther here, I should be counted censorious, and perhaps unjust, if I should enter into the unpleasant Work of reflecting, whatever Cause there was for it, upon the Unthankfulness and Return of all manner of Wickedness among us, which I was so much an Eye-Witness of myself; I shall conclude the Account of this calamitous Year therefore…
>
> A dreadful Plague in London was,
> In the Year Sixty-Five
> Which swept an Hundred Thousand Souls
> Away; yet I alive! (Defoe 2010, 212)

Interestingly, the prose writing ends in a poetic stanza that has been read as "an assertion of its miraculous survival" (Roberts in Defoe 2010, XXII). The fact of surviving amid the Great Visitation in 1665 may be considered as a small triumph over the Plague. On closer inspection, however, this self-assertion becomes questionable. The four lines mirror the very essence of the plague depiction: three-and-a-quarter lines cover the plague that devastated large parts of a city whereas only two-thirds of the last line are dedicated to the self who has the last word: the first word "away" conveys both the tremendous menace from which the lonely I escaped as well as its fierce resistance to it. Yet, it is hard to tell whether the last outcry shows the self-confidence of an individual who by chance defied the plague's threats or just stresses the abyss between the many dead and the few surviving bodies.[18] Intriguingly, the narrator's survival is already undermined by the editor who in a *Nota Bene* had informed the reader about the witness' burial place.[19] Thus, the benefit of having escaped an anonymous, collective death-by-plague seems only to have been a death marked by proper ritual and handling of the body.

---

18 Cf. Patrick Reilly, 39: "The contagion operates so efficaciously, however, that London's deliverance from the plague, as H.F. avers in the final pages of his journal, indeed rests upon a divine miracle." This is certainly true, but at the same time, the eventual disappointment does not leave any doubt about the fact that the many sufferings and victims had been "senseless."

19 "N.B. The Author of this Journal, lyes buried on that very Ground, being at his own Desire, his sister having been buried here a few Years before," 199.

Alessandro Manzoni or the Unreliability of the Eyewitness

In 1821, the Italian novelist and historian Alessandro Manzoni, inspired by the success of Walter Scott, started working on a historical novel in which the plague that devastated Milan in 1629–30 plays a pivotal role. His depiction differs from that of his three predecessors in many ways. For the first time, the plague is an integral part of a novel; the author, however, stresses the difference between the two chapters dedicated to the event and the fictional part. Moreover, Manzoni's narrator writes from a historical distance of two hundred years. Therefore, the inner detachment of the historian does not originate in an act of self-distancing nor can the narrator of the *Promessi Sposi* bring into play his first-hand knowledge. Interestingly, the issue of the eyewitness arises nonetheless.

Manzoni was initially disappointed with the first version of the novel *Fermo e Lucia* which circulated exclusively among his friends in 1823. The main critique seems to have been that he had not given a balanced representation of the many characters in the fictional plot and that the novel was overcrowded with historical digressions of varying lengths. In the new version which Manzoni drafted between 1824 and 1827, he revised the representation of the characters as well as the historical digressions. For instance, he moved the long description of the process of the "unguenti" (Anointments) to an appendix: *La Storia della Colonna Infame*. This second version of the novel, published under the title *I Promessi Sposi* in 1827, is not a purely historical novel. At the outbreak of the plague, Manzoni switches from the historical-fictitious plot to a historiographical discourse. In this sense, his novel is also a boundary-text as far as its adherence to genre rules is concerned. In contrast with the tradition established by the Scottish novelist, Manzoni makes his narrator explicitly step out of the ongoing storytelling in the chapters 31 and 32 and slip into the role of a historian who offers an archival reconstruction of the plague.[20]

Apart from the appendix to which the historical reconstruction in the novel explicitly refers its readers, it is in these two chapters that the value of personal testimony is questioned. According to the historian, the more he studied the chronicles as well as legal and administrative documents, the more he became aware of divergences and contradictions that eventually weakened his trust in eye-witness ac-

20 The plague does have an impact on the fictional characters too. According to Reilly, "[t]he aesthetics and the ethic in *The Betrothed*, then – i.e. Fra Cristoforo's (as well as the narrator's and Manzoni's) construct of destiny and the moral paradigm that informs it – do more perhaps to justify God's way to man than they do to illuminate the cause and nature of the plague or to mitigate the progress of its effects....Its [the plague's; fm] terror spreads unreined [sic!], and the human imagination seeks to explain aesthetically what it cannot comprehend intellectually: God. The plague may fell the blessed beside the damned, but by the sovereign God's grace the good shall be redeemed in heavenly embrace while the evil shall perish in hell. God selects, the plague is" (69–70).

counts. Whereas Defoe's first-person narrator happily engaged with a polyphony of testimonies, Manzoni's historian is puzzled by the conflicting and confusing picture that results from a comparative reading of the contemporaneous reports.[21] He does not reject one single testimony as unreliable, he rather concludes that witnesses' accounts do not coalesce into "history," he understands as a chain connecting causes to their effects. In other words, it is only from a historical distance that the records of contemporaries – however detached the voice of the author may sound and however controlled the composition is – can be pieced together in order to amount to what Manzoni calls "la storia della peste."

Whereas Boccaccio pointed at bestiality as a fundamental challenge to all human beings, Manzoni's depiction focuses on both, outstanding examples of human dedication as well as human failures. The issue of the eyewitness emerges within the reflection about the extent to which the people, most of all the governors and administrators, were to be held accountable for the plague's devastations. Manzoni, therefore, shifts the focus to the foolish reactions, to the voluntary blindness of contemporaries who prefer to deny reality – by not calling the plague by its name, and thereby contributing to its spreading. In particular, he pinpoints that even doctors and educated people who ought to have known better, fell victim to current irrational moods. In the novel, the historian alludes only briefly to the episode of the "unguenti" who had been suspected to infect the city with deadly poison and to the "terribile delirio" (Manzoni 2984, 539). He outlines that even skeptical contemporaries could not help believing in something highly unlikely (Manzoni 1984, 560). In contrast to Boccaccio, who used the device of an eyewitness to give credibility to something marvelous, Manzoni, as a historian, diagnosed – based on eye-witness reports – how easily contemporaries are entrapped by irrationality.

In the appendix dedicated to the trial against the "unguenti," he wants to prove that the high medical infection rate had been accompanied by an equally intense and perilous mental contamination. Whereas Piero Verri's reading of the case files pushed him into accusing the juridical use of torture as abuse, Manzoni came to the conclusion that even the judges had been affected by mental delirium. Significantly, he starts with the testimonies of three eyewitnesses who allegedly observed a man smearing a wall. He switches from the indirect to the eye-witness' direct speech in which the verbs "vedere" or "dare nell'occhio" occur three times.[22] He illustrates that

21 Cf. Alessandro Manzoni. 1984. *I promessi sposi. Storia milanese del secolo XVII scoperta e rifatta*, Mondadori, 525f: "Delle molte relazioni contemporanee, non ce n'è alcuna che basti da sè a darne un'idea un po' distinta e ordinata; […] In ognuna di queste relazioni […] sono omessi fatti essenziali [..] ci sono errori materiali […] In tutte poi regna una strana confusione di tempi e di cose; è un continuo andare e venire, come alla ventura, senza disegno generale, senza disegno nei particolari."

22 "Vide venire un uomo con una cappa nera, e il cappello sugli occhi, e una carta in mano, *sopra la quale*, dice costei nella sua deposizione, *metteua su le mani, che pareua che scriuesse. Le diede*

it does not require a very accurate reading of the testimonies to realize the extent to which the visual perception was marked by the current fear of anointers and that even the judges did not pay attention to the many inconsistencies. While Boccaccio's use of the eyewitness playfully alludes to the rise of a juridical means, Manzoni – consistent with his general critical reading of the ego-documents from the Milan plague – criticizes the practice by highlighting the ambiguity of first-person testimonials. Whereas he casts general doubts on first-person plague accounts in the novel, it is in the appendix that he contests the value of eye-witness testimonials. Like Boccaccio, Manzoni connects the reflection on the figure of an eyewitness to his main anthropological interest in plagues: the shortcomings of human perception and the looming menace of irrationality. In a nutshell, according to him, a contemporary is not able to detach himself from what is happening. Neither the personal testimonial nor the detached rendering of the plague offers a consistent and reliable narration of the epidemic.

Albert Camus or the Suspension of the First-Person Narrative

Similar to Alessandro Manzoni, the French author Albert Camus did not have any first-hand experience of a plague, even though in his homeland Algeria there were cases of contagious diseases. Instead, he learned from medical books and studied the ancient depictions. Unlike Manzoni, he did not take a historical interest in the plague. As far as we can tell from the surviving drafts of the first version, Camus did not plan to establish a first-person narrative. He rather wanted to give much space to the diary of a Greek and Latin teacher, Philippe Stephan, from which a narrator would have quoted large extracts. The extracts are filled with reflections upon a failed marriage and comments on the plague depictions of two ancient writers: Thucydides and Lucretius. The teacher seems to have been particularly interested in tracing the differences between a depiction by an eyewitness and a second-hand description. After the outbreak of a plague, the teacher would come to a better understanding of the two major plague tests.[23] Thus, in contrast with his first, highly acclaimed novel *L'Étranger* published in 1942, Camus did not pursue a rendering of the plague

nell'occhio che, entrando nella strada, si fece appresso alla muraglia delle case, e che è subito dopo voltato il cantone, e che a luogo a luogo tiraua con le mani dietro al muro. All'hora mi viene un pensiero, soggiunge, *se a caso fosse un poco uno di quelli che, a' giorni passati, andauano ongendo le muraglie, [...] et viddi, dice, che teneua toccato la detta muraglia con le mani.*" Alessandro Manzoni. 2020. *Storia della Colonna Infame*, Sellerio, 21.

23 Cf. Paul Demont. 2009. « *Le Journal de Philippe Stephan dans la première version de La Peste d'Albert Camus. Note sur une édition récente* ». *Revue d'histoire littéraire de la France*, Année 109, no. 3, 710–724.

from an exclusively subjective point of view. He established a third-person narration interspersed with long quotations from a diary.

These early drafts did not leave any trace in the final version of the novel *La Peste* of 1947. The character of the teacher disappeared, and the two ancient depictions are only hinted at once. Whereas the first version seems to have focused on psychological issues accentuated by the plague, in the final version Camus eliminated the topic of love. The plague became an allegorical tool[24] to speak and reflect on the impact of the German occupation on the French population and on possible forms of reacting and resisting it. Parallel to his new philosophical orientation, Camus did not so much outline the absurdity of the world than, in harmony with his essay *L'homme révolté*, plead for taking action and saving lives.[25]

La Peste starts as a chronicle about some events that took place in an unspecified year of the 1940s in Oran.[26] In the first paragraph, the chronicler does not even point to his being a citizen of the Algerian city. In the first chapter, the passive voice or, from the third paragraph on, the first-person plural prevails. Incidentally, contrary to Defoe's witness who is happy to join in with peers, in Camus' novel the first-person plural implies an imposed unity that, by the measures taken against the spreading of the plague, is separated from the rest of the world. Therefore, the pronoun "we" does not only express the suffering large group of those who feared falling victim to the plague, or already did, but most of all a community who is forced into exile. Whereas the witnesses of all the preceding plague writings were driven by the wish to convey their peculiar experience and knowledge to future generations, Camus' novel conveys an exceptional experience to those who live outside of Oran.

At the end of the first chapter, the narrator explicitly defines himself as a "chroniste" (Camus 1947, 13–14) because he limits his task to report what had happened during the epidemic, even if that what he must tell sounded contradictory and hard to believe. Intriguingly, the chronicler, in order to enhance his own credibility, places more confidence in the collective feeling of what is true than in relying on eye-witness testimonies: "il y a donc des milliers de témoins qui estimeront dans le cœur la vérité de ce qu'il dit" (Camus 1947, 14). In the following, the last paragraph of the first chapter, the chronicler calls himself a "narrateur" (Camus 1947, 14) who is not presented as an abstract entity or a merely literary voice, but as a character who lived in Oran during the plague. He justifies his narration by a series of coincidences that

24 This transformation is signaled in the novel's motto extracted from Defoe's *Serious Reflections*, the third volume of *Robinson Crusoe*, as has been pointed out by Cooper, 27.

25 Interestingly the reception of Camus' novel changed during the COVID-19-pandemic. It got almost rid of its clear political – antifascist – message and started being appreciated as one of the best, if not the most authentic representation of how people live and react to an epidemic.

26 Albert Camus. 1947. *La peste*, Gallimard, 11: "Les curieux événements qui sont le sujet de cette chronique se sont produits en 194., à Oran."

placed him at the core of the events and made him a collector of the reports of other citizens as well as the chance inheritor of some diaries or notebooks. Significantly, he does not tell his name, nor does he insist on his having been an eyewitness. He includes his own apparently mostly hearsay-based knowledge among some other oral and written testimonies in his account of the plague. The first chapter ends up alluding to a first-person narrator who does not only embrace other testimonies but also tries to suppress any personal features. By postponing the revelation of his identity, he leaves his readers in suspense. Significantly, he will not even use the first-person pronoun after having revealed his identity.

In the fourth chapter, this artificial suspension of the narrator's identity takes on a perplexing, if not an alienating form when the unnamed narrator brings a conversation to a halt:

> A ce point du récit qui laisse Bernard Rieux derrière sa fenêtre, on permettra au narrateur de justifier l'incertitude et la surprise du docteur, puisque, avec des nuances, sa réaction fut celle de la plupart de nos concitoyens. (Camus 1947, 41)

The narrator, who is the very doctor Rieux, transforms himself seemingly into a figure whose behavior at the first signs of the plague's outbreak he considers exemplary. Instead of retrospectively criticizing his own weakness and all-too-human impulse to ignore what was obvious, the narrator splits from his former self by placing it within a group that shows a broad range of similar behaviors. In other words, the narrator does not only transform himself into a quasi-aloof character but also into an "example." In this paragraph, the self-distancing seems to have entitled the narrator to be lenient with a form of blindness even if, to some degree, it had caused an important delay in taking measures to protect the population. Beyond that, it may be inferred from this voluntary objectification of the narrator that the horrible events cannot seamlessly be integrated into a personal biography. The plague causes a rupture that cannot be bridged.

At the beginning of the last chapter, the narrator presumes that it is time to reveal his own name. Although he continues to define the book as a chronicle, he explains why he had taken "le ton d'un témoin objectif" (Camus 1947, 272). Interestingly, he now defines himself as a contemporary who by chance had been placed at the center of the epidemic and has the intention to convey the many experiences without enhancing or distorting them. In other words, his objectivity stems from the decision to give space and voice to a plague-ridden community that is rigidly isolated from what had preceded and what would follow, and all that which is not part of it. The already mentioned hiatus, therefore, does not only concern the personal biography, it might also be specific to a world hit by the plague that by its nature suppresses subjectivity, individuality, and biographical continuity in its victims. In the following paragraph, conversely, the doctor evokes his being called to testify in the legal sense of the term. Thereby, the plague puzzlingly turns out to be a kind of crime in which the narrator bears witness in favor of the "victims" (Camus 1947, 273) as if he had been an onlooker.

At the end of the last chapter, when the moment in which the story ends overlaps with the very moment in which doctor Rieux decides to edit it,[27] the chronicle is suddenly changed into a commemoration of the plague's dead.[28] It is at this very moment that the narrator who always tried to keep himself at a distance acknowledges his isolation. The "chroniste" who in the first chapter is a happy member of the pre-plague city, appears as a nearly lone survivor, in the sense that he belongs to the very few who refuse to forget and to be carried along by the flow of life. Incidentally, this sensation may have been the reason why the novel starts with a completely detached voice of a chronicler. In sum, this twentieth-century novel, though being told by a fictional eyewitness and containing the writings of other eyewitnesses, is marked by a deliberate suspension or alienation of the first-person narrative. This is partly due to the voluntary act of attaining objectivity, but it may also be due to the trauma inflicted by both the devastation of the plague and by the subsequent forgetfulness and egoism of life. In other words, the novelist Albert Camus who brilliantly knew to deploy estranged first-person perspectives goes a step further by staging a first-person narrator who does not use the first-person pronoun. He is both inside and outside the plague-ridden community and goes on to stay even more isolated once the community is reunited with the rest of the world.

Conclusion

In conclusion, the plague writings from Thucydides to Camus showcase both the slow rise of the first-person perspective and a gradual movement from a historical or chronicle approach to a thorough fictionalization that, interestingly, does not completely abandon the original chronicle style. From the start, eyewitnesses emerge in plague writings, though initially only in isolated short passages. In both Thucydides and Boccaccio, these passages play an essential role inasmuch as they turn out to be

27 "Le docteur Rieux décida alors de rédiger le récit qui s'achève ici, pour ne pas être de ceux qui se taisent, pour témoigner en faveur de ces pestiférés; pour laisser du moins un souvenir de l'injustice et de la violence qui leur avait été faites, et pour dire simplement ce qu'on apprend au milieu des fléaux, qu'il y a dans les hommes plus de choses à admirer que de choses à mépriser" (Camus 1947, 279).

28 Famously, Shoshana Felman built her interpretation of Camus's La Peste as a literary testimony to the impact of the Holocaust on these last paragraphs of the novel from Albert Camus. Autumn 1991. "Postwar Writings, Crisis of Witnessing." *Cardozo Studies in Law and Literature*, vol. 3, no. 2, 197–242.

linked to what the plague description is meant to be about. Later, in Defoe's and Camus' novels, when the subjective perspective prevails, it does not manage to entirely pervade nor to dominate the narration of the epidemic. Whereas modern novels on war playfully experiment with the first-person perspective, a plague seems to set clear limits to the deployment of the first-person perspective.[29] Apparently, its overwhelming physical and mental impact continues to challenge the subject in the very act of narrating. The first-person narrator does not feel at ease with giving his own, naturally limited view of the disaster. Somehow the devastating and deindividualizing effect of the plague continues to beset any attempts to narrate epidemics. This is even true for fictional plague writings such as Camus' novel. The plague does not leave enough space for putting a first-person perspective center stage. Presumably, this situation will only change radically in the settings of science fiction novels that begin with the plague's aftermath. In the context of plague writings, personal experience remains a monolithic element in the narrator's life. Curiously, contrary to war novels, the plague writing does not feature the extent to which its victims cope with trauma after the disaster. The traumatization can be only sensed in the artificial suspension of the writer's identity as is the case in Albert Camus' *La peste* or in the strange opening of Defoe's Londoner self to its many peers, to the many other victims of the same plague. The eyewitness is certainly an important characteristic of plague writing. He can even evolve into a writer. Yet, he cannot access or build a place outside a plague-ridden world from which the traumatizing experience may be integrated into individual or collective development.

Bibliography

Boccaccio, Giovanni. 1903. *Decamerone*, translated by J. M. Rigg. https://www.brown.edu/Departments/Italian_Studies/dweb/texts/DecShowText.php?myID=d01intro&lang=eng.

Camus, Albert. 1947. *La peste*, Gallimard.

Cooke, Jennifer. 2009. *Legacies of Plague in Literature, Theory and Film*, Palgrave Macmillan.

Defoe, Daniel. 2010. *A Journal of the Plague Year*, Oxford UP.

Demont, Paul. 2009. "Le Journal de Philippe Stephan dans la première version de La Peste d'Albert Camus. Note sur une édition récente." *Revue d'histoire littéraire de la France*, Année 109, no. 3, 710–724.

29 Therefore, I do not agree with Elena Gomel's statement according to which "[w]riting becomes dying, not so much a means to survive as the endless postponement of the irreversible moment of death" (Gomel, 411).

Felman, Shoshana. 1991. "Crisis of Witnessing: Albert Camus' Postwar Writings." *Cardozo Studies in Law and Literature*, vol. 3, no. 2, 197–242.

Gomel, Elena. 2000. "The Plague of Utopias: Pestilence and the Apocalyptic Body." *Twentieth Century Literature*, vol. 46, no. 4 (Winter), 405–433.

Healy, Margaret. 2003. "Defoe's Journal and the English Plague Writing Tradition." *Literature and Medicine*, vol. 22, no. 1, 25–44.

Manzoni, Alessandro. 2020. *Storia della Colonna Infame*, Sellerio 62020.

Manzoni, Alessandro. 1984. *I promessi sposi. Storia milanese del secolo XVII scoperta e rifatta*, Mondadori.

Reilly, Patrick. 2015. *Bills of Mortality. Disease and Destiny in Plague Literature from Early Modern to Postmodern Times*, Peter Lang.

Reinhardt, Karl. 1966. "Thukydides und Machiavelli." *Vermächtnis der Antike. Gesammelte Essays zur Philosophie und Geschichtsschreibung*, edited by Karl Reinhardt, Vandenhoek & Ruprecht, 184–218.

Righi, Roberto. 2019. "Mediante specie: note a Francesco stimmatizzato." *Poesia e diritto nel Due – e Trecento italiano*, edited by Franziska Meier, Longo, 71–87.

Samuel Johnson's Dictionary. https://johnsonsdictionaryonline.com/views/search.php?term=.

Steel, David. 1981. "Plague Writing: From Boccaccio to Camus." *Journal of European Studies*, vol. 2, 88–110.

Thucydides. 2003. *The History of the Peloponnesian War*, translated by Richard Crawley. http://www.gutenberg.org/files/7142/7142-h/7142-h.htm#link2HCH0007.

On Washing One's Hands of it

Holmes, Semmelweis, Céline, and "Virality" as a Metaphor

Pierre-Héli Monot

> If Plato and Aristotle wrote on politics, it was as though they were laying down rules for a madhouse.
> *Pascal*, Pensées *(256), 167*[1]

Infodemic

The early phase of the COVID-19 crisis (2020–2021) provided a rare opportunity to test, under real-life conditions, many of the popular politological concepts that have characterized the last decade: "populism," "fake news," "echo chambers," "polarization," "conspiracy," "post-truth," "post-democracy," "biases," "bubbles," etc.[2] This lexicon is, remarkably, equally established in both scientific and colloquial discourse and is hence not a *sociolect* in the narrow sense of the term, i.e., a dialect whose extensive use could be predominantly attributed to specific social actors defending specific epistemic positions or pursuing specific interests: it seems to have, if not explanatory value, at least a broadly recognized descriptive power. Critics are nevertheless quick to point out the severe deficiencies of each of these concepts. "Populism," for instance, often entails the delegitimization of progressive movements whenever it is used to critique reactionary ones. This lexicon also appears to be broadly tautological, which raises persistent demarcation problems: certain utterances, ranging from the most disheveled speculations to Colin Powell's 2003 speech at the United Nations, have been *simultaneously* described as "conspiracy

1 My translation from H. F. Stewart's Cambridge University Press edition of the French original text (Pascal 2013, 93).

2 This project has received funding from the European Research Council (ERC) under the European Union's Horizon 2020 research and innovation program (grant agreement No 852205). This publication reflects only the author's view, and the Agency is not responsible for any use that may be made of the information it contains.

theories," "fake news," "post-democratic," "post-truth," and "biased" (Rimbert 2021, 21). Additionally, as a historically determined set of epistemic tools, this lexicon seems not only to create as many political problems as it claims to solve, it also boldly attributes agency to information. Finally, these terms also elude a crucial strategic and anthropological ambiguity: Should we willingly dispense with the notion of rational, or at the very least *reasonable* social actors when we attempt to explain how misinformation "spreads" among populations? If so, would this not preemptively negate all attempts to cure the body politic of its disorders? Rhetorical questions aside, a healthy public sphere now often seems to be predicated not on the presence and agency of rational social actors, but on the absence of misinformation among epistemically passive populations.

These apparent contradictions have become entrenched in public discourse since the beginning of the COVID-19 pandemic. They have also marked some of the prominent attempts by supranational organizations to address the risk posed by misinformation to public health. These risks are, in fact, real and empirically supported. Since 2020, the World Health Organization has for instance drawn on the neologism "infodemic" in order to "immunize the public against misinformation" concerning the nature of and therapeutic approaches to the COVID-19 virus. It has advocated a seven-step program to "flatten the infodemic curve": Ssnsibly, populations are instructed to always "[a]ssess the source," "[g]o beyond headlines," "[i]dentify the author," "[c]heck the date," "[e]xamine the evidence," "[c]heck [their] biases" and, if none of this helps, to "[t]urn to fact-checkers" (World Health Organization 2020). The term "infodemic" itself was coined in 2003 during a previous epidemic: The SARS "infodemic" was – and ostensibly still is – a cocktail of "a few facts, mixed with fear, speculation and rumor, amplified and relayed swiftly worldwide by modern information technologies" (Rothkopf 2003). The term suggests that information spreads like pathogens do, but also, perhaps inadvertently, that pathogens spread like information. The project of "immunizing the public against misinformation" (World Health Organization 2020) is hence a multifaceted enterprise: it implies the mutual convertibility of epistemic and medical goods, of knowledge and health. Its *explicit* locus is hence not language, but politics.

There is, in fact, a lot of truth to this metaphor: misinformation kills, and empirical studies abundantly demonstrate its enormous social cost (Lee, Sun, Yang et al. 2022; Lyu, Zheng, Luo 2022). Most prominently, unvaccinated patients are significantly more likely to either die or need long-term treatment after a COVID-19 infection (Kuodi et al. 2022; Xu et al. 2021). In what follows, however, I will argue that such public relations efforts are not only laudable and necessary, but also terminologically misguided and historically insensitive. While they conflate epidemiological and informational phenomena *metaphorically*, they cannot exclude the possibility of *literal* readings of this conflation. By way of a detour through literary history, I will argue that individual and collective social actors should strive to ascertain the social cost of the metaphors they use when they pursue socially beneficial aims.

My general argument is twofold. First, the conflation of medical and informational discourses depends on a historically variable social acceptance of metasocial and metacommunicational metaphors as policy-carriers: under specific political circumstances, populations may in turn dismiss or reject the metaphorical nature of this conflation and either *literalize* or *personalize* this conflation itself. I draw on an extreme historical example to substantiate this risk: the transformation of mutually dependent discourses on viral contagion and rational public debate, beginning with Oliver Wendell Holmes, Sr.'s writings on puerperal fever in the 1850s up to Louis-Ferdinand Céline's twin involvement with epidemiology and antisemitic pamphleteering in the interwar period. My aim in doing so is not only to spell out a recent chapter in the history of "virality" in a *longue durée* history of metasocial and metacommunicational metaphors, but also to suggest a possible, additional discursive context for the alarming increase in scapegoating, antisemitic beliefs, and political irrationality since the beginning of the COVID-19 pandemic (European Commission 2021). My second argument is that these metaphors place the burden of informational responsibility upon populations while simultaneously depriving them of the means to bear this burden *rationally*: empirically speaking, misinformation does not spread like pathogens, and pathogens do not spread like misinformation; populations are hence encumbered with a conceptual apparatus that obfuscates the effective vectors and multiplicators of misinformation. In what follows, I outline the progressive literalization of a medical metaphor and, in turn, some of the social consequences of this momentous shift.

Holmes

In 1855, Oliver Wendell Holmes, Sr., not quite a Boston Brahmin yet and mostly noted for his occasional poetry and anti-abolitionist sentiments, published *Puerperal Fever as a Private Pestilence*, the first of his two major medical pamphlets. Holmes wrote against the "stale philology of the word *contagion*" (emphasis in original; Holmes 1855, 7) and levelled a harsh accusation against the medical profession. The spread of postpartum infections among the public was a not only a "*Pestilence*" in the Latinate sense of the term (i.e. a "plague"), it was also more specifically a "*Private*" pestilence because it engaged the *moral responsibility* and *professional ethics* of every individual medical practitioner: "Whatever indulgence may be granted to those who have been the ignorant causes of so much misery," the pamphlet argued in its concluding paragraph, "the time has come when the existence of a private pestilence in the sphere of a single physician should be looked upon not as a misfortune but a crime" (Holmes 1855, 57). Holmes had, in fact, correctly identified the main vector of contagion: doctors would not wash their hands between visits to patients, nor after dissecting corpses, and would hence expose women in childbirth to the spread of "inflammation." These women did not merely die – they were "poisoned in some way by their medical attendants" (Holmes 1855,15).

While smallpox had been a pathology of the Early Republic, creating antagonist reading publics, dividing the early American public sphere into warring factions, and falling upon "communities" rather than the body politic *in toto* (Gross 2020), the puerperal fever was a pathology that seemed strangely attuned to the contradictions of Jacksonian Democracy. Vexing questions kept arising in learned treatises and lecture halls: the puerperal fever was a disease that could either take quasi-epidemic proportions, or befall an individual practitioner whose daily visits would henceforth be followed by a cortege of hearses – why? It was a disease that fascinated the prudish obstetricians of New England (the "Synod of Accoucheurs," as Holmes nicely puts it [7]), yet failed to elicit any systematic scientific investigation – how? It was, finally, a disease whose etiology could simultaneously be established with clarity and casually brushed aside by the most famous practitioners of the era – on which grounds? Here, the medical profession turned to profane sociology; doctors belonged to the affluent class, after all, and "a gentleman's hands are clean," as Charles D. Meigs famously concluded (Meigs 1854, 104).

Yet Holmes's main point lies elsewhere. A gentleman's hands not only explore abdominal cavities, but they also receive the fruits of scholarly pursuits – babies, books. Holmes warns "the Medical Students into whose hands this Essay may fall" against the undue authority of their genteel professors. Students "naturally have faith in their instructors, turning to them for truth, and taking what they may to choose to give them; babes in knowledge, not yet able to tell the breast from the bottle, pumping away for the milk of truth at all that offers, were it nothing better than a Professor's shrivelled forefinger [sic]" (Holmes 1855, 8).

The principles of Holmes's maieutics are plain. Both the denial of valid scientific results by dominant actors in the medical field and the active dissemination of dated or fraudulent medical opinions among the wider public have tangible effects on patients. Doctors should hence acknowledge the fact that the circulation and evaluation of any scientific hypothesis about midwifery engages their ethical responsibility. In practice, however, they reject this responsibility and philologize about contagion instead. Hence, it is of vital importance – to patients, first and foremost – that public discourse be subjected to both reasoned enquiry and the critique of those official institutions that remain impervious to rationally argued hypotheses. Scientific communication in a nominally scientific but effectively genteel medical field must necessarily entail metacommunication: at the very least, professional medical readers must be reminded that their evaluation of the proposed measure – washing one's hands – *will* have medical and ethical consequences. The assumed distinction between the public sphere on the one hand, and social history in its most corporeal form on the other, is hence strictly artificial: "better that twenty pamphleteers should be silenced, or a many professors unseated, than that one mother's life should be taken" (Holmes 1855, 23). Henceforth, whenever contagion occurs, it *must* breed contrition.

In *Puerperal Fever as a Private Pestilence*, Holmes framed an appropriate readerly disposition: the reader, once reminded of the dysfunctionality of the medical field and of the soundness of Holmes's main argument, should approve of the proposed hygienic measure. Holmes's text was hence not a "pamphlet" in the modern, largely polemical understanding of the term: he assumed that a rational, structured investigation of contagion must carry a force of conviction to which few of his colleagues would remain impervious. He was wrong.

From Semmelweis to Céline

In 1924, Louis-Ferdinand Céline submitted his doctoral thesis to the Medical Faculty of Paris. A short, highly dramatized biographical narrative, Céline's dissertation recounts Ignaz Semmelweis's study of puerperal fever while working as an assistant in Vienna's General Hospital from 1847 onwards. Céline narrates Semmelweis's dismissal on the grounds of having advocated the practice of washing hands with chlorinated lime in order to avoid cadaveric contamination, Semmelweis's proscription from the medical profession, his subsequent nervous breakdown and eventual death in a Viennese mental asylum. Within a span of ten years, and 5800 kilometers apart, Holmes and Semmelweis had come to the same conclusions, and had done so independently from one another: puerperal fever spreads for no more sensational a reason than doctors neglecting to wash their hands.

Céline's *Semmelweis*, his first published work, is not only valuable for its literary style – it is available in paperback and is considered an integral part of Céline's literary oeuvre –, but also for its wild distortion of Semmelweis's life. "Holmess, O. W. [sic]" is duly listed in Céline's trim bibliography. Like Holmes before him, Céline begins by chastising the medical treatises published by Semmelweis's predecessors, the "symphony of words which surrounded the whole problem of infection in all its complexities. This battle of words was almost interminable. It became a play of talent to explain death by 'thickened pus,' 'benign pus' or 'laudable pus'" (Céline 2020, 87). Yet if philology can never be medicine, if etymology can never be etiology, and if all hopes for a nominalist understanding of "contagion" and "disease" must be abandoned, the pursuit of medical knowledge and the fate of patients nevertheless remain inextricably entwined with the publication and fair assessment of research results. In Céline's narrative, Ignaz Semmelweis eventually becomes a martyr to Viennese medicine: the chief physicians and clinic directors "were not merely blind, unfortunately. They revealed themselves at the same time loud-mouthed and lying, and above all stubborn and wicked" (Céline 2020, 134).

Incidentally, Céline's reinterpretation of the life of Semmelweis is also a comment on Holmes's pamphleteering activities on puerperal fever, which Céline repeatedly draws on in his study. In *Semmelweis*, – against all historical data – Céline progressively turns his subject into a pamphleteer. While he shows a young Semmelweis reflecting at the outset of his career upon the uselessness of "polemics" (101), his final years are spent hanging up "manifestos" in the streets of Vienna: "Fathers," Céline transcribes, "do you know what it means to call a doctor or a nurse to your pregnant wife's bedside? It means you willingly put her at deadly risks, which are so easily avoidable etc." (Céline 1999, 134).[3] None of this ever occurred. In Céline's *Semmelweis*, the endemic shortcomings of medicine necessarily lead to polemical responses.

In the 70 years that separate Céline's dissertation from Holmes's and Semmelweis's work, a significant shift has hence occurred: for Céline, pamphleteering is now the only appropriate response to defective public and professional deliberation. Doctors have failed to become more conscientious; in turn, medicine – "medicine… this shit," as the opening chapter of *Death on Credit* famously puts it (Céline 2022, 3) – has remained impervious to rational argument. The study of contagion hence remains pointless as long as it dispenses with a reflection on the only appropriate vector of true knowledge among "stubborn and wicked" officials: the pamphlet. As long as women die as a result of medical negligence, there will always be *official culprits* and *officious texts*. Conversely, in a functional society, pamphleteering (and, for Céline, literature in general) are never necessary. In a dysfunctional society, literature is merely palliative; pamphleteering alone is therapeutic.

Céline

In the twenty years that followed his dissertation, the theme of contagion reappeared at every turn of Céline's professional and literary career. In 1925, he published a treatise on the use of quinine in the treatment of malaria and took up a position as secretary at the Institute for Hygiene and Epidemiology at the League of Nations, on whose behalf he visited Canada, Cuba, several African countries, as well as the Ford plants in Detroit. After his return to France, he was first employed in a working-class clinic of Clichy in 1928, then set up a private practice in suburban Meudon. Céline would remain a doctor for the remainder of his professional life: "I wanted to do something that was medical, I enjoyed it. I enjoyed it for a long time. I was a

3 My translation of the French original. This passage is missing from the current English translation (Céline 1999, 113).

doctor for 35 years. I enjoyed treating a varicocele, I enjoyed toying around with a case of measles, I thought it was very good" (my translation, Céline 1959).

In 1932, Céline published *Journey to the End of the Night* to critical acclaim. A communizing, if not an unequivocally communist novel, it was followed by *Death on the Instalment Plan* (1936), in which the same narrator, now a doctor, recounts his near-proletarian youth in Paris. In 1936, Céline visited Leningrad and, barely two months later, published the anticommunist *Mea Culpa*, the first of his four antisemitic pamphlets, in which he jointly attacked "the Jews," the French bourgeoisie (an "infection"), and the Soviet regime (again, an "infection").[4] Here, Céline would first present the rudiments of his post-communist anthropology: "Man is, after all, 'human' just about as much as a chicken is a flyer. When a hen gets a good swift kick in the tail, [she] flops right back down to resume pecking at her own dung. That's her nature and her ambition. For the rest of us, in human society, it is exactly the same. ... For this very reason, a Revolution should only be judged twenty years after it has occurred."[5] For the remainder of his literary and political career, Céline would renounce the very last rudiments of humanism that could, here and there, still be detected in his first two novels.

Between 1937 and 1941, Céline would go on to publish three further antisemitic pamphlets: *Trifles for a Massacre* (*Bagatelles pour un massacre,* 1937), *School for Corpses* (*L'École des cadavres*, 1938), and *A Fine Mess* (*Les Beaux draps*, 1941); all three contain explicit calls for the assassination of the *entirety* of Jewish population in France. A fanatical supporter of the German occupation and without any doubt the most vocal antisemite among French collaborationist writers, Céline would far exceed his own previous rhetorical violence in his short-form writing (cf. Tettamanzi 127–142). These four texts, whose brutality remains unmatched in collaborationist literature, are also, along with Émile Zola's *J'accuse...!* (1898) and Victor Hugo's *Napoléon le Petit* (1852), the most notorious pamphlets in the French literary tradition.

Céline's polemical writings have been barred from publication in France since 1945 and have lost none of their obscenity.[6] In all of Céline's pamphlets, and most explicitly in *School for Corpses*, Pasteur is made to assist Semmelweis in the quest for an "aseptic" body politic. I quote with discomfort from this chaotically organized, 130-page text:

---

4 I am correcting the English translation, which translates "infection" as "scourge" (Céline 2020, 24).

5 I am making slight corrections to the faulty English translation of the last sentence (Céline 2020, 46).

6 According to Céline's wishes, his widow has been opposed to the republication of his pamphlets since 1945. The texts themselves are neither censored, nor illegal.

> Does a surgeon make a distinction between good germs and bad ones? ... Everything about a germ is mysterious, like everything about a Jew. ... You can't afford to let in a single dangerous germ, or a single dangerous Jew onto the operating table. No one knows what will happen, before all this, how would you deal with a germ or a Jew which was seemingly harmless? All of Pasteur's opponents weren't completely stupid, or in bad faith. A few of them made very honest efforts in incorporating new pasteurization techniques into their surgery. They didn't think they needed to sterilize their instruments more before operating. They thought they'd sterilized them perfectly, all in good faith, they'd heated them for a good few minutes, like a boiled egg, for two or three minutes, ten minutes maximum. The results were devastating. "Mr. Pasteur is a charlatan!" His aseptic technique is a farce. ... (Céline 2012, 486)[7]

The equation of germs and "Jews" had, of course, been a staple of nationalist rhetoric in Europe since the 1890s, a prominent trope in the history of French anti-Judaism and antisemitism (Golsan 2010, 136), and a key rhetorical device of National Socialism, beginning with Adolf Hitler's programmatic writings of the mid-1920s (David 2012, 12). Yet Céline's polemical writings amend this grim tradition by returning to an argument first developed in *Semmelweis* and by implicating the "philological" dispositions of his colleagues:

> It took Pasteur ten years to explain the difference between 3-minute sterilizations and 20-minute sterilizations to the most intelligent race on Earth. ... For these eminent Latinist brains, the word "sterilization" was enough. They'd got this before! They knew about this! It's just boiling, right? ... As long as you have the word: "boiling"? We boiled them well enough? That's the most important bit! Pasteur was condemned by the Latinist, verbose French Academy of Medicine, the moment the word was uttered, he was fucked. They repeated everything, all forty academicians. That was it. If it didn't work, too bad! The Latins, the Latinists only have faith in words, that's it, it's not them that use words, it's the words that use them. They believe in words, that's it. They think that the world is a word, Jew is a word, sterilization is a word, that everything falls into place with words, with one word, with one proper word, with a happy word. They come up with happy, verbose solutions, they don't know any other solutions. (Céline 2012, 487–488)

The "purification" of the body politic advocated by Céline implies the "purification" not of language itself, but of its social uses. Dominant actors in the medical field take philological liberties with technical nouns: they subject medical language to a profane interpretation and equate "sterilization" (a precise technical process) with

---

7 All excerpts from Céline's School for Corpses are derived from an amateur translation by Szandor Kuragin posted online. I correct the translation whenever needed using Régis Tettamanzi's edition of Céline's pamphlets. https://schoolforcorpses.wordpress.com/.

"boiling" (its colloquial *near*-equivalent). Academicians negate, in other words, the distinction between a technical and a non-technical use of language. Yet Céline's insists that his linguistic critique also applies to the social composition of the medical profession itself. Medical doctors and Academicians hence systematically deny both textual and "racial" differences and thereby pursue "systematic bastardisation" (Céline 2012, 365). Their readers, the "impassioned readers of the great, optimistic Jewish press," consequently succumb as much to the homology of technical and profane language, as to the adequation of Frenchmen and Jews: "Homology! Paris the ghetto! Kosher meat for free!" (365). They are bad readers; hence, they will make bad murderers – and vice versa. In fact, for Céline as much as for the German occupation forces and the French collaborators, non-verbose "solutions" must necessarily be non-verbal ones.

Crucially, for Céline, these Academicians are also Jews: "Doctors Kalmanovitch, Oppman, Rougès, Lecain, Bli, etc. (all Jews), the main people behind all of it" (Céline 2012, 508).[8] The distinction between discourse and disease is now abolished and will remain so until 1945. At the intersection of verbose communication and viral contagion, at this critical point of indistinction, Céline erects a figure that personalizes the mutual convertibility of epistemic and medical threats – "the Jew." He is, for Céline and his hundreds of thousands of readers, both the *vector* by which misinformation spreads among the body politic and the *content* of contagion itself, i.e., he is simultaneously disease, disinformation, homology, and "bastardization": "We will all become Jewified, unrecognizable, even by our origins, we will be homogenized, infected by the Jews" (Céline 2012, 456). Pamphleteering, by mere reversal, becomes the vector of discursive and corporeal health.

From the Operating Table to the Public Sphere

The case of Céline is admittedly the most extreme of examples. The salient facts of Céline's pamphletary work – its antisemitism, its repetitiousness, its explicit calls for the assassination of approximately 320,000 Jewish men, women, and children – have not only attracted universal condemnation, but they have also come to function as historical signposts in much of the recent memorial work in France. Let us then approach the problem from another angle and focus on current discussions of "virality" as an object of both public health and public discourse.

In recent years, calls to regulate information and truth claims in the public sphere have increased in frequency and vehemence. Opponents to the legal

8 Or again: "trade union members, doctors, dentists; pharmacists never mention their origins due to shame, no doubt. They've all suppressed their origins. Dentists, doctors and surgeons weren't born anywhere" (Céline 2012, 455).

containment of "fake news" have pointed out the antidemocratic nature of these proposed regulations. They have often done so in bad faith. The problem, according to these somewhat minoritarian voices, is not that the legal prosecution of "lies" or "misinformation" would be tantamount to censorship (it would not: in fact, the current legislation in most Western countries already allows for many of the containment measures present in most projected laws against "fake news" and misinformation). The problem is rather that the social construction of "truth" or "information" is often *itself* the object of public contestation. According to these positions, curtailing this specific discursive agency would, in effect, amount to a significant breach of democratic sovereignty. On the opposite side, supporters of such regulatory measures rightly point out that the COVID-19 pandemic has made it plain that the social cost of misinformation *can* be measured in human lives.

Among the several models that attempt to explain the spread of misinformation among the public, "virality" has achieved a particular status as what Hans Blumenberg once described as an "absolute metaphor," i.e., one that has become autonomous from the contents its originally sought to illustrate (Blumenberg 2010, 4). "Virality," like "the naked truth," "the book of nature" or "the body politic," obscures the very concepts it draws on and conceals the empirical incompatibility of informational and viral propagation; as such, an absolute metaphor is not only a figure of speech, but also, alas, a disfigurement of thought. Other entries in the current politological lexicon share a similar linguistic fate. The inherently metaphorical concepts of "biases" and "echo chambers," for instance, are routinely used both to describe the properties of technological infrastructure (for instance the segmentation of internet publics through search algorithms and the emergence of fragmentary communities of information) *and* to describe the ideological dispositions of populations in liberal, democratic societies (for instance when an utterance is criticized or excluded from the public sphere on account of its "bias"). The double valence of these concepts is significant in itself. Because "biases" and "echo chambers" simultaneously refer to apperceptive dispositions and to the technological infrastructure through which these apperceptive dispositions are made public, critical engagement with these terms tends to conflate ideology and technology, when in fact a conceptualization of this overlap itself (of *ideological* "biases" and *technological* "echo chambers," for instance) is needed. Absolute metaphors hence pose a threat to the epistemological and deliberative standards of liberal democracies whenever they thoroughly obscure the semantic realms they originally sought to bring together *rhetorically*.

Meanwhile, it is difficult to shield calls to "immunize the public against misinformation" from the risk of literal readings. After all, "virality" has become one of the structuring metaphors – and, in equal measure, structuring literalisms – of modern public health management and information theory alike. It has crowded out older figurative motifs – "to spread like wildfire," "to disseminate," "to become common currency" – and seems to have brought a near-hegemonic Foucauldian tradition in the humanities to turn its coat, give in to analogical reasoning, and actively conflate blatant political irrationality with mental illness: political opponents, both reactionary and progressive, now belong to the "lunatic fringe" (whether this profane diagnosis is accurate or not is entirely beside the point; I am drawing attention the power of metaphors to essentially *nullify* dominant intellectual traditions and to overturn even the most dogmatic readings of "biopower," "discipline," "dispositifs" and other critical potboilers).

Yet it would be misleading to single out organizational discourse as the sole, or even main vector by which "virality" has gained credence in recent years. In fact, internet culture has long developed its own profane theory of cultural transmission which reproduces a similar conflation of pathology and discursivity. The concept of the "meme," which loosely derives from evolutionary biology, is an eminent case in point. It extrapolates from evolutionary genetics to argue that culture be best understood as a series of units of cultural transmission which actively cannibalize users in order to compete with other cultural units. In this particularly crude theory of culture, information itself is endowed with agency: a snippet from a movie, an image, but also Homer's *Odyssey*, eating with a fork, not wearing a hat in a church, or a way of cooking pasta are "memes" precisely because they gained supremacy over other units of culture. The eerie terminology at play in this subfield – "cultural parasites" (Dennett 2007, 81), "mind viruses" (Aunger 2007, 602) – emphasize both that cultural units, not people, are agential and that "virality" remains the covert paradigm operating in "meme" theory. Here, populations ("users") are but passive carriers of culture: their agency in selecting, evaluating, sharing or not sharing cultural units is, at best, treated as an epiphenomenon in scholarly accounts of "viral" phenomena (Nahon and Hemsley 2013, 60). Internet "virality" and "meme" theory, as analytic concepts, hence merely duplicate the very conflation of medical and informational "contagion" they sought to escape in the first place. Both hence fall short of the humblest demands for critical reflexivity.

One fact, however, is well established: in the overwhelming majority of instances, information does not "go viral" – whatever the validity of this metaphor. In fact, the chances of information "going viral," i.e., of being shared with very high intensity beyond its original communicational setting, are infinitesimal. If information did spread across the public sphere with a frequency anywhere resembling that of pathogens, "viral" discourse would be endemic and crowd out all other possible types of information and communication. Conversely, if pathogens behaved like information, the risk of contagion events and epidemics ever occurring would be negligible.

Recent epidemics and pandemics clearly show this is not the case. We are hence faced with an interesting contradiction. On the one hand, political irrationality, scapegoating, and disinformation are on the rise. On the other, prevalent absolute metaphors give a poor account of informational and pathogenic propagation and simultaneously present specific, historically identified political risks. In other words, Semmelweis and Holmes were right, Céline's pamphletary conflations were not, COVID-19 and disinformation kill, vaccination is effective in preventing contagion, *and* information does not spread like pathogens. It would hence seem to be of vital importance to escape the deadlock of figurative language and to return, instead, to actionable and more carefully rational accounts of how populations communicate or miscommunicate on the threats they face.

Key Points

Let me simplify my argument somewhat and outline five key points. The first is that the very need for any kind of institutional storytelling involving a metaphorical "discursive contagion" or "infodemic" is doubtful. What knowledge or kind of knowledge is secured by equating the spread of pathogens and the spread of information *about* these pathogens, no matter if this information is correct or incorrect? The need for such a narrative superposition (of disease and discourse *about* disease) is nevertheless supported by a large portion of the public and by supranational institutions, both having devoted significant resources – labor, attention, and capital – to the narrativization of what, until recently, was taken to be an unavoidable, if regrettable consequence of an open public sphere. I would argue that the social risks derived from this rhetorical conflation outweighs its purported benefits.

My second point is that, for all practical concerns, at least some of the measures proposed by these supranational health organizations in order to contain misinformation remain valid, if in a much narrower sense than originally proposed. Assessing the sources, going beyond headlines, checking the date, examining the evidence: this is all very sound advice. This leaves out two important subproblems, however. The first is that these measures are inadequate to identify misinformation with sufficient reliability and, conversely, may miscategorize factual statements as fraudulent ones. A few paradigmatic examples immediately come to mind. Chelsea Manning's 2010 release of classified information through the WikiLeaks platform, for example, would fail to meet all seven criteria and pass the seven-steps test, even though the status of the leak as valid "information" has been thoroughly ascertained since (Maxwell 2019). Yet the source, publication date, and supporting evidence of the documents could not be assessed by the general public, the author of the leak was anonymous, biases could merely be postulated, etc. The second subproblem derives from the first: the cases in which these steps would be able to reliably identify misinformation are also precisely the cases where they would be either superfluous, or unable to reach their target users. In fact, blatant misinformation is usually suspicious for other reasons: it often negates basic empirical observation (Kumkar

2022). Conversely, the negation of basic empirical observation by users is unlikely to be corrected by "fact checkers" and an examination of "biases."

My third point is that the "infodemic" metaphor remains helpful, provided we turn it on its head: populations may be "immunized" against misinformation *even though* misinformation does not spread like a virus. In social psychology, for instance, "inoculation theory" has empirically demonstrated that resistance to influence and persuasion can be induced by exposing populations to "weakened" versions of discursive threats (for instance political misinformation or marketing campaigns): "Preemptive exposure to weakened challenging content motivates a process or processes of resistance to future exposure to stronger challenging content" (Compton, 4295). The analogical reasoning that motivates inoculation theory is glaring, yet is does not entail the kind of social costs "virality" does. Empirical studies seem to corroborate one essential observation: populations and individuals, once alerted to the dangers and sensuous seductions of "challenging content," may in turn treat "stronger challenging content" with "boosted attitude certainty" and without "dampen[ed] reactance" (Compton, 4297).

My fourth point is that this kind of mechanical, reactive handling of "challenging content" nevertheless sits uneasily with the main tenets of a robust democratic culture. The point is hence both constative and normative: this is not really what we need, this is not really what we should want. In fact, enabling good "reactance" to challenging texts and statements was once the goal of higher education. Enabling citizens to deal rationally, critically, and collaboratively with complex material remains an essential competence in democratic societies. Yet these are not only competences: they are also historically constituted "values" or social norms that can be explicitly defended as such. Facilitating access to the tools that make goods such as "truth" and "information" available to all would amount to explicitly postulating the value of these goods in themselves. We should therefore abandon formalist descriptions of a "good public sphere" and "public rationality" and uphold these goods for what they are: historically constituted, unequally distributed, but also more equally distributable values that are dependent on historically constituted, unequally distributed, but also more equally distributable *competences*. The erosion of higher education curricula, along with the sweeping technological transformation of the past decade (Rothkopf's "modern information technologies" discussed in the first section of this essay), have arguably played a significant role in the erosion of public discourse itself. Yet if universities are the central purveyors of epistemic tools in Western democracies, the place of the humanities in higher education is wholly paradoxical: they are under tremendous pressure to make essential tools available to the population while being deprived of the material means to do so *in full recognition of their political import*. I wish to suggest that a radical reconsideration of the role and value of such competences would make the further legal regulation of truth claims in the public sphere less urgent.

Finally, as a general rule of thumb, and by way of conclusion, metasocial and metacommunicational metaphors should be avoided whenever their efficiency depends on their public perception *as metaphors*. The social acceptance of metasocial metaphors (i.e., the social tolerance for figurative statements that pertain to society itself) is historically and situationally variable; this variability itself should be subjected to a careful risk assessment, especially – and this should go without saying – when previous iterations have led to the identification and scapegoating of minorities. The responses to Céline's activity as a pamphleteer between 1937 and 1941, for instance, convey a general impression of the wide variety of possible public perceptions in a given historical situation. Some, like future Nobel Prize winner André Gide, insisted on the metaphorical and comedic nature of Céline's "Jew": in fact, for Gide, the "semitic question" had not even been touched upon in *School for Corpses* (Gide 1999, 302). Others telephoned the publisher of the pamphlets to express their outrage at Céline's literal calls for the assassination of approximately 320,000 men, women, and children. A few more straightforward opponents openly challenged Céline in bars and restaurants: "Hey Céline, my name is Cohen. Fuck you!" (Alliot 2021, 401, my transl.).

European Research Council
Established by the European Commission

Bibliography

Alliot, David, editor. 2021. *D'un Céline l'autre*, Bouquins.

Aunger, Robert. 2007. "Memes." *The Oxford Handbook of Evolutionary Psychology*, edited by R. I. M. Dunbar, Louiss Barrett, Oxford UP, 599–604.

Blumenberg, Hans. 2010. *Paradigms for a Metaphorology*, Cornell UP.

Bourdieu, Pierre. 1997. *Pascalian Meditations*, Stanford UP.

Céline, Louis-Ferdinand. 2022. *Death on Credit*, translated by Ralph Manheim, Alma Books.

Céline, Louis-Ferdinand. 2012. *Écrits polémiques*, edited by Régis Tettamanzi, éditions 8.

Céline, Louis-Ferdinand. 1959. Interview with Louis Pauwel, June 19, 1959. https://www.youtube.com/watch?v=4hjtjZYXXic.

Céline, Louis-Ferdinand. 2020. *Mea Culpa & The Life and Work of Semmelweis*, Sunwise Books.

Céline, Louis-Ferdinand. 1999. *Semmelweis*, Gallimard.

Compton, Josh. 2021. "Threat and/in Inoculation Theory." *International Journal of Communication*, vol. 15, 4294–4306.

David, Christian S. 2012. *Colonialism, Antisemitism, and Germans of Jewish Descent in Imperial Germany*, U of Michigan P.

Dennett, Daniel C. 2007. *Breaking the Spell: Religion as a Natural Phenomenon*, Penguin.

European Commission. 2021. "The Rise of Antisemitism Online During the Pandemic: A Study of French and German Content," edited by the Institute for Strategic Dialogue, online. https://op.europa.eu/en/publication-detail/-/publication/d73c833f-c34c-11eb-a925-01aa75ed71a1/language-en.

Gide, André. 1999. *Éssais Critiques*, Gallimard.

Golsan, Richard J. 2010. "Antisemitism in Modern France: Dreyfus, Vichy, and Beyond." *Antisemitism: A History*, edited by Albert S. Lindemann and Richard S. Levy, Oxford UP, 136–149.

Gross, Andrew. 2020. "Vaccination, Inoculation, and Franklin's Grief." *American Counter/Publics*, edited by Ulla Haselstein, Frank Kelleter, Alexander Starre, and Birte Wege, Universitätsverlag Winter, 137–158.

Holmes, Oliver Wendell, Sr. 1855. *Puerperal Fever, as a Private Pestilence*, Ticknor and Fields.

Kuodi, P., Y. Gorelik, H. Zayyad et al. 2022. "Association between BNT162b2 vaccination and reported incidence of post-COVID-19 symptoms: cross-sectional study 2020–21, Israel." *npj Vaccines*, vol. 7, 101. https://doi.org/10.1038/s41541-022-00526-5.

Lee, S. K., J. Sun, S. Jang et al. 2022. "Misinformation of COVID-19 Vaccines and Vaccine Hesitancy." *Scientific Reports*, vol. 12, 13681. https://doi.org/10.1038/s41598-022-17430-6.

Lyu, Hanjia, Yihe Zheng, Liebo Luo. 2022. "Misinformation versus Facts: Understanding the Influence of News regarding COVID-19 Vaccines on Vaccine Uptake." *Health Data Science*. https://doi.org/10.34133/2022/9858292.

Kumkar, Nils C. 2022. *Alternative Fakten: Zur Praxis der kommunikativen Erkenntnisverweigerung*, Suhrkamp.

Meigs, Charles D. 1854. *On the Nature, Signs, and Treatment of Childbed Fevers; in a Series of Letters, Adressed to the Students of His Class*, Blanchard and Lea.

Nahon, Karine, Jeff Hemsley. 2013. *Going Viral*, Polity Press.

Maxwell, Linda. 2019. *Insurgent Truth: Chelsea Manning and the Politics of Outsider Truth-Telling*, Oxford UP.

Pascal, Blaise. 2013. *Apology for Religion: Extracted from the Pensées*, Cambridge UP.

Rimbert, Pierre. 2021. "La main prise dans le pot à bobards." *Le Monde diplomatique*, 21.

Rothkopf, David J. 2003. "When the Buzz Bites Back." *The Washington Post*, May 11, 2003, online. https://www.washingtonpost.com/archive/opinions/2003/05/11/when-the-buzz-bites-back/bc8cd84f-cab6-4648-bf58-0277261af6cd/.

Tettamanzi, Régis. 2001. "Les Pamphlets de Céline et "l'invasion juive" en médecine." *Actualité de Céline*, edited Alain Cresciucci, Du Lérot éditeur, 127–142.

World Health Organization. 2020. "Immunizing the public against misinformation." https://www.who.int/news-room/feature-stories/detail/immunizing-the-public-against-misinformation.

World Health Organization. 2020. "Let's flatten the infodemic curve." <https://www.who.int/news-room/spotlight/let-s-flatten-the-infodemic-curve>

Xu S., R. Huang, L. S. Sy et al. 2021. "COVID-19 Vaccination and Non–COVID-19 Mortality Risk – Seven Integrated Health Care Organizations, United States, December 14, 2020–July 31, 2021." *MMWR Morbidity and Mortality Weekly Report* 2021/70, 1520–1524. http://dx.doi.org/10.15585/mmwr.mm7043e2.

The Lockdown Diary
Crisis in Corona Fictions

Yvonne Völkl

Introduction[1]

After the outbreak of COVID-19 in China and Italy, the WHO officially declared this health crisis as a worldwide pandemic on March 11, 2020. The ensuing pandemic crisis management and the measures to break the chain of infection and subsequently relieve the burden that was placed on healthcare systems disrupted the social life of whole populations in an unprecedented way. Many governments worldwide implemented a partial or full lockdown (cf. Dunford 2020; Ritchie et al. 2020) and urged their citizens to "stay at home unless [there was the] need to go out for certain reasons, such as going to work, buying food, or taking exercise" (Collins 2022).[2] Especially throughout the first collectively shared lockdown experience, which was largely believed to be a one-time event in the early stages of the pandemic, repercussions in the cultural realm regarding the reception as well as the production of fictional narratives could be observed (cf. Research Group *Pandemic Fictions* 2020; Nesselhauf 2023).

On the one hand, it was possible to discern a rapid increase in the reception of "pandemic fictions" (i.e., fictional narratives relating to historical or fictitious epidemics or pandemics). During the first lockdown, a new interest emerged, for example, in literary classics, such as Giovanni Boccaccio's *Decamerone* or Albert Camus's *The Plague*, which were broadcasted for collective consumption via the Internet (e.g., #Décaméron-19, #lirelapeste) and the radio (e.g., Camus' 1947 classic was read on

1 Acknowledgments: This research was funded by the Austrian Science Fund (FWF: P 34571-G) and was inspired by the observations my colleagues Julia Obermayr, Elisabeth Hobisch, Albert Göschl, and I made during and after the COVID-19 induced lockdown in the spring of 2020.

2 In addition to national lockdowns in which entire business sectors (e.g., restaurants, shops, cinemas, libraries) as well as educational institutions and nursing homes were closed, other mitigation measures such as border closings, travel restrictions, physical distancing mandates, or mouth and nose coverings, were also implemented on an international scale.

Austrian radio station FM4, was sold out in many bookstores, and even had to be reprinted by publishers). Even the French president and other politicians encouraged their fellow citizens to read while staying at home (cf. Stemberger 2021, 10–11). Furthermore, an increase in the consumption of cinematic pandemic fiction was observed; on the video-streaming platform Netflix, movies such as *Outbreak* (1995) or *Contagion* (2011) were among the frequently most watched films in March 2020 (cf. Clark 2020; Mann 2020).[3]

On the other hand, after the declaration of the COVID-19 pandemic and the implementation of the first lockdowns and other mitigation measures, authors and filmmakers – both professionals and non-professionals – began to produce their own fictional narratives about this specific time (cf. Guyenne 2021). These new "Corona Fictions" integrate contemporary media and political discourse on the pandemic crisis and reactivate structures and elements of pre-existing pandemic fictions, such as the classic "outbreak narrative" (Wald 2008) or themes of fear and anxiety (cf. Research Group *Pandemic Fictions* 2020, 322f.; Hobisch et al. 2022, 201). They direct the focus toward the COVID-19 crisis from a variety of perspectives and use different genres and media formats for this purpose.[4] The first Corona Fictions mainly emerged as music videos (cf. Obermayr and Hobisch 2024), web and TV series (cf. Mateos Pérez 2021), as well as in prose and poetry anthologies (cf. Völkl 2025). In addition, among the immediate responses to the implementation of the first lockdown, the number of public diaries, so-called "lockdown diaries," has mushroomed (cf. BnF 2021, 13; Fleury and Gateau 2022; Gammel and Wang 2022; Obergöker 2020; Schafer 2022; Stemberger 2021, 41–42; Yang 2021).

In this chapter, I start from the hypothesis that these publicized diaries, were produced at the beginning of the COVID-19 induced lockdown due to their positive

---

3 Other well-known examples of pandemic fictions in Western culture include the biblical passages which infer that God punishes the people by sending a plague, the first medical eyewitness report by Thucydides, and the fictitious eyewitness account given in *A Journal of the Plague Year* (1722) by Daniel Defoe. More recent works also can be categorized as examples of pandemic fictions, such as the Canadian series *Épidémie* (2020/2021) or José Saramago's novel *Ensaio sobre a Cegueira* (1995) (cf. Research Group *Pandemic Fictions* 2020, 322–323; Hobisch et al. 2022, 192). Regarding the role of the eyewitness in pandemic fictions, cf. Franziska Meier's contribution in this collection.

4 A diverse corpus of Corona Fictions produced in the Romance languages can be accessed via the Corona Fictions OA bibliographic database (cf. Hobisch et al. 2021-2025). This material tends to appear in short, often collaborative formats and genres in early audiovisual and written Corona Fictions. Such tendencies "can be attributed to the demands of our social media-driven world, which prefers quick media [...] formats and genres, on the one hand, and to the sense of community that is created and strengthened by working together (although mostly remotely) on a common music, film, or book project, on the other [...]" (Völkl 2025, 92).

effects on the mental well-being of both their producers and audiences.[5] Thus, in the following, I investigate how diaristic narration strengthens the resilience of those who create them and examine how resilience-strengthening capacities are transferred through the lockdown diaries to the audience.

Drawing on socio-psychological studies about trauma and resilience (e.g., Cyrulnik 2002; id. 2013; Engelhardt 2005; Ford 2009; Kast 1990), I elucidate psychological effects provoked by the crisis discourse that evolved in the political arenas and media during the early stages of the COVID-19 pandemic. I also briefly outline reasons why some people seem to be more resilient than others in crisis situations and explain why (self-)narration is a useful coping strategy to which people are drawn to in and after unsettling experiences. Subsequently, the chapter addresses the subject of the lockdown diary and illustrates the extent to which diaristic narratives have opened up possibilities to increase resilience among those who produced (i.e., narrated) and those who received (i.e,. read, watched or listened to) them during the first lockdown, citing – besides earlier studies on the topic – two striking examples of diaries created in the context of the European lockdowns that were explicitly addressed at an audience and also reference mental and physical health aspects. The first one is the Spanish *Diario de estar por casa, o "Mis conversaciones con un murciélago"* (*Diary of Being at Home, or "My Conversations with a Bat"*) by Fernanda Krahn Uribe, who published her "graphic diary" on her Facebook page. The second example is a personal lockdown diary in the French language by Prune Antoine, published under the English title *#My Funny Quarantine* on the public blog of the author.

I equally regard both Krahn Uribe's auto-fictional diary and Antoine's (allegedly) factual blog diary as literary works. These and other lockdown diaries can be interpreted as "literarizations of life" (cf. Görner 1986, 31), since from a narratological perspective diaristic narration – like any other form of "cultural fact- and worldmaking" (Nünning 2023, 78) – involves "selection, deletion, abstraction, weighting and ratings of relevance, configuration, ordering, and emplotment, and, last but not least, the choice of point of view and the arrangement of perspectives" (ibid.).[6] The

5 Although the reactions of the audience to lockdown diaries were both positive and negative, this article places a focus on the potentially positive effects. In France, for instance, the diaries of renowned authors Marie Darrieussecq and Leïla Slimani provoked an intense and black-hearted debate on social media, unearthing a deeply rooted hatred of the Parisian elite and bourgeoisie as well as misogynistic attitudes within certain sections of society (cf. Obergöker 2020; Stemberger 2021, 42–43).

6 Ansgar Nünning (2023, 68) bases his profound reflections on the relevance of narratological considerations concerning writing as one of the most powerful ways of cultural fact- and worldmaking "on the insight that the chaotic events of a crisis like the COVID-19 pandemic or a war, for example, can only be made accessible and communicated in society after such chaotic happenings have been transferred into writing and comprehensible stories. This,

fact that the lockdown diaries were publicly disseminated on online platforms and thereby intentionally produced for an audience is just another factor that comes into play here (cf. Ainetter 2006, 31–34; Görner 1986, 37; Kalff and Vedder 2016, 235–236).

Pandemic Discourse and Management: Psychological Effects and Responses

At the beginning of the pandemic, political and "media reports embedd[ed] the [...] global challenge of the COVID-19 pandemic in terms (and therefore also logics) of crisis when referring to it as 'corona crisis'" (Research Group *Pandemic Fictions* 2020, 322) and used military metaphors to "trigger change in beliefs and behaviour in terms of undertaking specific measures" (Silaški and Đurović 2022, 275) in an attempt to counter the spread of the pandemic.[7] This sort of crisis discourse in the political management of illnesses is not new; it has been used for centuries as demonstrated, for example, by Susan Sontag (1978, 65–66) and Richard Gwyn (2002, 110–111). In fact, whether a situation is perceived as unsettling depends largely on the extent to which it is communicated as critical or life-threatening. Undeniably, using military metaphors increases the threatening dimension of an illness through its "ability to arouse people into a state of fear and preventive activity, to mobilise against an emergency" (Gwyn 2002, 110). While a heightened awareness may indubitably be beneficial to encourage individuals in joining the collective fight against a specific threat, it may also be detrimental to the individual's health and well-being. In fact, experiencing a life-threatening situation and being exposed to a (long-lasting) crisis discourse, may jeopardize the perception of being able to shape one's life independently. In other words, experiencing the loss of individual autonomy – a value that is held very high in Western cultures – may stoke fears and anxieties (cf. Kast 1990, 16) and, at worst, may cause (re)traumatizing effects (cf. Ford 2009, 34).[8]

---

again, requires narratives and rhetorical strategies, which are by no means inherent to the events or facts as such but are imposed on them by the forms of the narrative discourse which functions as a shaping pattern." Further discussions and explanations regarding the complexity, multidimensionality, and historicity of the notion of "fact" can be found in Susanne Knaller's interdisciplinary volume on *Writing Facts* (2023), in which Nünning's text also appeared.

7 For an overview of the public debates and language use in different countries during the first year of the pandemic, cf. the edited volumes of Musolff et al. (2022) or Blumczynski and Wilson (2023).

8 E.g., in her autobiographical account, Régine Robin (2020) – historian, novelist, translator, and professor of sociology – described the sudden lockdown, which she experienced in Paris, as having triggered her trauma as a Jewish child in Paris during World War II. She was not only triggered by the heavy restrictions of free movement, but also by the war rhetoric of French

In the spring of 2020, the COVID-19 pandemic was not only accompanied by a crisis discourse that metaphorically framed the invisible coronavirus as a deadly "threat" or "enemy," but also by general lockdowns and other mitigation measures, such as border closings and distancing mandates.[9] Early on, psychologists and psychiatrists (cf. Ansermet 2020; Cottin 2021; Render Turmaud 2020; Tourette-Turgis and Chollier 2020, 195) perceived this crisis management strategy, which was applied transnationally at the beginning of the pandemic, as a traumatic rupture of life. The measures caused a lack of self-determination and generated great amount of uncertainty regarding how life will continue. This situation thereby exhibited all of the components of a trauma.

Previous socio-psychological studies on trauma and resilience show that some individuals survive the same crisis better than others (cf. Engelhardt 2005; Kast 1990; Cyrulnik 2002; id. 2013; Ford 2009, 60–94). Among many other factors (e.g., personal or environmental), the varying effects of traumatic experiences are attributed to the degree of resilience of individuals. Resilience in this sense is understood as "the process and outcome of successfully adapting to difficult or challenging life experiences, especially through mental, emotional, and behavioural flexibility and adjustment to external and internal demands" (APA 2022). Numerous innate and acquired factors strengthen resilience and "contribute to how well people adapt to adversities, predominant among them (a) the ways in which individuals view and engage with the world, (b) the availability and quality of social resources, and (c) specific coping strategies" (ibid.).

One significant coping strategy that can activate and even increase resilience is the act of narration – all the while recognizing that also personal (e.g., age, physical condition) and environmental factors (e.g., living conditions, income) as well as other coping strategies (e.g., relaxation techniques, eating meals on a regular basis, or taking breaks of negative news) have an influence on an individual's resilience capacities. The testimonial narrative (as product of this narration) is a means of establishing a logical and coherent narrative link between different (traumatic) experiences and events in one's life. At the same time, it is a means of bearing witness to the crisis and remembering what has happened – both for oneself and for posterity. In other words, trauma and resilience studies associate the act of narration with therapeutic, testimonial, and commemorative functions (cf. Cyrulnik 2002, 110; id.

politicians and in media, their infantilization of adult citizens, media censorship as well as people's reactions to the crisis discourse (e.g., panic buying or a climate of denunciation).

9 Although the distancing practices called upon in the course of the pandemic management were mostly referred to as "social distancing," they fundamentally aimed at the body and are therefore more accurately described as "physical distancing" (cf. Klein and Liebsch 2020; ead. 2022).

2004, 194; id. 2005, 49; Herman 1992; Pennebaker 2004; Tourette-Turgis and Chollier 2020).

Diaries represent such individual testimonial accounts of events that interrupt daily life in a striking way. By making notes daily, the diary keeper can record impressions which impact their life so much faster than under normal circumstances (cf. Boerner 1969, 17). From a historical point of view, the use of the diary to bear witness to a crisis is not unusual. An increase in the number of published diaristic narratives was observed at the beginning of World War I and at the end of World War II; thus, diaries written in the 20th century have been considered as a "medium of crisis" (cf. ibid., 63). Generally speaking, this increasing use of the diary may be explained by examining the crises that affected the subjects; these, in turn, are linked to the political and historical past, to war, dictatorial regimes, or strong restrictions on possibilities of free self-expression (cf. Kalff and Vedder 2016, 239–240). In summary, the traumatic scope of experiences and events that affect individuals plays a crucial role, encouraging them to take up pen and paper or, today, move to the keyboard and monitor.

Diaristic Narration during the First Lockdown

As indicated in the introduction, diaristic narration and diaristic narratives proved to be very popular at the beginning of the pandemic crisis.[10] Their self-denomination mostly as "lockdown diary" (*journal de confinement* in French and *diario de confinamiento/cuarentena* in Spanish[11]) reveals that these narratives are situational products born out of the health crisis, such as the diaries produced during World Wars I and II, which would not exist without these unsettling events. As products of the first general lockdowns, they share the chronological structure of the entries, which are assigned to a specific date or day, thereby bringing some kind of order into this unprecedented and unsettling time.

Many diaristic narratives produced during this period appeared in a written form and were published either analogue or digitally in newspapers, anthologies, blogs, or on social media platforms as also observed by Jonas Nesselhauf (2023, 344–345). Numerous audiovisual lockdown diaries also exist, including the Spanish sitcom *Diarios de la cuarentena*, broadcasted as a kind of *docu-ficción* on public TV

10 In France, e.g., the Bibliothèque nationale de France, the Association pour l'autobiographie and other institutions collected and archived digital diaries of the first lockdown (cf. BnF 2022; Schafer 2022, 185). The Corona Fictions Database (cf. Hobisch et al. 2021-2025) also exhibits a large number of lockdown diaries in various languages

11 Although both Spanish terms refer to the lockdown phase, "confinamiento" has widely been used in Spain while "cuarentena" has been more prevalent in Latin American countries (cf. Pineda 2021).

during the first lockdown in Spain; audio podcasts, such as the *Journal de confinement* created by Lebanese-Canadian writer and stage director Wajdi Mouawad; or danced video podcasts, such as the one produced by choreographer Maud Contini based on Prune Antoine's readings of her blog diary. As argued above, they can be interpreted as conscious "literarizations of life" (cf. Görner 1986, 31) since every writing and storytelling process – be it fictional or factual – "is a performative act that constructs and establishes the very facts that texts seem to merely represent" (Nünning 2023, 54).

Previous research on lockdown diaries indicates that they serve the above-mentioned therapeutic, testimonial, and commemorative functions which explains their phenomenal popularity. However, the terminology used by researchers has sometimes differed, with additional functions being highlighted, such as enhancing agency or community-building.

In "Online Lockdown Diaries as Endurance Art," Guobin Yang (2021), for example, investigated lockdown diaries produced in the city of Wuhan, which was the first city to be sealed off abruptly on January 23, 2020, to mitigate the spread of the coronavirus. Yang interprets the writing and online posting of lockdown diaries practiced during this early phase as "acts of *personal* agency in an otherwise contingent, uncontrollable reality, one that depended on the ability to make this repeated gesture in a consciously collective context – in this case, social media [italics in the original]" (ibid., 2). The public sharing of the lockdown diaries and the interactions that subsequently occurred between diary keepers and readers, enabled them to develop a "sense of community" (ibid., 3). Therefore, Yang understands the online lockdown diaries as an "art of endurance" (ibid., 7) or a way to more effectively cope with the lockdown since no one knew at the time that this lockdown in the city of Wuhan would last for 76 days until April 8, 2020.

In "'Why Has the Outbreak Turned so Deadly?': Diary from a Quarantined City," Irene Gammel and Jason Wang (2022) regard the lockdown diary as "pivotal tool during crisis," situated "at the intersection of the diaristic truth-telling, traumatic narrative, history, and the pandemic," and remark that it shares "key features with the traditional diary such as its focus on truth-seeking fueled by frankness" (ibid., 29). Moreover, they interpret the lockdown diary as "an 'outbreak narrative,' whose rhetorical and narrative goal is the containment of a pandemic" (ibid., 30), thereby also bestowing a certain agency upon the diary keeper. The focus of their analysis is directed toward the most famous and one of the earliest examples of the lockdown diary: Fang Fang's *Wuhan Diary* (2020). The renowned Chinese novelist documented her observations and reflections during the first Chinese lockdown from the inside of the quarantined city on the social media platforms Weibo and WeChat. Her diary entries were read, shared, and (both positively and negatively) commented upon by millions of followers in real-time. Shortly after the end of the lockdown in Wuhan, they were published in the form of a book, which was translated into 18 languages (cf. ibid., 28). Gammel and Wang also emphasize the therapeutic and testimonial functions of Fang's lockdown diary by indicating that its writing and posting served the author "[a]s a self-reflexive way of coping by bearing testimony during a historic moment" (ibid., 28). The cathartic function of Fang Fang's inner "urgency of communicating" (ibid.) is also highlighted by Martina Stemberger (2021) in her literary history of pandemics where she quotes directly from the German edition of the *Wuhan Diary*, "'Ich konnte nur jeden Tag schreiben, schreiben, schreiben...', [...]; literarische 'Anstrengung, mir selbst freien Atem zu verschaffen', die auch 'anderen beim Atmen' zu helfen erlaubt [...]" (38).[12] Fang's aspiration to support her readers with her diaristic narration is also signaled here.

The last study mentioned in this context is the analysis of French online lockdown diaries by Cynthia Fleury and Valérie Gateau (2022). In "Récits et fonctions psychiques de la narration dans les journaux de confinement," they describe four writing functions (i.e., sharing, cathartic, imaginative and political, and historicizing) for three different groups of diary keepers (i.e., general public, health care workers and their patients, and intellectuals). The public mainly used the sharing function of diaristic narration, which resembles the community-building function in that these diary writers mostly attempted to reduce their loneliness by sharing their daily lives with their readers and proclaiming their solidarity with others to "hold on" during the lockdown. For healthcare workers and their patients, diaristic testimonial narration served a cathartic function. It enabled them to describe the challenging aspects of care during lockdown and the suffering experienced by caregivers. It also highlighted the sense of solidarity that emerged between caregivers and patients. Intellectuals, as the third group of diary writers, had recourse mainly to the imaginative and political functions of the lockdown diary. These functions are similar to the agency function, as they called for more united political and democratic responses to the crisis. Finally, all of the groups investigated had recourse to the historicizing function of the testimonial narrative, by which the individual stories are inscribed into the collective history, thereby one day taking on commemorative function.

In the following, two examples of online lockdown diaries, which explicitly address aspects of mental and physical health, will be given in order to illustrate how – on a thematic and formal-aesthetic level – lockdown diaries open up possibilities for increasing the well-being and resilience of the diary keepers and their recipients.

12 "'I could only write, write, write every day...'; literary 'effort to give myself free breath' that also allows 'others to breathe'" (author's translation).

Diario de estar por casa

The first of the two examples of diaristic narratives developed in the context of the first European lockdowns in spring 2020 is the auto-fictional lockdown diary of the Austrian-based and Chilean-born author Fernanda Krahn Uribe, published under the title *Diario de estar por casa, o "Mis conversaciones con un murciélago"* (*Diary of Being at Home or "My Conversations with a Bat"*). This "graphic diary" with handwritten pages and colored hand drawings tells the exceptional lockdown encounter between a single middle-aged woman and her strange visitor – an elderly bat – in the style of a serialized story. Starting from March 15, 2020, Krahn Uribe published one diary page per day on the social media platform Facebook over 40 days, then also longer diary entries at increasingly irregular intervals until July 12, 2020. The entries clearly show aspects of (emotional) support as well as enjoyment in their production and as the author describes in her preface,[13] her diaristic creation was, in fact, all about "priorizando el disfrutarlo antes que crear algo 'perfecto.'"[14]

The first diary entry was written on "Domingo 15 de marzo 2020" and introduces *in medias res* the female first-person narrator and protagonist, who spends the lockdown alone in her apartment and can be interpreted as the author's *alter ego*. She addresses the readers directly in an informal style, telling them both timidly and excitedly that she has recently noticed something strange on her coat rack during a meditation practice: there, where her umbrella usually hangs, she has discerned a bat. While she was frightened at first and thought she was hallucinating, she admits to having entered into a dialogue with this bat in the next day's entry. In the subsequent conversation with the animal, which extends over several months, the readers accompany the narrator and learn about her and, nearly simultaneously, about the life of this bat named Yi Qui, who is already several hundred years old. Yi Qui "tells" her about the plague he experienced in 17th century Italy, emphasizing the terrible circumstances under which his human friends survived this epidemic at the time. This "eyewitness account" of a previous epidemic adjusts the narrator's perspective of the world as it reminds her (as well as the readers) that deadly epidemics have been omnipresent throughout history and that, even in times of crisis, there are always ways to maintain one's agency.

The conversation between the narrator and Yi Qui, during which he relates his adventures and those of his friends during the plague, is occasionally interrupted by the depiction of the narrator's mental and physical well-being during the lockdown. On the one hand, her emotional distress to this entirely new situation be-

13 This (textual) preface was appended to the subsequent manuscript of the graphic diary, which Fernanda Krahn Uribe kindly made available to the author of this chapter for research purposes, and which forms the basis of the present analysis.

14 "[H]aving fun rather than creating something 'perfect'" (author's translation).

comes apparent through vivid drawings ranging from nightmares to hysterical crying, or through the narrator's confession that she finds online teaching very stressful. On the other hand, coping strategies for this exceptional situation are presented in addition to the illustration of the narrator's meditation practice at the beginning of the graphic diary: these drawings show the narrator how she accesses social resources by talking on the phone with her friends or taking part in an online yoga class. Other drawings, in turn, show her taking a walk, doing gardening activities, or refraining from reading apocalyptic news before she goes to bed to avoid having nightmares.

Generally, the changing well-being of the protagonist in this exceptional situation is underpinned by a nuanced artistic depiction of both her good and poor states of mind. For example, while the depictions of her nightmares are represented through a chaotically arranged interplay of scribbled handwriting and color-intensive hand drawings in the March 20 entry, the depictions of her coping strategies are pastel-colored and the handwritten text and drawings are rectilinear and more evenly distributed in the March 18 entry. However, the longer the lockdown and the conversation with Yi Qui lasts, the more the narrator is absorbed and distracted by his story. On a formal level, this is noticeable in that Yi Qui's story becomes more and more central by literally taking up more and more space in the diary entries, while references to her own life and well-being become shorter and shorter as the graphic diary (i.e., as time) advances.

The animal interlocutor, which is not accidentally a bat – after all, the political and media discourse also initially circulated the accusation that the coronavirus originated from either bats or pangolins – can be interpreted as a zoomorphological fear of the virus, which seems otherwise invisible. However, the bat not only metaphorically stands for the fears that the pandemic discourse, the lockdown, and the ensuing additional mitigation measures bring to light; it simultaneously represents the "cure" to it. Through her constant conversation with the bat, the narrator is not only distracted from and can forget about her negative feelings; she also confronts her fears as she gradually becomes aware of them and can finally free herself from them. As a result, at the end of the graphic diary, the bat leaves, but promises to come back, thereby reminding the fact that the emergence of epidemics and pandemics is rather normal in the course of human history.

#My Funny Quarantine

The second exemplary lockdown diary created in the context of the first European lockdowns is the French-language blog with the English title *#My Funny Quarantine* written by the Berlin-based writer and journalist Prune Antoine over a period of 28 undated days, starting with *Jour #Un* (Day #One) to *Jour #Vingt Huit* (Day #Twenty-eight), concluding with *fin* (the end). Although the personal diary usually is of a private nature and not intended for publication, Antoine already had defined a specific purpose and, therefore, also had an audience in mind when narrating and posting it publicly. As insinuated by the title and revealed in the meta-reflexive passage of the fourth day, Antoine's motivation for its creation is geared towards providing enjoyment for her quarantine blog readers. She directly addresses them in a formal style, as evinced in the passage "[S]i cela peut vous amuser, vous distraire, cela sera ma modeste contribution à cette expérience collective que nous traversons"[15] (Jour #4). Moreover, Antoine addresses her audience from the perspective of a freelancer and mother, describing the disturbing effects on the individual and the collective experience of the mostly unprecedented restrictions to the freedom of movement. She evokes, for example, the hardships associated with being confined around-the-clock to a small city apartment with her partner and child and addresses her experience of the chaos the COVID-19 crisis has brought to European societies in general. She also writes about the consequences of the crisis management for women in particular, such as experiencing cabin fever or mental overload when together 24/7 with her family; or falling into the traditional female roles of housewife and mother as childcare centers and schools stayed closed.

On a formal level, the experience of confusion and disorientation is related by the seemingly erratic associations and loose paragraphs, which are conveyed in an informal style. This style is endowed with words and phrases in German and English, as well as with French argot, such as *meuf* (Fr.) for *femme* (Fr.) (woman) or *reum* (Fr.) for *mère* (Fr.) (mother). Moreover, at the beginning, Antoine has a hard time finding an appropriate expression for the new situation, writing "[c]omme vous tous, je m'apprête à vivre un truc d'ouf, 24/7 avec mon mec et ma fille à la maison pour une durée indéterminée, confinés *inside* comme des bâtonnets Findus, [...] [italics in the original]"[16] (Jour #1). Readers not familiar with these languages, registers, or cultural references – and thus left only understanding half of what is said – receive a comprehensible impression of her troubled state of mind through the hindered reading. Other readers may be confirmed in their own feelings about the lockdown experience and exhilarated by the frank choice of words used to express those feelings. Especially the metaphoric comparison with the French fish-stick brand called Findus illustrates Antoine's feelings of helplessness and powerlessness towards the lockdown situation.

---

15 "If it can amuse you, entertain you, it will be my modest contribution to this collective experience we are going through" (author's translation).

16 "Like all of you, I'm about to go through something crazy, 24/7 with my boyfriend and my daughter at home for an indefinite time, confined inside, like Findus fish sticks" (author's translation).

Prune Antoine also regularly refers to the crisis discourse in the political arena and media channels. She contrasts, for example, the haunting war rhetoric used by the French president, which mainly triggered fear, with the unemotional rhetoric used by the German chancellor, who attempted to invoke a collective sense of responsibility.[17] The fear-generating nature of the crisis discourse is placed in the foreground through the use of repeated quotations of official infection statistics and mortality statistics, as well as the use of sensational quotes from politicians and media representatives in both countries. Antoine also openly relates that she feels distressed by the macabre statistics and scary reports. Like the narrator of the graphic diary, she soon realizes that the only way to overcome her feelings of paralysis and fear is to reduce media consumption, which she announces by making an open call for "Débranchons"[18] (Jour #5).

One distinct characteristic of diaries is their continuous chronological progression, usually headed by exact date specifications as in the case of Krahn Uribe. Prune Antoine's blog diary, however, lacks any date references. Her only attempt to keep track of this exceptional period, consists in the sequential numbering of the entries, headed with *Jour #1*, *Jour #2*, etc., and occasional references to the months of April or May and the spring season within the entries. The longer the lockdown lasts and the more her routine in the private sphere becomes monotonous, she manifestly loses sight of how the days pass by: "[J]e ne sais même plus quel jour nous sommes"[19] (Jour #10). From the tenth day on, she writes only every second day, meaning that the blog entries are reduced by half. Such a cognitive change in the perception of time also becomes evident in Krahn Uribe's graphic diary, when, after about a month, the narration of the events that occur over several days or even weeks is contracted. In other diaristic narratives, the sense of time dissolves almost completely; this occurs, for example, when entries suddenly start lacking date indications and are only entitled "Sunday" or "morning," as in the case of the short diaristic lockdown story "La vida en cuarentena" (Engl. *Life in Lockdown*) by Maria del Rosario Lara (2020).

Concluding Discussion

Due to the sudden, massive appearance of diaries in the wake of the first COVID-19-induced lockdown in various countries in spring 2020, this chapter drew on trauma

17 For an analysis of the different communication strategies used by German, French, and Spanish politicians and media representatives at the beginning of the COVID-19 pandemic, cf. Schmelzer (2020).

18 "Let's disconnect" (author's translation).

19 "I don't even know what day we have" (author's translation).

and resilience studies in order to find explanations for the popularity of the lockdown diary. As was resumed from previous studies on lockdown diaries (cf. Yang 2021; Gammel/Wang 2022; Gleury/Gateau 2022) and could be demonstrated on the basis of two lockdown diaries' examples, the diaristic narration largely directed the focus of the audience toward the depiction of the narrator's experience of not being allowed to leave the home, as well as the depictions of the negative effects on the mental and physical health resulting from the sudden and unprecedented disruption of everyday life and their responses to it. By narratively formulating individual and collective anxieties, stressors, and coping strategies, the diary keepers engaged in a narrative process of shaping, translating, and containing this first shared lockdown experience for themselves, their audiences, and for posterity. Thereby, these diaries fulfil a testimonial function for their contemporaries and will assume commemorative function for future generations who wish to learn more about the lockdown experiences from a personal perspective. Furthermore, the act of narration enabled the authors to relativize the threatening nature of the crisis, shifting the audience's focus away from their emotional distress and feelings of helplessness towards their (i.e., the narrator's and the reader's) own ability to act. In the preface of her *Diario de estar por casa*-manuscript, Fernanda Krahn Uribe even describes her diaristic narration explicitly as a consciously adopted coping strategy:

> [Durante el confinamiento] [m]e amenazaba una avalancha de temores, preocupaciones y demás elementos del bloque del boicot interior, ese que conozco bastante bien y que tanto me paraliza. [...] [El murciélago] significó la salvación de una depresión en ciernes. A partir de ese día, se reactivó en mi interior el espíritu de la niña que fui.[20] (Krahn Uribe, preface)

Starting to narrate on a daily basis and describe what was going on inside her fulfilled a personal therapeutic function. It not only allowed her to introduce structure into her monotonous lockdown days and distract her, but also helped her to regain some form of agency in a time in which self-determination and any sense of certainty about the future was scarce.

Manifold lockdown experiences throughout all social groups are reflected in the large pool of lockdown diaries. Some of these diaries were produced, as illustrated by the two diaristic examples given, by single women, mothers, and migrants, but also by healthcare workers and members of minority groups, whose perspectives were

---

20 "During the lockdown, I was threatened by an avalanche of fears, worries, and other elements of the inner boycott, the one I know so well and that paralyzes me so much. The bat meant salvation from a beginning depression. From that day on, the spirit of the girl I used to be, was reactivated inside me" (author's translation).

largely absent from the political and media crisis discourse in spring 2020. This diversity of the diary keepers and their respective lockdown situations (in the two examples given: living alone vs. living together with the family) enabled the recipients to recognize or even identify themselves with the authors and their situations. It enabled them to see that they are not alone with their emotional responses to the lockdown situation; that others are suffering as well, maybe suffering differently or even more. This recognition thereby opened up the possibility for (more) mutual understanding, acts of solidarity, and social cohesion. Moreover, the reception of the lockdown diaries allowed the readers to see how others had coped with similar situations and to receive impulses that they could use to strengthen their own resilience.

Concurrently, we must not forget the motto of ancient poet Horace, that literature should not only be instructive, but also entertaining for its audiences (cf. *Ars poetica*, v. 333). This entertaining or distracting aspect was also explicitly addressed by Prune Antoine and given as the reason for her lockdown diary *#My Funny Quarantine*. Although she was well aware that this unprecedented situation might (re-)traumatize some people, she wanted to alleviate their destiny with her diaristic narrations. In this sense, similarities between Antoine's diary and Krahn Uribe's diary become apparent: the conversation between Krahn Uribe's narrator and the old bat distracted and relieved her as well as the readers. Both lockdown diaries thereby also fulfill a therapeutic function for their audiences.

To conclude, one can argue that, indeed, the lockdown diaries of the first COVID-19 induced lockdown strengthened the well-being of both their producers and recipients in multiple ways, thus, being one explanation for their popularity in this exceptional and unprecedented time.

Bibliography

Ainetter, Sylvia. 2006. *Blogs – Literarische Aspekte Eines Neuen Mediums: Eine Analyse Am Beispiel Des Weblogs Miagolare* 5, LIT.

American Psychiatric Association (APA). 2022. "Resilience." *APA Dictionary of Psychology*. https://dictionary.apa.org/resilience.

Ansermet, François. 2020. "Entre Vie Et Mort: Destin De La Pandémie." https://www.puf.com/actualites/La_collection_Questions_de_soin_sengage.

Antoine, Prune. 2020. *#My Funny Quarantine*. Blog diary. https://plumaberlin.com/2020/03/01/my-funny-quarantine/.

Blumczynski, Piotr, and Steven Wilson, editors. 2023. *The Languages of COVID-19: Translational and Multilingual Perspectives on Global Healthcare*, Routledge.

BnF. 2021. "L'épidémie De COVID Et Le Premier Confinement: Un Parcours Guidé Dans Les Archives De L'internet." https://www.bnf.fr/fr/parcours-guides-archives-de-linternet#step19.

Boerner, Peter. 1969. *Tagebuch*, J.B. Metzler.

Clark, Travis. 2020. "The Movie 'Outbreak,' About a Deadly Virus, Is Now One of Netflix's Most Popular Titles in the US." *Insider*, March 13, 2020. https://www.businessinsider.com/coronavirus-outbreak-one-of-netflixs-most-popular-movies-2020-3?r=DE&IR=T.

Collins Dictionary. 2022. "Lockdown." https://www.collinsdictionary.com/dictionary/english/lockdown.

Contini, Maud, and Prune Antoine. 2020. "Jour 1 # Podcast Dansé / Prune Antoine Chronique Et Voix." *Podcast dansé*. https://www.youtube.com/watch?v=4EGPCH_bdMY

Cottin, France. 2021. "La Pandémie Présente Toutes Les Composantes Du Traumatisme." *Le Monde*, April 15, 2021. https://www.lemonde.fr/planete/article/2021/04/15/la-pandemie-presente-toutes-les-composantes-du-traumatisme_6076929_3244.html.

Cyrulnik, Boris. 2002 [1999]. *Un Merveilleux Malheur* 78, Jacob.

Cyrulnik, Boris. 2004. "La Mémoire Traumatique." *Jeunes, Ville, Violence: Comprendre, Prévenir, Traiter*, edited by Norbert Sillamy, 194–201, Questions contemporaines, L'Harmattan, 194–201.

Cyrulnik, Boris. 2005 [2002]. *Le Murmure Des Fantômes* 163, Jacob.

Cyrulnik, Boris. 2013. "La Résilience: Un Processus Multicausal." *Revue française des affaires sociales*, vol. 1, no. 1–2, 15–19.

Dunford, Daniel et al. 2020. "Coronavirus: The World in Lockdown in Maps and Charts." *BBC News*, April 7, 2020. https://www.bbc.com/news/world-52103747.

Del Rosario Lara, Maria. 2020. "La Vida En Cuarentena." *La Vida En Tiempos Del Coronavirus: Antología*, edited by Guadalupe Avalos, s.l. Nordlys Publicaciones, 43–53.

Diarios De La Cuarentena. Series. Spain: Morena Films, 2020. Weekly Sitcom. https://www.rtve.es/alacarta/videos/diarios-de-la-cuarentena/.

Engelhardt, Dietrich von. 2005. "Coping." *Literatur Und Medizin: Ein Lexikon*, edited by Bettina von Jagow and Florian Steger, Vandenhoeck & Ruprecht, 159–163.

Fang, Fang. 2020. *Wuhan Diary: Dispatches from a Quarantined City*, Harper Collins. Collection.

Fleury, Cynthia, and Valérie Gateau. 2022. "Récits Et Fonctions Psychiques De La Narration Dans Les Journaux De Confinement." *Revue française d'éthique appliquée*, vol. 12, no. 1, 87–100. https://doi.org/10.3917/rfeap.012.0087.

Ford, Julian D. 2009. *Posttraumatic Stress Disorder. Scientific and Professional Dimensions*, 1st edition, Elsevier.

Gammel, Irene, and Jason Wang. 2022. "'Why Has the Outbreak Turned so Deadly?': Diary from a Quarantined City." *Creative Resilience and COVID-19: Figuring the Everyday in a Pandemic*, edited by Irene Gammel and Jason Wang, *The COVID-19 Pandemic* series, Routledge, 27–38.

Görner, Rüdiger. 1986. *Das Tagebuch: Eine Einführung*, Artemis-Einführungen 26, Artemis.

Guyenne, Lisa. 2021. "Au royaume du Covid, L'écriture est reine." *France Culture*, February 14, 2021. https://www.radiofrance.fr/franceculture/au-royaume-du-covid-l-ecriture-est-reine-4900080.

Gwyn, Richard. 2002. *Communicating Health and Illness*, Sage.

Herman, Judith Lewis. 1992. *Trauma and Recovery: The Aftermath of Violence – from Domestic Abuse to Political Terror*, 13th edition, Basic Books.

Hobisch, Elisabeth, Yvonne Völkl, and Julia Obermayr. 2021–2025. "Corona Fictions Database." *Zotero Group Library*. https://www.zotero.org/groups/4814225/corona_fictions_database/library.

Hobisch, Elisabeth, Yvonne Völkl, and Julia Obermayr. 2022. "Narrar la pandemia. Una introducción a formas, temas y metanarrativas de las Corona Fictions." *Pensamiento, Pandemia y Big Data: El impacto sociocultural del coronavirus en el espacio iberoamericano*, edited by Ana Gallego Cuiñas and José A. Pérez Tapias, de Gruyter, 191–211.

Horace. 19BC. *Ars Poetica*. https://www.thelatinlibrary.com/horace/arspoet.shtml.

Kalff, Sabine, and Vedder Ulrike. 2016. "Tagebuch Und Diaristik Seit 1900: Einleitung." *Zeitschrift für Germanistik*, vol. 2, no. 26, 236–242.

Kast, Verena. 1990 [1987]. *Der schöpferische Sprung: Vom therapeutischen Umgang mit Krisen*, 5th edition, Walter.

Klein, Gabriele, and Katharina Liebsch. 2020. "Herden unter Kontrolle: Körper in Corona-Zeiten." *Die Corona-Gesellschaft: Analysen zur Lage und Perspektiven für die Zukunft*, edited by Michael Volkmer and Karin Werner, transcript, 57–65.

Klein, Gabriele, and Katharina Liebsch. 2022. "Ansteckende Berührungen: Körper-Ordnungen in der Krise." *Covid-19: Sinn in der Krise: Kulturwissenschaftliche Analysen der Corona-Pandemie*, edited by Jan Beuerbach, Silke Gülker, Uta Karstein, and Ringo Rösener, de Gruyter, 133–147.

Knaller, Susanne, editor. 2023. *Writing Facts: Interdisciplinary Discussions of a Key Concept in Modernity*, transcript.

Krahn Uribe, Fernanda. *Diario De Estar Por Casa, O "Mis Conversaciones Con Un Murciélago."* Graphic diary. Facebook page of the author and copy provided by the author.

Mann, Court. 2020. "Coronavirus Side Effect: The Movie 'Contagion' Is Super Popular Again." *Deseret News*, March 10, 2020. https://www.deseret.com/entertainment/2020/3/10/21172795/contagion-movie-where-to-watch-stream-download-free-coronavirus-covid-19-cinemax-hulu-amazon-prime.

Mateos Pérez, Javier. 2021. "Narrativas Televisivas En Contexto De Crisis. El COVID-19 En Las Series De Ficción Televisiva Española." *IC*, no. 18, 131–153. https://doi.org/10.12795/IC.2021.I18.08.

Mouawad, Wajdi. 2020. *Journal De Confinement.* Podcast. https://www.colline.fr/spectacles/journal-de-confinement-de-wajdi-mouawad.

Musolff, Andreas, Sara Vilar-Lluch, Kayo Kondo, and Ruth Breeze, editors. 2022. *Pandemic and Crisis Discourse: Communicating COVID-19 and Public Health Strategy*, 1st edition, Bloomsbury Academic.

Nesselhauf, Jonas. 2023. "Viral Narrations: Aesthetic Knowlegde and the Co-presence of a Pandemic." *Pandemisches Virus – nationales Handeln. Covid-19 und die europäische Idee*, edited by Dominik Brodowski, Jonas Nesselhauf and Florian Weber, Springer, 331–351.

Nünning, Ansgar. 2013. "Wie Erzählungen Kulturen Erzeugen: Prämissen, Konzepte Und Perspektiven Für Eine Kulturwissenschaftliche Narratologie." *Kultur – Wissen – Narration: Perspektiven Transdisziplinärer Erzählforschung Für Die Kulturwissenschaften*, edited by Alexandra Strohmaier, transcript, 15–53.

Nünning, Ansgar. 2023. "Writing as a Cultural Way of Fact-Making. Modest Reflections on the Genesis, Role, and Status of Facts." *Writing Facts. Interdisciplinary Discussions of a Key Concept in Modernity*, edited by Susanne Knaller, transcript, 53–84.

Obergöker, Timo. 2020. "Les Journaux De Confinement De Leïla Slimani Et De Marie Darieussecq – Histoire D'un Malentendu." *PhiN-Beiheft*, no. 24, 371–382.

Obermayr, Julia, and Elisabeth Hobisch. 2024. "Uplifting Corona Fictions: Interdisciplinary Perspectives on Representations Encouraging Well-Being in Music Videos." *Re:visit. Humanities & Medicine in Dialogue* 3, 75–97.

Pennebaker, James W. 2004. *Writing to Heal: A Guided Journal for Recovering from Trauma & Emotional Upheaval*, New Harbinger.

Pineda, Luis Gabriel. 2021. "Confinamiento Y Cuarentena." Lengua Suelta. Aprendemos español. https://www.lenguasuelta.com/palabras-confinamiento-y-cuarentena/.

Render Turmaud, Danielle. 2020. "Trauma of Pandemic Proportions." *Psychology Today*. https://www.psychologytoday.com/us/blog/lifting-the-veil-trauma/202003/trauma-pandemic-proportions.

Research Group *Pandemic Fictions*. 2020. "From Pandemic to Corona Fictions: Narratives in Times of Crises." *PhiN-Beiheft* no. 24, 321–344. http://web.fu-berlin.de/phin/beiheft24/b24t21.pdf.

Ritchie, Hannah, Edouard Mathieu, Lucas Rodés-Guirao, Cameron Appel, Charlie Giattino, Esteban Ortiz-Ospina, Joe Hasell, Bobbie Macdonald, Diana Beltekian, and Max Roser. 2020-. "Policy Responses to the Coronavirus Pandemic." https://ourworldindata.org/policy-responses-covid.

Robin, Régine. 2020. "La Réactivation D'un Traumatisme De Guerre: Paris Confiné." *Récits Infectés*, edited by Léonore Brassard, Benjamin Gagnon Chainey, and Catherine Mavrikakis, s.p. Montréal.

Schafer, Valérie. 2022. “Préserve-Moi ! Des Journaux Intimes À Ceux De Confinement Dans Les Archives Du Web.” *Le Temps des médias*, vol. 38 no. 1, 175–194. https://doi.org/10.3917/tdm.038.0175.

Schmelzer, Dagmar. 2020. “New We. Die Diskursive Performanz Gesellschaftlichen Zusammenhalts in Corona-Zeiten – Ein Deutsch-Französisch-Spanischer Vergleich.” *PhiN-Beiheft* no. 24, 129–148. http://web.fu-berlin.de/phin/beiheft24/b24i.htm.

Silaški, Nadežda, and Tatjana Đurović. 2022. “From an Invisible Enemy to a Football Match with the Virus: Adjusting the Covid-19 Pandemic Metaphors to Political Agendas in Serbian Public Discourse.” *Pandemic and Crisis Discourse: Communicating COVID-19 and Public Health Strategy*, edited by Andreas Musolff, Sara Vilar-Lluch, Kayo Kondo, and Ruth Breeze, 1st edition, Bloomsbury Academic, 271–284.

Sontag, Susan. 1978. *Illness as Metaphor*, Farrar, Straus and Giroux.

Stemberger, Martina. 2021. *Corona im Kontext: Zur Literaturgeschichte der Pandemie*, Narr Francke Attempto.

Tourette-Turgis, Catherine, and Marie Chollier. 2020. “L’impact Psychosocial Du (Dé)Confinement : Repenser L’accompagnement De La Population Générale En Période De Crise.” *Psychotropes*, vol. 26, no. 2, 191–207. https://doi.org/10.3917/psyt.262.0191.

Völkl, Yvonne. 2025. “Corona Fictions Anthologies. On the Compilation of Hispanophone and Francophone Corona Fictions During the First Lockdown.” *Coming to Terms with a Crisis. Cultural Engagements with COVID*, edited by Martin Butler, Sina Farzin, Michael Fuchs and Fabian Hempel, transcript, 91–113.

Wald, Priscilla. 2008. *Contagious: Cultures, Carriers, and the Outbreak Narrative*, Duke UP.

Yang, Guobin. 2021. “Online Lockdown Diaries as Endurance Art.” *AI & Society*, 1–10. https://doi.org/10.1007/s00146-020-01141-5.

Improper Bodies
Narrations of Immunity

Jan Hinrichsen

"Do I contradict myself?
Very well then I contradict myself,
(I am large, I contain multitudes)"
Walt Whitman [1855][1]

"Either immunology is not about the self,
or, if it is about selfhood then that self is
not cartesian"
A. David Napier[2]

"Science Fiction": A Story of mRNA-Cyborgs[3]

June 2021: According to my faded yellow vaccination card, I am immune. At least partly. However, it makes a vast difference whether my partly vaccinated body is located in Austria, where I work, or Germany, where I live. According to Austrian regulations, twelve days after my first shot, I am free of the obligation of getting regular antigen screenings, free to breathe potentially contaminated air and to touch my own face again unencumbered by a facial mask. In Germany, however, I still pose an imminent risk to society (paradoxically: especially returning home from Innsbruck, since German officials have defined Austria a designated risk zone)

1 Walt Whitman: Song of Myself [1855], Walt Whitman. 2004. *Leaves of Grass*, Bantam Dell, 23–76.

2 David Napier (2012): "Nonself Help: How Immunology Might Reframe the Enlightenment," *Cultural Anthropology* 27, 1, 122–127, here 125.

3 This chapter is based on my praxiographic research on the production of immunity in a clinical trial of an mRNA vaccine against COVID. A first draft was presented in the research colloquium of the Department of Medical Ethics and History of Medicine of the University Medical Center Göttingen. I want to thank my colleagues and the editors of this volume for thorough and productive feedback. A very special thanks is owed to Monique Scheer and Helen Franziska Veit for their critical reading and insightful and inspiring comments.

and will continue to do so until 15 days after my second *jab of Comirnaty. In other words: once according to EMA*[4] *and STIKO*[5] *recommendations, BioNtech's*[6] *instruction leaflet and the processual and preliminary results of uncounted clinical trials, the titer of antibodies against Corona-virus' spike antigen in my blood has reached a sufficient level to be considered immune against COVID. Immune, as in: equipped with a body capable of profoundly responding to viral contamination while in the best case – the jury is still out on this – not posing a threat of infecting others but at least contributing to national (!) herd immunity.*[7]

Depending on geographical and temporal contingencies, I am an mRNA-cyborg: "my" "natural" immune system is enhanced by a biotechnological miracle that represents no less than the promise of salvation: "health-giving information" (CureVac: n.d.)[8] *(something like: "the Gospel"), – as CureVac, a leading figure in this emerging field of biotechnology, advertises its mRNA-technology – had been implanted into my body to stimulate the production of my body's "own medicine." The gospel's stirring touch of my innermost is meant to result in self-contained and self-sustained invulnerability. In less sublime, no less miraculous words: I was injected with a very small dose of messenger ribonucleic acid fresh from the RNA-printers at BioNtech, formulated in lipidnanoparticles, which simultaneously stabilize the delicate RNA, prevent my body from allergic reaction to RNA-proteins, ensure the passage of the "healing information" into my cells, and serve as an adjuvant, triggering the immune system. This recombinant mRNA strand (that is: "artificial," even though in the world of biotechnology it makes no sense to speak of artificial as opposed to "natural") codes for coronavirus' spike antigen sequence. Reduced to pure yet crucial information, it simultaneously* is *and* is not *viral matter; as a "messenger" this sequence serves as a blueprint for my body's protein factories, the ribosomes, that translate the "construction plan" into the production of oodles of spike antigens. These are nonetheless equipped with the agency of triggering the immune system's production of antibodies specific to my DIY-Spike-antigens, thus hindering a (fatal) outbreak of disease in the likely case of infection and storing this "response-ability" in ingenious memory cells for an uncertain future. The result is immunity against COVID – as we know by now: a delicate, at best transient but most certainly highly inconclusive phenomenon.*

My awareness of being immune, however, took time to sink in, and was fully realized only after it had been partially suspended in the bureaucratic act of crossing the border back to Germany. What I, instead, had been well aware of, also through a handwritten slip of paper cover-

---

4 European Medicines Agency.

5 *Ständige Impfkommission* at the Robert Koch Institute, Germany. The STIKO issues recommendations on vaccines, vaccination practice and protocol.

6 The mRNA-based vaccine Comirnaty (or: BNT162b2) was developed and is produced in a cooperation between the biotech company BioNtech and the pharmaceutical company Pfizer.

7 The "herds" in "herd immunity" are predominantly nationally defined ones.

8 CureVac imagefilm: https://www.curevac.com/en/about-us/ [09.06.2023]. Note: in the German version of the image film the formulation "heilsame Information" (curative, healing) is used, while in the English version employs the rather technical notion of "health giving information."

ing the syringe, was that I was administered "BioNtech off-label": the outcome of quarrels over the legal amount of vaccine doses drawn from one vial. A disinfectant was wiped over my exposed arm, my flesh was pinched by a gloved hand in a cubicle, separated from the public by a green curtain granting isolation for the intimate act to come. The needle punctured me, tearing a hole, tiny yet considerable, into the barrier that I was accustomed to embody: my skin, which, as I had once learned to feel, separated me from the outer world and everybody in it. Almost painlessly, a colorless liquid was released into the muscle tissue of my left, passive arm, meant to trigger, or better: constitute, another embodied barrier: my immune system.

"Please sit down in the resting zone for 15 minutes," I heard the doctor say. The signs there, however, recommended 20–30 minutes and together with the sudden awareness of paramedics, defibrillators, and shock stretchers inhabiting the repurposed exhibition hall, I realized how utterly vulnerable I am to my own immune system and the power invested in it to let me live or push me into the horrors of anaphylaxis. I made sure I waited 30 minutes, pondering existence, shock, and the suspicious absence of hand sanitizing stations in the waiting room. I left, as mechanical pain was spreading in my cyborg arm. Only back in the city, I thought for the first time: I am immune; my body has been turned into a biotechnological machine granting and taking care of my invulnerability, by a biotechnological machine whose marvelous purpose is to turn "nature" into a biotechnological machine.

Complicating Narrations: The Social Life of Immune Systems

In many regards, the great story that is the coronavirus pandemic conflicts with the hitherto success story of biomedical interventions, especially the superiority of vaccinations over other forms of mitigating the devasting effects of pandemics – the proverbial "biggest success of western medicine" (Thiessen 2017). The teleology of vaccine development in the 2020s – a bona fide "science fiction" (Haraway 2016, 1991a, 1991b) of the supremacy of biomedical reason imbued with the sterile aesthetics of late modern (bio)technology and featuring scientists molded to the cast of Silicon Valley's tales of technological hegemony – has, by now, given way to intricate stories of the vulnerability of our late modern, globalized, and technologized modes of existence. If these modes of existence had once thrived on the belief in a general immunity to the perils of infectious disease, coronavirus has exposed the utter contingency of that very immunity, both figuratively and literally. The pandemic thus tells different stories of the limits of technological immunization against critical threats on a societal-semiotic level as well as of the limits of biomedical immunization against the coronavirus on a corporeal-material level; these two aspects are intertwined in the practice of vaccination.

Through the pandemic we learned to think of immunity as an extremely contingent phenomenon. It is contingent on the velocity of vaccine research and production, on progress in emerging biotechnology, on political decisions, medical discourse (informing or counteracting those decisions), medial discourse (commenting all of the former), time (between spring 2021 and spring 2023, the equitation of "having been vaccinated" and "being immune" has dissolved), and on national borders (different countries had different liberties adhering to the vaccination status). In short: immunity appears not only as a biological or bodily feature but rather as a sociocultural category. And as such, it is dependent on meaning, on discourse, or – simply – narrations of immunity.

However, many of the alternative stories about immunity that have emerged during the pandemic seem incompatible with classic narratives of the immune system, in public discourse and not least in cultural anthropology as the discipline concerned, among other things, with quotidian representations. In other words: coronavirus has fundamentally challenged cultural anthropological approaches to immunity as well their underlying theories of the body. At the same time, those cultural anthropological approaches have laid the groundwork for other narratives of immunity. The argument unfolded in this chapter is as follows: immunity, especially as perceived by cultural anthropological studies, used to speak in terms of "modern" concepts of the body and the individual. They are modern in a Latourian sense (1993) insofar as they render the function of the immune system to be keeping the demarcations of the body and the individual intact (Brown 2019; Cohen 2009). In this light, the immune system is the body's (and therefore nature's) apparatus to defend an individual's physical integrity (ibid.). It is, however, not only the novel coronavirus that complicates the inherent modernity of immunological thought. It is furthermore the very practice of vaccination against COVID that demands a reconceptualization of the "social life" of immune systems and their inherent relationality underpinned by biotechnological reason and practice.

To achieve this reconceptualization, this chapter revisits seminal conceptual approaches to immunity from medical anthropology, the history and philosophy of the body, the history of science, as well as political theory to identify the actors, plots, and plot twists they offer for the complicated stories about immunity that "have never been modern" (Latour 1993) and presumably never will be. It sets out with a reading of Barbara Duden's feminist-phenomenological history of the body and her insistence on the disembodying nature of abstract immunological discourse. In stark contrast to this, cultural anthropologist Emily Martin analyzes the cultural logics of this very immunological discourse and its potential for informing popular discourse on post-Fordist bodies, highlighting the cultural meanings of the immune system, while failing to acknowledge the practical embodiment of immune systems. Nevertheless, these accounts underscore the paradigm of "self-non-self discrimination" as the purported telos of immune systems and thus the "modern" axioms of immunology as seen by its interpreters in the social and cultural sciences. These can also be traced to a political theory of immunity as suggested by philosophers Roberto Esposito and Peter Sloterdijk. By help of feminist science and technology scholar Donna Haraway's work, and drawing on suggestions of immunologist Niels Kaj Jerne, the inherent contradictions of the cultural logics of immunity are mapped out, a reading of the immune- as a commune-system (Cohen 2009) is proposed, and its active role in the constitution of equally contradictory bodies and subjects is analyzed. These are "response-able" (Haraway 2016) body-subjects, that challenge conventional and fundamental conceptualizations of responsibility, solidarity, and autonomy manifest in vaccination policies and the practice of immunization.

The complicated stories unfolded in this chapter are ironic, metaphoric and contradicting – they are SF in Haraway's notion:

> SF is a sign for science fiction, speculative feminism, science fantasy, speculative fabulation, science fact, and also, string figures. Playing games of string figures is about giving and receiving patterns, dropping threads and failing but sometimes finding something that works, something consequential and maybe even beautiful, that wasn't there before, of relaying connections that matter, of telling stories in hand upon hand, digit upon digit, attachment site upon attachment site, to craft conditions for finite flourishing on terra, on earth. (Haraway 2016, 10)

In this light, narrations of the immune system are not mere representations of medical or even natural facts, nor are they simply about language. As the argument will show, narration is a practice[9] and practice is a nexus of "sayings" and "doings" (cf. Schatzki 1996, 89), that is: a way of practically relating to, enacting, – or simply: being – our body (cf. Mol 2002). They are, ultimately, semiotic-material practices (Haraway 1991a, 1991b) active in the constitution of bodies and subjects.

Bipod Immune Systems

Historian Barbara Duden expresses her outrage about having been told to identify herself with her "immune system" (Duden 1997, 260)[10]:

> I am no more a writing surface, cinema screen, or political manifesto than I am an immune system. I am not ready to identify what many researchers today call "my body as the carrier of cultural encoding and the projection surface of social constructs" with that tangible and palpable self with which I have familiarized myself in women's history. (Duden 1997, 262)

---

9 Or: "language game," as Wittgenstein (1953) would have it, who will, as the narrations unfold, make multiple (and somewhat surprising) appearances.

10 All quotes from Duden 1997 are my translations from her German original.

Duden understands the trajectory of a history of the body in analyzing "past and present "embodied" certainties, hence in denaturalizing and historicizing cultural perceptions and conceptualizations that are inscribed into the body and appear there as ineluctable, natural facts" (Duden 1997, 262). Consequently, Duden asks how a "cultural construct" becomes "flesh" (263), a subjective, tangible and inhabitable body. Paradoxically, however, Duden renders the immune system as the mere discursive reduction of living and feeling persons to "a function notation, to a system [...], that annuls [them]." Accordingly, referring to the "system under the skin" is the epitome of "total disembodiment" (Duden 1997, 272). The immune system, she argues, is not tangible, not perceptible, and, therefore, not subjective flesh: it is the forced – but ultimately impossible? – embodiment of complex, uninhabitable abstracta. In this logic, immunologic discourse alienates us from our flesh. Discourse, as it appears for Duden, is the opposite of flesh: "non-flesh" that has no business under our skin.[11]

Cultural anthropologists would beg to differ wondering what it is we embody if not abstract and complex concepts. What part of our body is unmediated and concrete? And isn't this precisely what Bourdieu's theory of habitus and hexis (Bourdieu 1987, 97–121; 1977, 78–95), or, for that matter, the history of the body (Sarasin 2003, 2001), have taught us? Why should "heart" and "head" (Duden 1997, 272) be less defined by cultural representation and therefore less abstract than, say, T-helper cells, B-lymphocytes, or macrophages? What is more, aren't the pandemic experience, having grown up in the times of HIV/AIDS, vaccination against measles or tetanus, or the consumption of lemon juice when faced with a common cold, specific ways of practically relating to, embodying, and *doing* the immune system? Aren't using condoms, being identified by a yellow vaccination card, submitting your body to a clinical trial study, or discussing your Comirnaty-induced side-effects or superpowers[12] with friends ways of making the "abstract" system concrete, tangible, palpable? Shouldn't one, therefore, ask *how* the immune system is embodied *in practice*, how having and embodying an immune system is part of the late-modern condition of what it *is* to be a subject and a body (cf. Martin 1994; 1990)? Shouldn't one take the immune system as the central arena of answering the question "of what 'health' is, what it includes, what a body is made up of, what a person is made up of [...], what disease

11 It is insightful how Duden, scrutinizing immunological discourse, involuntarily reproduces immunological arguments of the integrity of flesh/proper bodies threatened in their integrity by an improper "outside." Her alienation argument is, in *sensu stricto*, an immunological argument; the flesh and the subject that are threatened with annulment are "immunological."

12 A participant of one of the first clinical trials for a COVID vaccine told me about his children's reaction to his being vaccinated with an untested mRNA vaccine. They were exhilarated by the idea of their father acquiring superpowers and becoming "something like Spiderman."

is, and how the terms in which people come to understand themselves yield particular answer to questions like these," as was the way paved by cultural anthropologist Emily Martin (1994, xiv)?

Duden shares Martin's assumption that the immune system gives "a novel, corporeal, hence consistent expression to epochal sensitivities in late 20th century" (Duden 1997, 264). Yet, instead of insisting on immunology's disembodying discourse, Martin wants to inquire how the immunological discourse generates "our taken-for-grantedness about the body" (Martin 1994, xiii). She analyzes how "[t]hat what goes to make up a person in these times [of the AIDS pandemic; JH] is being reconfigured" (Martin 1994, xvi) by a shift from the hygienic logic of polio in the 1950s to an "immuno-logic" (my term; JH). This shift was brought about by the first successful vaccination against polio and fully realized during the heyday of the HIV/AIDS pandemic. Doing so, she shows how immunologic discourse links up to or interacts with the logic of "flexible specialization" (Martin 1994, 40) of late capitalism, thus constituting flexible subjects in post-Fordist bodies as complex, and ultimately open-ended systems governed by the invocation of their self-responsibility.

However, immunity's power to constitute and govern subjects and bodies, to Martin, stems predominantly from the power of language, of metaphor. Very much in line with Susan Sontag's work on "illness as metaphor" and on AIDS (Sontag 1978; 1989), Martin's interest is exclusively in *representations* of the immune system[13]: representations in media, scientific, and lay discourse, as well as their underlying and emerging cultural grammars defined by the logics of late capitalism. She meticulously reconstructs how her interlocutors *make sense* of their own immune system and how they *perceive* of it, how immunological discourse is imbued with the vocabulary of flexible accumulation and vice versa. But she disregards what the immune system *is*, or what it *does*.[14] She scrutinizes *understandings* of the body and what it *means* to be a subject. Thus, the constitution of subjects, to Martin, owing to post-structuralism and the linguistic turn, is nothing but a language game[15]; she has no

---

13 Hence, *Flexible Bodies* (1994) is, by and large, a collection of inquiries into the "immune system as seen by XYZ."

14 As a result, Martin pays astonishingly little attention to the fact that the majority of her interlocutors share the conviction that their immune system "does" something or acts self-sustained, respectively. Moreover, even though she wants to scrutinize the taken-for-grantedness of the body, Martin widely disregards her interlocutors' insistence on the body as something that belongs to them individually. From the perspective of a history of the body, however, it is precisely this notion of "I *have* a body," which is in need of explanation (Sarasin 2001) and, thus, hardly to be taken for granted.

15 Consequently, also Martin's view on biopolitics is about the power of representation: "Accepting vaccination means *accepting* the state's power *to impose a particular view* about the body and its immune system" (1994, 194; my emphasis).

interest in the (multiple) ontologies of the immune system let alone their embodiment or, simply, what it *is to be* a late modern subject.

Bodies at War

In all fairness to Martin: one can hardly overestimate the power of language, narrative and metaphor in immunology – not least because the discipline of immunology itself has embraced that very notion of language and metaphor more often than not. Historians of immunology such as Anderson et al. (1994) accuse Martin and Haraway for having reduced immunological discourse to the metaphor of self-nonself discrimination and for thereby having omitted the situatedness and location of that metaphor. Nonetheless, it is worthwhile taking a look at the language game of self v. nonself that immunology and its interpreters have played: immunology appears as "the science of self/nonself discrimination" (Klein 1982) – a significant part of the history of immunology (written from within or from outside the field) revolves around this notion, either underpinning or undermining it. Ample debate has gone into the question of what the immunological "self" is, and whether the immune system's function is to either recognize self (and therefore nothing else; with "nonself" posing a problem for not being recognized) or to recognize "nonself" (and therefore being blind to self). Usually, the concept of tolerance is used to explain why immune response is only triggered by "foreign" entities.

Albeit a shortsighted vantage point (as Anderson et al. [1994] elaborate in their "Unnatural History of the Immune System"), the "science of self/nonself discrimination" renders immunology inherently "modern-" The immunological self is impregnated with modern conceptualizations of subjectivity and personhood (Cohen 2009). Immunity, thereby, serves as a way of thinking about integrity and differentiation as it distinguishes elements that sustain integrity from those which are threatening it. Thus, it is seen a boundary concept: it draws a seemingly clear boundary between inside and outside, between "proper" ("eigentlich" or one's own) and "improper" ("uneigentlich" or common) (Esposito 2011), between individual and environment, between self and nonself. "At the heart of the immune system is the ability to distinguish between self and nonself. Virtually every body cell carries distinctive molecules that identify it as self" (Schindler 1988 in Martin 1990, 411). In this light, "self" is the body, its material, its produce; "nonself" are the contagious entities – pathogens, viruses, antigens: they are contagious because they are nonself, they are nonself because they are contagious.

The juxtaposition of self and nonself as a conflicting relationship is at the heart of immunological thought – or at least its cultural theoretical readings: in 1881, immunology's founding father Elie Metchnikoff "deduces an entirely new way to perceive how organisms coexist and thereby ushers biological 'immunity' into the world as an organismic form of 'defense'" (Cohen 2009, 2). To Cohen, this is, however, "a classic example of [...] *action under the form of description*. In other words, by construing his experimental protocol as an intrusion, Metchnikoff *enacts* it as such and then reasons that, however the larva reacts, this reaction represents the intrusive catalyst's logical antithesis" (ibid.; my emphasis). These "defensive poetics of modern medicine" (206) render the function of immunity to demarcate the boundaries of our bodies, to render them other-than-environment and to vigorously keep these borders intact. The immuno-logical body is a "nation-state" with clear borders to the outside and gendered division of labor on the inside (Martin 1990, 416) "at war." As the body's armament immune systems counter attacks from a threatening, contagious outside. This is based on binaries such as "purity/normality" and "contamination/pathological," which have been analyzed by cultural anthropologist Mary Douglas (2001 [1966]) as a crucial structure of Western thought and which sociologist Bruno Latour (1993) regards as the fundamentals of a "modern" epistemology. From this perspective, immune response is an act of literal dis-infection, of purification,[16] and thus a way of relating to and ensuring us of our selves. In the words of phenomenologist Jean-Luc Nancy's reflections on his heart transplant and the need to suppress his immune function in order to "tolerate" the donor heart: "if you weaken the immunity, you also weaken the identity" (Nancy 2000, 35; my translation, JH), or so "the moderns" have us believe. In this light, immunity is the epitome of the "modern" integrity of the body – its apotheosis, even (Cohen 2009) – and the individual.

Uncommon: Proper Bodies

This invocation of the individual is also at the heart of philosopher Peter Sloterdijk's (2015) concept of immunization, which, to him, is equivalent to individualization and particularization. It is the technique of creating spheres of one's own (cf. Esposito's idea of the "proper") in order to make the (naturally) hostile environment breathable, livable, inhabitable. With the aid of, for example, air conditions – a prototypical immunization technique for Sloterdijk (71–106) – the *common* air is conditioned, particularized and individualized into individual atmospheres, inhabitable spheres of breathing. In the postmodern condition, this notion of shared spheres is more and more compartmentalized, privatized and individualized; bigger spheres evaporating into smaller and smaller, non-communal ones: "foams."[17] This opposi-

16 Another one of Latour's concepts.

17 Sloterdijk's body of work on the matter is titled "Schäume," which translates to "foams." The notion of spheres of breathing being more and more compartmentalized could be witnessed during the pandemic: Individual households were treated similar to "shared immune systems," thereby freeing their members from the obligation of wearing facial masks. The lat-

tion of immunity and community is interpreted by philosopher and political theorist Roberto Esposito (2011) as the epitome of subjectivity and integrity. To him, *immunitas* is to be freed from social obligation ("munus"); immunitas is "proper", "un-common" (Esposito 2011, 5–6), one's own, whereas *communitas* refers to social obligation, the common, the improper (ibid.). This opposition is alive today in concepts such as political or legal immunity. Martin demonstrates how immunity had once exclusively referred to the individual's capacity of warding off the state (as in being exempt from obligation[18]) and only in the 19th century acquired the meaning of warding off disease (Martin 1994, 193; Cohen 2009, 1–31).

Seen from this perspective, immunity is embodied *noli me tangere*, the capacity of being "untouchable," unaffectable, and the blueprint of modern subjectivity and corporeality: one subject in one body, a literal "in-dividual," rendered by and able to draw a clear-cut boundary between "me"/"my body" and the Other. This immuno-logical self is located in an invulnerable castle-body confined and rendered by a boundary (the skin?), whose disturbance can exclusively be conceptualized in the realm of the pathological: as wounding, violation, infection or disease. As signifiers of life's vulnerability, these disturbances are commonly thought of as opposed to and restraining human agency and, consequently, as counterproductive of subjectivation (Asad 2003). However, what if one were to think about the constitution of subjects and bodies, of subject-bodies and their agency, not from the vantage point of self-determination and self-containment, but, as Asad and others suggests, from their very vulnerability? How modern, how "proper" would they be?

Donna Haraway's work – pioneering in "post-alienation" and "post-representation" thinking and in the critical analysis of the social making of the body in technoscience – is instructive for understanding the precarity and impurity of the process of the constitution of subjects and bodies. To Haraway (1991a), the cyborg – that I have become through being vaccinated and yet simultaneously always have been – is an impure and improper body. It has never known pure, proper substance from which it could have deviated and from which abstract discourse it could have been alienated it in the first place. Accordingly, concepts such as immunology or the immune system in technoscience are not a mere representation of a pre-existing body but "a plan for meaningful action to construct and maintain the boundaries for what may count as self and other in the crucial realms of the normal and the pathological" (Haraway 1991b, 204). From this vantage point, immunological discourse is neither a mode of disembodiment (as it is for Duden), nor is the immune system a representation signifying what bodies mean, how they are perceived of and thought about

ter, in turn, can be seen as the pinnacle of the individualization of breathing/breathable air in the pandemic (Hinrichsen 2021).

18 Note that immunity, from Latin: *immunitas*, bears the original meaning of being exempt of military service.

(as for Martin). As an "elaborate icon for principal systems of symbolic and material 'difference' in late capitalism" (Haraway 1991b, 207), the immune system is a material-semiotic actor, an epistemic object, active in the constitution of bodies. "Organisms are made; they are constructs of a world-changing kind. The construction of an organism's boundaries, the job of the discourses of immunology, are particularly potent mediators of the experiences of sickness and death for industrial and post-industrial people," she argues (Haraway 1991b, 208). That means: because bodies are *made*, they need an agency that makes them. Because they are not stable, not self-evident, they need boundary work. The immune system accomplishes that. With Haraway, the immune system is a practical relation, a *way of being a body*. Inquiry into immunology, thus, tells us not how bodies are seen, but rather what they *are and how they are made*. And if bodies are made, this making (and doing) renders bodies fundamentally vulnerable and precarious.

This vulnerability and precarity, however and much in line with an ethics of care, is, according to Esposito, the crucial element for understanding immunity. He, accordingly, analyzes the dialectic of the "protection and negation of life" that underlies the logic of immunity: in order to protect life, the practice of vaccination introduces something into the organism, that is, in essence, harmful – a negation of a life that is protected by that negation. In his analysis, contagion, impurity, or infection are not so much threatening life (and immune systems prevent that threat) as they are constitutive for life itself to flourish: to be immune is therefore to be utterly vulnerable in the first place; along the same lines, Nik Brown borrows from Mary Douglas and argues "purity is danger" (Brown 2019, 215). From this perspective, immunity is less a closure and confinement of life into a body/individual of integrity, than it is an essential opening to the world.

Emily Martin draws on Ludwik Fleck (1980 [1935]), an immunologist responsible for one of the earliest, yet most influential works on the social – which to him, *avant la lettre*, also means the practical – construction of scientific facts, to argue for a relational understanding of immunity: "Instead of the organism as a self-contained independent unit with fixed boundaries, [Fleck] proposed a 'harmonious life unit', which could range from the cell, to the symbiosis between alga and fungus in a lichen, to an ecological unit such as the forest" (Martin 1990, 420). Immunity from this perspective, refers less to "modern" self-contained subject agents confined in "modern" individual bodies than it points to precarious bodies in "naturecultures" (Gesing et al. 2019; Haraway 2016; 2003; Tsing 2015)[19] or, in the words of Esposito,

19 The concept of "naturecultures" leaves behind conceptualizations of "nature" and "culture" as two separated epistemological and ontological spheres and instead scrutinizes their binarism by stressing the fundamental relationality of "nature" and "culture," albeit critically analyzing the knowledge practices that are involved in letting them appear as two realms.

to the "endless contagion that combines, overlaps, soaks, coagulates, blends, and clones bodies" (2011, 151).

If "endless contagion" is the name of the game and if, furthermore, "contamination [i]s collaboration" (Tsing 2015, 27), then immunity is not the demarcation of rigid borders. Immune systems are not defense apparatuses shielding a self-contained subject-actor from the world around him/her. On the contrary, they are "not a minor part of naturecultures [and] they determine where organisms, including people, can live and with whom" (Haraway 2003, 31). Immune systems are, following from this, apparatuses of sensibilization and "response-abilization"[20] towards a world that is not simply an "Other," but intertwined with us, connected, and corresponding – in and by this enmeshedness, and in the endless contagion, the binarisms of self and other, of individual and society, body and technology, nature and culture, are troubled and undermined: "[S]taying alive – for every species – requires liveable collaboration. Collaboration means working across difference, which leads to contamination. Without collaborations, we all die" (Tsing 2015, 28). And it is precisely here, that immune systems engender – or rather "render capable" (Haraway 2016, 16) – bodies, selves, environments, and (significant) others (Haraway 2003).

"I Contain Multitudes", or: the "Commune System"

The armored bodies, inhabited and constituted by warring T-killer-cells, macrophages and antibodies as the classic representations of immunity have undergone ample critique (Napier 2012; 2002; Haraway 1991b; Martin 1994; 1992; 1990; Moulin 1989) – not only by feminist critical theory, science and technology studies, and anthropology, but especially by immunologist thought itself. It has questioned the very notion of "self v. nonself", as well as its diffusion into a lopsided picture of immunological reason.

A most radical requiem – and quite a literal one, as he had, in a manner reminiscent of Wittgenstein,[21] declared the pending "end of immunology"[22] a few years before – came from Danish immunologist Niels Kaj Jerne. His "idiotypic network theory" declared the "completeness" of the immune system. This means "that the

20 This is in reference to Haraway's (2016) notion of "response-ability."

21 Wittgenstein famously declared that, having written his first book, he had solved all the problems of philosophy. Not quite as bold as Wittgenstein, Jerne's "end of immunology" is not the end of his Wittgenstein moves: in his Nobel price acceptance speech, Jerne inquired into the "generative grammar of the immune system" in an attempt to "establish an analogy between linguistics and immunology" (1993, 211). Immunology, a "language game" after all?

22 Jerne declared in 1969: "[I]mmunology will be completely solved within 50 years from now" (quoted in Anderson et al. 1994, 575).

immune system can respond, by formation of specific antibodies, to *any molecule existing in the world*, including [...] to molecules that the system has never before encountered" (Jerne 1993 [1984], 220; my emphasis; JH). How is this possible? In short: "[T]he immune system of a single animal, after producing specific antibodies to an antigen, continues to produce antibodies to the idiotopes of the antibodies which itself has made" (Jerne 1993 [1984], 216). The body produces antibodies to its own antibodies, against which it produces antibodies, which trigger the production of antibodies.... Completeness is endlessness. To Jerne, this not only makes obsolete the differentiation between "recognizing" (the antigen) and "being recognized" (by the antibody) (219), but furthermore results in an enormous repertoire, exceeding 10,000,000 in variety, of antibodies *of any specificity* in the body present all the time. That means 3000 antibodies to *every single possible* antigenic combination of proteins. Jerne: "Antibodies are not echoes of the invading antigen, but were already available to the animal in its repertoire of B cells *before the antigen arrived*" (222; my emphasis; JH). In Jerne's theory, the immune system is a "self-centred," closed, and yet endless network, all the while it already contains the entire world, it "contain[s] multitudes" (Whitman 1855, 76).[23]

If recognizing and being recognized is the same thing, a self can't be distinguished from the outer world. It contains this outer world, is made up of it, made up of "atoms belonging to me as good as to you," as the poet of a self which has never been modern, Walt Whitman, would say (ibid.). If this self "contains multitudes," it is, thus, not a self, at least not in a Cartesian sense (Napier 2012, 125), but at best a contradictory one.[24] To such a self – as to the cyborg – the skin is not a clearly rendered boundary. And if David Napier is right, then the modern cosmology of immunity is unhinged and the immune system – the apotheosis of modern castle-subject-bodies – becomes apparent as its own contradiction: the *commune system*. "How different might we live in the world imagining that our 'commune system' mediated our living relations with and in the world?" (Cohen 2009, 281).

Outlook: Improper Bodies, Commons, Responsibility.

From the perspective of a self-declared mRNA cyborg, "immunity" is neither a biological, nor physical, let alone corporeal phenomenon. Furthermore, vaccination – as the practice of making subjects and bodies – is the literal incorporation of (bio)technology. This sheds light on the pressing question, posed by cultural

---

23 It appears, Jerne was not just Wittgensteinian, but also Whitmanian, a truly postmodern romantic.

24 "Do I contradict myself? / Very well then I contradict myself, / (I am large, I contain multitudes)" (Whitman 1855, 76).

anthropologists Niewöhner, Kehl, and Beck (2008) of "how culture gets under the skin,"[25] whereas at the same time it complicates the notion of "culture" and skin as the apparent barrier between the body and the environment "under" which culture has to "get" in the first place is scrutinized. From the perspective of an anthropology of knowledge and science, immunity and the immune system, thus, inform us of how bodies are made social(ly), that is how they are both constituted and inhabited as social entities, utterly precarious and contingent and thus responsible for one another. Finally, given that those immune systems serve as the primary target of the global response against the COVID pandemic and, accordingly, vaccination as the embodiment of (governmental) technology, the immune system not only appears as the neuralgic center of the biopolitical governing of life (Esposito 2011). Furthermore, it allows for conclusions about what the body of biopolitics *is*, how bodies are made into political matter, how they are made to respond to and align with – and become! – technologies of government, paradoxically *because* immunity turns the individual body into a common, social good, a social apparatus, responsible for itself *and others*. If immunity is investigated at the intersection of organism and technology, subject and society, biology and culture, the immune system becomes manifest as the very interface of those categories. It is the very practice of vaccination – injecting an epistemic object, mRNA strands "packed in" lipidnanoparticles, into the muscle tissue – that, in one and the same process, underlines the binary character of these categories, while it simultaneously complicates, discards, overthrows and re-negotiates it. What is more, in the way I don't simply "have" or "own" a body, I don't simply "have" an immune system, but rather in processes of acquisition, manipulation, and inhabitation, my immune system, my body, as well as the "I" are co-constituted.

My inquiry into "how culture gets under the skin," how skin-enclosed bodies are made social(ly), and how these bodies become the arena for the biopolitical response to the COVID pandemic draws on the concepts of Donna Haraway to understand how the immune system makes a body/subject "response-able." That is: how bodies and subjects are "rendered capable" (Haraway 2016, 16), granted agency and assigned responsibility, while and by being sensitized for their environment. What, therefore, "gets under the skin" by way of vaccination is biotechnology as aggregated social knowledge, as material form social practice coagulates into. What is embodied – in the most literal sense: becoming body or corporeal "nature" – is political reason and its efforts of governing "life itself" (Rose 2001); is economical reason with biotechnology as an arena of both venture capitalism and state intervention; is, first and foremost, social knowledge, concepts, and norms: the differentiation between the normal and the pathological, definitions of what health and what disease is. And it

25 My translation of the German title of their book *Wie geht Kultur unter die Haut?*

is, ultimately, morality and ethics[26]: who is responsible for whom and what, who and what is deemed vulnerable and in need of protection, whose deaths are grieveable and whose lives are disposable (Butler 2006). Consequently, what is embodied by the act of vaccination are the sociomaterial epistemologies of what life is and what it is to live one, what a body is and what it is to have one, what a subject is and what it is to be one, what society is and what it is that it is made up of. With this embodiment, the immunized subject-bodies are invoked as "response-able" (Haraway 2016) yet "improper," "common" (Esposito 2011) subject-bodies to whom normative invocations of social responsibility and mutual care are – both implicitly and explicitly – addressed. In the course of this, immune systems become the central arena of the negotiation of the most fundamental issues of bio- and medical ethics: autonomy, responsibility, and solidarity.

Read in this way, immunity ultimately leaves behind its "modern" veneer. The immune system does not produce self-sufficient, self-contained subject-actors confined in bodily boundaries, which are clearly distinguished from the outside world; immunity is not about rational and self-responsible agents withdrawn from the social and its affordances, but on the contrary: it is about precarious multitudes in naturecultures, which are constitutively vulnerable – as Haraway says: "Life is a window of vulnerability. It seems a mistake to close it" (1991b, 224).

Immunitas and *communitas* are inversed or they fall into one and drift – like all modern phantasmas and metaphors of immunology and its dichotomies – into a zone of indistinguishability ("common immunity" (Esposito 2011, 165–177), when "being immune" becomes a "social" obligation (think of the discourse on mandatory vaccinations etc.) – social in every sense of the word: its epitome is herd immunity. *Communitas* and *immunitas* are interdependent; we remain healthy because we are vulnerable.

How precarious our existences are, how much we can only live in society, has been shown to us every day by the COVID-19 pandemic. Because we are constitutively vulnerable, we are dependent on each other and because we are dependent on each other, we are vulnerable. That is the most crucial assumption of an "ethics of care" (Butler 2006, Ferrarese 2016, Laugier 2016, Mol 2008); if we are dependent on each other, "we owe each other everything," as anthropologist Marcel Mauss (1990 [1950], 77) would say. Vaccination – as was clearly communicated in the German sphere at least – is then an act of solidarity and the recognition of a mutual obligation; and, thus, it is not surprising that the countless vaccination campaigns and appeals rarely omit the moral imperative. Vaccination, as the German Red Cross advertised on twitter and in a brochure, is "love" (DRK Kreisverband Müggelspree e.V. 2021). Seen from this perspective, protecting oneself with a vaccination is a service

26 Didier Fassin: "When biomedicine speaks the truth it also speaks morals" (quoted in Cohen 2009, 269).

to society, an act of charity and altruism (*Nächstenliebe* (EKMD n.d.) – and this is yet another allusion to the new "gospel."

Somewhat less sacred: the immune system becomes the field of negotiation of community and the common good. The analysis of its "sayings" and "doings" (cf. Schatzki 1996, 89)[27] – that is: of its *practical* negotiation – shows how bodies become political objects as well as subjects, a political issue as well as matter in its material sense identified by way of a yellow vaccination card or an electronic vaccination certificate. In other words: it shows how immunity turns the supposedly individual body into a social one, a social body through and through, responsible for itself and the others.

As vaccines engender response-able bodies, the immune system becomes a commons – which is astonishing given the fact that this is in no way true of the vaccines themselves. The biotech giants steadfastly refuse to make the vaccines royalty-free; the vaccines themselves are not public domain, not a creative commons, but hard-fought, hard-currency commodities that enable our freedom and make us immune by denying others, for example the countries of the global South, their immunity.

To conclude: as vaccines produce response-able bodies, the immune system becomes a commons. A response-able subject with a "commune system" is not a modern subject for whom responsibility was an indication of self-assertion. A response-able subject *is* a semiotic-material relation, situated and embodied. A response-able body is not a modern body whose boundaries are clearly defined, which belongs to us and vice versa, but also a semiotic-material relation, situated and embodied. It is an improper body, a social body, a common body; and as such it is never "immune" in the common sense.

Bibliography

Anderson, Warwick, Myles Jackson, and Barbara Gutmann Rosenkrantz. 1994. "Toward an Unnatural History of Immunology." *Journal of the History of Biology*, vol. 27, no. 3, 575–594. http://www.jstor.org/stable/4331331.

Asad, Talal. 2003. *Formations of the Secular: Christianity, Islam, Modernity*, Stanford UP.

Bourdieu, Pierre. 1977. *Outline of a Theory of Practice*, Cambridge UP.

Bourdieu, Pierre. 1987. *Sozialer Sinn: Kritik der theoretischen Vernunft*, translated by Günter Seib, Suhrkamp.

Brown, Nik. 2019. *Immunitary Life: A Biopolitics of Immunity*, Palgrave Macmillan.

Butler, Judith. 2020. *Precarious Life: The Powers of Mourning and Violence*, 1st edition, Verso.

---

27 This is yet another Wittgenstein move: Schatzki's approach to "Human Activity and the Social" is, as promised in the title, decidedly "Wittgensteinian."

Cohen, Ed. 2009. *A Body Worth Defending: Immunity, Biopolitics, and the Apotheosis of the Modern Body*, Duke UP.

CureVac. N.d. "About Us: Spotlight on CureVac." Imagefilm. https://www.curevac.com/en/about-us.

Douglas, Mary. 2001 [1966]. *Purity and Danger: An Analysis of Concept of Pollution and Taboo*, reprint, Routledge.

DRK Kreisverband Müggelspree e.V (@DRKmüggelspree). 2021. "Warum lohnt es sich, sich impfen zu lassen? Und warum engagieren sich manche, um die Impfkampagne zu unterstützen? Das erfahrt ihr in unserer Broschüre (...) #ImpfenIstLiebe." *Twitter* June 21, 2021. https://twitter.com/DRKmueggelspree/status/1406926495633846278?cxt=HHwWjMC51bGMtIYnAAAA.

Duden, Barbara. 1997. "Das 'System' unter der Haut. Anmerkungen zum Körpergeschichtlichen Bruch der 1990er Jahre." *Österreichische Zeitschrift für Geschichtswissenschaft*, vol. 8, no. 2, 260–273.

Esposito, Roberto. 2011. *Immunitas: The Protection and Negation of Life*, Wiley.

Evangelische Kirche in Mitteldeutschland EKMD. n.d. "Material für die Öffentlichkeitsarbeit." https://www.ekmd.de/service/onlinebestellen/ekmshop/plakat-impfen-ist-naechstenliebe-a4.html#gallery.

Ferrarese, Estelle. 2016. "Vulnerability. A Concept with Which to Undo the World As It Is?" *Critical Horizons*, vol. 17, no. 2, 149–159. https://doi.org/10.1080/14409917.2016.1153885

Fleck, Ludwik. 1980 [1935]. *Entstehung und Entwicklung einer wissenschaftlichen Tatsache: Einführung in die Lehre vom Denkstil und Denkkollektiv*, Suhrkamp.

Gesing, Friederike, Michi Knecht, Michael Flitner, and Katrin Amelang, editors. 2019. *NaturenKulturen: Denkräume und Werkzeuge für neue politische Ökologien*, Edition Kulturwissenschaft 146, transcript.

Haraway, Donna J. 1991a. "A Cyborg Manifesto: Science, Technology, and Socialist-Feminism in the Late Twentieth Century." *Simians, Cyborgs, and Women. The Reinvention of Nature*, Routledge, 149–182.

Haraway, Donna J. 1991b. "The Biopolitics of Postmodern Bodies: Constitutions of Self in Immune System Discourse." *Simians, Cyborgs, and Women. The Reinvention of Nature*, Routledge, 203–230.

Haraway, Donna J. 2003. *The Companion Species Manifesto: Dogs, People, and Significant Otherness*, Prickly Paradigm Press.

Haraway, Donna J. 2016. *Staying with the Trouble: Making Kin in the Chthulucene. Experimental Futures*, Duke UP.

Hinrichsen, Jan. 2021. "Regime Des Atmens Und Die Sorge Um Immunität. Kulturtheoretische Sondierungen." *Hamburger Journal für Kulturanthropologie (HJK)*, no. 13 (July), 382–92. https://journals.sub.uni-hamburg.de/hjk/article/view/1761.

Jerne, Niels K. 1993 [1985]. "The Generative Grammar of the Immune System. Nobel Lecture, 8 December 1984." *Nobel Lectures. Physiology or Medicine 1981–1990*, edited by Tore Frängsmyr and Jan Lindsten, World Scientific Publishing Co, 211–225.

Klein, Jan. 1982. *Immunology: The Science of Self-Nonself Discrimination*, John Wiley.

Latour, Bruno. 1993. *We Have Never Been Modern*, Harvard UP.

Laugier, Sandra. 2016. "Politics of Vulnerability and Responsibility for Ordinary Others." *Critical Horizons*, vol. 17, no. 2, 207–223. https://doi:10.1080/14409917.2016.1153891.

Martin, Emily. 1990. "Toward an Anthropology of Immunology. The Body as Nation State." *Medical Anthropology Quarterly*, New Series, vol. 4, no. 4, 410–426. DOI: http://www.jstor.org/stable/649224.

Martin, Emily. 1992. "The End of the Body?" *American Ethnologist*, vol. 19, no.1, 121–140. DOI: https://www.jstor.org/stable/644828.

Martin, Emily. 1994. *Flexible Bodies: The Role of Immunity in American Culture – from the Days of Polio to the Age of AIDS*, Beacon Press.

Mauss, Marcel. 1990 [1950]. *Die Gabe: Form und Funktion des Austauschs in archaischen Gesellschaften*, translated by Eva Moldenhauer, Suhrkamp.

Mol, Annemarie. 2008. *The Logic of Care: Health and the Problem of Patient Choice: Health and the Problem of Patient Choice*, Routledge.

Mol, Annemarie. 2002. *The Body Multiple: Ontology in Medical Practice*, Duke UP.

Moulin, Anne Marie. 1989. "The Immune System: A Key Concept for the History of Immunology." *History and Philosophy of the Life Sciences*, vol. 11, no. 2, 221–236. DOI: https://www.jstor.org/stable/2333034.

Nancy, Jean-Luc. 2000. *Der Eindringling: Das fremde Herz/L' Intrus*, translated by Alexander García Düttmann, Merve-Verlag.

Napier, A. David. 2002. *The Age of Immunology: Conceiving a Future in an Alienating World*, U of Chicago P.

Napier, A. David. 2012. "Nonself Help: How Immunology Might Reframe the Enlightenment." *Cultural anthropology: Journal of the Society for Cultural Anthropology*, vol. 27, no.1, 122–137. https://doi:10.1111/j.1548-1360.2012.01130.x.

Niewöhner, Jörg. 2015. *Wie geht Kultur unter die Haut? Emergente Praxen an der Schnittstelle von Medizin, Lebens- und Sozialwissenschaft*, edited by C. Kehl and S. Beck. VerKörperungen/MatteRealities – Perspektiven empirischer Wissenschaftsforschung 1, 1st edition, transcript.

Rose, Nikolas. 2001. "The Politics of Life Itself." *Theory, Culture & Society*, vol. 18, no. 6, 1–30. https://doi.org/10.1177/02632760122052020.

Sarasin, Philipp. 2001. *Reizbare Maschinen: Eine Geschichte des Körpers 1765–1914*, Suhrkamp.

Sarasin, Philipp. 2003. *Geschichtswissenschaft und Diskursanalyse*, Suhrkamp.

Schatzki, Theodore R. 1996. *Social Practices. A Wittgensteinian Approach to Human Activity and the Social*, Cambridge UP.

Sloterdijk, Peter. 2015. *Luftbeben: An den Quellen des Terrors*, Suhrkamp.
Sontag, Susan. 1978. *Illness as Metaphor*, Picador.
Sontag, Susan. 1989. *AIDS and its Metaphors*, Picador.
Thießen, Malte. 2017. *Immunisierte Gesellschaft: Impfen in Deutschland im 19. und 20. Jahrhundert*, edited by A. Nützenadel, G. Budde, D. Gosewinkel, P. Nolte and H.-P. Ullmann, Kritische Studien zur Geschichtswissenschaft 225, 1st edition, Vandenhoeck & Ruprecht.
Tsing, Anna L. 2015. *The Mushroom at the End of the World: On the Possibility of Life in Capitalist Ruins*, Princeton UP.
Whitman, Walt. 2004 [1855]. "Song of Myself." *Leaves of Grass*, Bantam Dell, 23–76.
Wittgenstein, Ludwig. 1953. *Philosophical Investigations*, Basil Blackwell.

Social and Historical Narratives

Visually Narrating Disease?

Syphilis in the German Public Sphere During the Early 20th Century

Victoria Morick

In the early 20th century, the venereal disease (VD) syphilis was often perceived as a major concern for German public health (Laukötter 2021, 50). At the time, an increasing amount of social, political, scientific, and economic resources were invested to educate the general public about diseases and hygiene. This led to the development of various new forms of medical communication – among which VDs were a recurrent subject. The foundation and institutionalization of the German Hygiene Museum Dresden (*Deutsches Hygiene-Museum Dresden*, DHMD) between the 1910s and 1930s were deeply intertwined with these tendencies. Combining resources and interests of a variety of actors, it soon became a key player in popularizing scientific knowledge and mediating between public, scientific, and political spheres (Steller 2014, 9–12). The museum tried to circulate various kinds of educational materials among large parts of the population. For example, around 1925, it published a series of slides or diapositives *(Lichtbildreihe)* on the reciprocities between social conditions and the spreading of VDs (Bethke 2007, 89).[1]

This series includes a picture of a woman and a man talking to each other in the streets (Fig. 1). Even though the exact date of the depiction's origin remains unknown, given the broader historical context, the protagonists' clothes and body language indicate that we see a well-dressed bourgeois man as well as a woman with a rather open body language and clothes that probably hinted at a lower, non-bourgeois class (Bethke 2007, 75–76). They do not touch, but their shadows overlap. The caption added in an explanatory text reveals further details: "Syphilis transmission through intercourse with prostitutes."[2] Contemporary viewers potentially

1 The original German title of the series is *Soziale Bedingungen der Geschlechtskrankheiten* (Social conditions of VDs). The diapositives made of glass were presented to larger audiences through projection. All pictures can be looked up on the museum's website (Deutsches-Hygiene Museum Dresden (DHMD), n.d.). I am grateful to the Image Department of the DHMD for kindly making several images available for this chapter.

2 "*Soziale Bedingungen der Geschlechtskrankheiten.*" n.d. DHMD 2002/282.

recognized the woman's profession based on their established viewing practices (Bethke 2007, 76). In any case, the caption adds information regarding a VD to the picture that might otherwise remain obscure or might not be part of its viewers' perceptions. The (textual) link between the visually depicted situation and syphilis expresses a moralistic syphilis narrative that framed prostitutes as spreaders of the disease and a potential menace to male citizens – a prominent narrative during the 19th and early 20th century (König 2014, 52–53).

Fig.1: Syphilis transmission through intercourse with prostitutes / Syphilis-Übertragung durch den Verkehr mit Dirnen, Deutsches Hygiene-Museum; DHMD 1999/1641

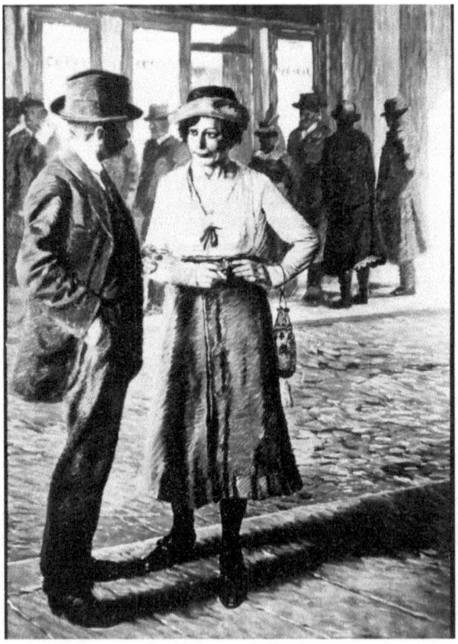

The depiction was, however, used for the slide series around 1925 – and since around 1900, various actors (at least officially) tried to change the disease's perception from a moralistic towards a more pragmatic approach (Sauerteig 2001, 78).[3] The state, physicians, and other institutions like the DHMD tried to inform more openly about this formerly "shameful" illness. One oftentimes expressed goal was to spread "objective" medical knowledge (Gertiser 2015, 16). VDs were increasingly considered

3 Yet, this did not mean that the connection to prostitution was erased completely. The approaches on combatting STDs differed and some of them were more pragmatic than other ones. On the strands combatting VDs in detail cf. Sauerteig 2001.

a medical as well as a social problem. Thus, many actors also meant to convince of a "healthy" lifestyle following certain (sexual) norms. This included new perspectives on syphilis, but also (partly adjusted) already existing ones as well as moral references (Sauerteig 2001, 79–81).

In this changing context, the choice of this particular image without explicit visual reference to syphilis might still seem confusing: Why was it used to inform about the disease? This question is the starting point for the analysis of two educational slide series on VDs provided in this chapter. The aim is to trace how disease and related ideas were visually rendered into a narrative about syphilis that was designed to reshape and "de-moralize" the public's perception. The analysis tries to not only identify which knowledge(s) and (ideological) views expressed themselves in the images, but further intends to examine the narrative potential of the slides to impact their audience. As illustrated by Fig. 1, this includes social ideas and narratives: did the new campaigns lead to less moral implications in practice? What emotions were addressed?[4] What role did disease and the "infected" body play?[5] In what way were (potentially) infected or infectious people, medical experts, and other groups presented as characters of a story?

In pursuing this aim, my main argument is that, even though the campaigns officially encouraged a less moralistic discourse on syphilis and rather new visual tropes and characters were part of the slide series, a more fitting description for this example would be a moral re-coding of already existing narratives in which one moral narrative was gradually supplanted by another. As shown in the course of this chapter, this process was correlated with essential changes: the increasing importance of the medical expert, changing scientific knowledge, and the opening of the human body to the objectifying medical gaze. The entire *Volkskörper* ("national body") including all classes was now presented as endangered.[6] However, class boundaries remained intact. I will further argue that the shift helps explain changes in public education, as members of the higher classes could not be treated by prohibition and

4 Here I am referring to works on the history of emotions; for an introduction, cf. Matt and Stearns 2014; Plamper 2015. Following Ute Frevert, I assume that emotions can be influenced by media. Also, emotions must be looked at in social contexts and their social patterns must be taken into consideration as well (Frevert 2020, 11, 22).

5 On an underlying level, as Philipp Sarasin's approach to the history of the body implies, this also includes the analysis of the social construction of body images, the body's coding in narrative discourses, related pictures and the role of syphilis depictions for the creation of collective identities (1999, 447): how did the "syphilitic body" differ from "ideal" or "healthy normal" bodies?

6 The term *Volkskörper* comes along with difficult ideological implications as it later became a crucial part of the national socialists' ideology. It referred to biological, racial traits and was included in the concept of "national community" or *Volksgemeinschaft* (Wildt 2014).

police force like prostitutes but required other forms of treatment, e.g., campaigns presenting their desired action framework.

My analysis is based on the theoretical premise that pictures have a generative competence and shape the perception of reality (Paul 2014). Thus, when looking at the construction of narrations about disease, supplementary to text analysis, visual material must be considered. Images do not simply illustrate, but also produce knowledge and meaning. I mainly follow Sturken's and Cartwright's ideas on the "Practices of Looking," arguing that negotiating the meaning of images is a process that includes reading visual signs as conventions. Images can be decoded "by interpreting clues pointing to intended, unintended, and even merely suggested meanings" (2009, 26).[7] Viewers are actively engaged in producing meaning. Pictures can be an additional part of narrations, e.g., as a representation of a series of events and also in terms of ideological narrative. Moreover, especially the impact of (visual) mass media should be considered (Hall 2006).

For my analysis, the DHMD's series #40 ("The Social conditions of VDs") on the reciprocities between social conditions and the spreading of VDs and series #10 ("*Die Geschlechtskrankheiten*"/"The VDs") on VDs in general are the main references.[8] Both were published during the 1920s, a crucial time for public health educational campaigns mostly including visually attractive material (Weindling 1989, 409–410). Despite their impact on the contemporary discourses on VDs, visual media have only been insufficiently included in research so far.[9] The museum's slide or diapositive series offer profound insights into educational campaigns on VDs and are suitable examples to analyze narrations of pandemics as they used an upcoming visual medium consumed by many people. The series enable us to trace how slides and variants of visualizations work together in creating stories about disease, but also in trying to influence the public narrative of syphilis more generally. Even though the narrative potential of the slides is limited and one can argue that they often represent a status rather than a developing story just like other pictures (Gossmann

7 Referring to Stuart Hall, they argue that all images are part of encoding and decoding processes in their production respectively their viewing (Sturken and Cartwright 2009, 72). Cf. Hall 2006.

8 Series 10 is also accessible on the museum's website (Deutsches-Hygiene Museum Dresden (DHMD), n.d.).

9 However, the importance of visual material in negotiating VDs around 1900 has been continuously pointed out (cf. Sauerteig 1999; Ellenbrand 1999; König 2014; Pietzrak-Franger 2017). Various publications even focus on visual material like movies on VDs (cf. Laukötter 2021; Gertiser 2015), or the museum's exhibitions and slide lectures more generally also hinting at VDs (cf. Weinert 2017; Steller 2014; Bethke 2007; Brecht/Nikolow 2000). These studies serve as points of reference for this paper providing a basis for the missing analysis of further widespread visual media like slide series. Additionally, the (German) context of public health education and visual media must be considered (cf. Gossmann 2022; Serlin 2010).

2022, 267–269), there are exceptions formed through picture sequences giving them a narrative frame (Bethke 2007, 19). Also, the depictions aimed to encourage viewers' imagination since they are not neutral representations, but subjects of looking practices (Cooter and Stein 2010, 172). Thus, despite these limitations, the series as a whole and its sequences offer insights into examining the presented syphilis narrative, its main characters, and plots.

To analyze the visual narratives, this paper proceeds in three steps: a brief reconstruction of perspectives on syphilis and the related educational campaigns will provide historical context information necessary to assess the ideological changes between the turn of the 20th century and the 1920s. Afterwards, I will briefly introduce the slide series and address the major, often overlapping themes, focusing on syphilis and public health. Finally, the paper concludes by analyzing the two series' narrative potential and the narratives of syphilis they created.

Syphilis and Educational Campaigns

In the early 20th century, VDs were part of the urban world and people were familiar with their visible symptoms (Laukötter 2021, 50). Syphilis, in particular, was increasingly prominent in social and public health debates, partly because several statistics since 1900 had shown increasing rates of infections. The First World War contributed to this trend (Quétel 1990, 176), intensifying the debate. Until the turn of the 20th century, syphilis was commonly associated with sin, guilt, and prostitution (König 2014, 52). Thus, a main strategy to combat the disease was to control prostitutes. Yet, around 1900, syphilis was also increasingly connected to the "moral decline" and "degeneration" of (urban) society in a more general sense potentially leading to national, military, and even "racial" decline.[10] In addition to criticizing prostitution, further arguments became crucial, for example criticism of urban life, moral changes, alcoholism, the delayed marriages of the upper class, and declining birthrates (Sauerteig 2001, 76–78). At the same time, medical knowledge changed. For example, the pathogen that causes syphilis was "discovered" in 1905, a blood test was introduced in 1906, and treatment options for the disease – which may affect almost the entire body if untreated – changed around 1910 (Laukötter 2021, 52–53).

Reacting to these tendencies, some educational measures were already implemented before the war and kept expanding after 1918 (König 2014, 57–59). Hygienic public education (*Hygienische Volksbelehrung*) in general became a new systematic

10 On "eugenic" and "racial" associations, cf. Weindling 1989. Legal debates about the question how to combat VDs were ongoing and the Act for Combating VD (*Reichsgesetz zur Bekämpfung der Geschlechtskrankheiten*) was not passed until 1927 (Sauerteig 2001, 78).

state intervention strategy at the time (Gossmann 2022, 2). When discussing education about syphilis, the idea of "demoralizing" the disease that spread since the 1880s and the introduction of new tropes have to be taken into account (König 2014, 54). The innovative VD campaigns of the early 20th century challenged the old perspectives: Instead of simply controlling prostitutes medically, they aimed at raising awareness among the entire population and addressed all social classes as potentially threatened by the disease (Sauerteig 2001, 80). In this context, Malte König argues that a certain "fear" of syphilis changed around 1914: while its moral dimension diminished, partly due to the introduction of the category of "innocent sufferers," this very development also led parts of the population to fear the disease who formerly felt unthreatened. This fear was used by campaigns to convince infected people to get treated in spite of possibly still existing feelings of shame (2014, 74).[11]

Many campaigns were conducted with the aim of informing the public medically about the dangers of VDs and spread hygienic education, e.g., about prophylaxis. For instance, around the turn of the century, many doctors supported premarital chastity and fidelity within marriage (Sauerteig 1999, 280). Also beyond VD campaigns, the population was frequently asked to follow a (supposedly) medically proven healthy lifestyle with "personal and public health" as a new norm seemingly replacing moral and religious ideas – as Alfons Labisch argues, health became the "neutral" ideal of daily life. From a contemporary perspective, this allowed to proclaim a certain lifestyle as the only correct one (1986, 275–279). In case of syphilis, (sexual) morality remained connected to a healthy lifestyle (Sauerteig 2001, 81–83).

Changing the Narrative? Slide Lectures on VDs

VD campaigns made use of new media to transfer pictures that had oftentimes been created in scientific processes into the public sphere.[12] Among these new educational methods employed by the DHMD were two slide lectures on VDs.[13] For the

---

11 The interests and discussions of the various groups involved in VD campaigns, the design of the various campaigns, the new tropes that were introduced, and the broader debates about VDs cannot be discussed in detail in this chapter. For more details, see, e.g., König 2014, Sauerteig 2001, Gertiser 2015. As the term "health" and the nature of a venereal disease suggest, discussions about syphilis can also be connected to increasing discussions about the human body in general, e.g., regarding its productive contribution to economy, or as an object of care and scientific interest. On these discussions about the body in general, see Weinert 2017, 3.

12 On this topic of popularization of scientific knowledge in general and with a focus on pictures cf. Daum 1998; Hüppauf and Weingart 2009; Nikolow and Bluma 2015.

13 On the history of the DHMD, cf. Steller 2017. So far, only little research on the museum's slide series and diapositives has been published (cf. Bethke 2007). Slide series 40 was published in two versions including 58 and 70 pictures, respectively. In this article, the focus will be one

lectures and other projects, the museum worked together with other key players in combatting VDs, for example the Society to Combat Venereal Disease (*Deutsche Gesellschaft zur Bekämpfung der Geschlechtskrankheiten*, DGBG).[14] In general, the various slide lectures offered by the DHMD reached wide audiences; the museum sold about 700.000 pictures between 1923 and 1930 (Bethke 2007, 47). The two series' pictures on VDs were likely combined from different sources and exhibit a variety of visualization methods (Bethke 2007, 89). Besides that, there is little information about their distribution and impact.

Presentations were supposed to be accompanied by a lecture. As supporting material for presenters, the museum provided a caption and description for each individual picture. As Berit Bethke argues, series 40 on social conditions of VDs is exemplary for the task of public education: in the beginning, it uses statistics to make references to scientific authorities, it then picks up the medical gaze, e.g., through microscopic pictures, moulages, photographs and drawings (2007, 96). The second series on VDs is structured similarly and often includes the same depictions. Within the series, each visual format had to fulfil a certain function: as it is also the case for exhibitions, slides showing statistics represented scientific relevance, bacteria supported belief in germ theory, and moulages showed symptoms in a shocking manner (Brecht and Nikolow 2000, 513).

The images were only projected for a limited amount of time, so they had to be concise, clear, and use well-known patterns to communicate their content (Bethke 2007, 19–20). Similar to other educational measures, as we cannot recreate the processes of inscription and transcription that took place during the presentations, we cannot trace viewers' exact reactions and emotional responses (Cooter and Stein 2010, 173). The material only represents what the creators wanted viewers to see.

---

the second, shorter version. The list including all pictures of the longer series suggests many similarities and also hints at a publishing date around 1925 (*Soziale Bedingungen* n.d.; Vereinsnachrichten 1925, 84–85). On the presumed years of publication, cf. Bethke 2007, 89. The exact date of publishing remains unclear for series 10 as well. Traces of this series and series 40 can be found in a catalogue from 1926 (*Der hygienische Lehrbedarf* 1926). Series 10 (*Die Geschlechtskrankheiten* n.d.) includes 70 slides. VDs are also part of a third series of slides, series 41 on the "Sexual Question of the Youth" (*Sexuelle Frage der Jugend*; Bethke 2007, 52).

14 At least for the short version of series 40, it is known that the dermatologist Eugen Galwesky, leading member of the DGBG and a doctor, was also involved. He connected the museum, the DGBG, and medical expertise (Bethke 2007, 89). On Galwesky, cf. Scholz 2009. It is also possible that the Reich Committee for hygienic public education (*Reichsausschuss für hygienische Volksbelehrung*) was financially involved since it often financed the production of such slides (Gossmann 2022, 96–97).

Introducing New Characters, or: Why Everyone Could be Affected by VDs

Statistics were a common method in educational campaigns such as exhibitions and used to visualize the social relevance of health (Nikolow 2006, 266). Thus, it does not seem surprising that both picture series on VDs begin with statistical charts. They range from bar and line charts to tables, allowing viewers to immediately make a connection to the "objective scientific gaze." As an addition, they often include textual elements and sometimes even illustrated drawings of the people referred to, ensuring the reader's "correct" understanding. Content-wise they cover, among others, the spread of venereal diseases in urban environments, numbers of lodgers (*Schlafgänger*) in cities, the rates of VD's spread among men and women, and among different age groups. Series 10 also includes the spread of VDs and the mortality rate of people infected with syphilis.[15] Such statistics communicated tendencies in public health and the "dramatic" numbers they include underline the urgent need to react in order to save the public. At the same time, they confronted viewers from all classes with their individual connections to society, showing everyone could potentially be affected by VDs (Nikolow 2006, 277).[16]

In this process, social and moral issues often played a prominent role putting certain factors and groups into focus: VDs were presented as a rather urban phenomenon, and the problem especially of young people being infected is highlighted which was a contemporary trend as well (Sauerteig 2001, 76). In the slide series, in addition to these topics, decreasing morals and living conditions, alcohol consumption, and unemployment are mentioned as further problems in one of the statistics' descriptions for the oral presentation. This is also the case for the army around the war that was traditionally connected to VDs (*Erläuterungen* n.d., 5).

Moreover, discourses on gender are integrated into the slides' statistics: while the numbers of infections among women are mostly presented as slightly lower than among men, statistical depictions of women are more prevalent and diversified. In

---

15 Cf. "*Verbreitung der Geschlechtskrankheiten in 30 deutschen Großstädten.*" N.d. DHMD 1999/1605; "*Schlafgänger in Großstädten.*" N.d. DHMD 1999/1618; "*Verbreitung der Geschlechtskrankheiten (Stockholm 1913 bis 1919).*" N.d. DHMD 1999/1606; "*Verteilung der Geschlechtskrankheiten auf die verschiedenen Lebensalter.*" N.d., DHMD 1999/1607; "*Vergiftete Jugend.*" N.d. DHMD 1999/1608; "*Verbreitung von venerischen Krankheiten.*" N.d. DHMD 1999/982; "*Sterblichkeit der Syphilitiker, nach den verschiedenen Krankheiten geordnet.*" N.d. DHMD 1999/1032.

16 This goes along with the contemporary definition of venereal diseases as a *Volkskrankheit*. Around 1900, the term indicated "[...] that everybody, whether woman, man or child, and whether bourgeois, worker or farmer, was threatened by infection according to germ theory. At the same time, [...] each individual was supposed to protect themselves from infection and illness and in so doing contribute to the so-called *Volksgesundheit* (health of the people or nation) [...]" (Brecht and Nikolow 2000, 518–519).

these gendered depictions, lower class women are more commonly depicted, although bourgeois women are not completely excluded from potentially being infectious in all slides. For example, one slide in series 40 ranks groups of women that were most "dangerous" to men.[17] The question of how these women were infected or which men typically infected women was not a concern; only women are explicitly mentioned as being infectious. The listing includes foremost prostitutes, but also other professional women with a working-class background, who had been frequently added to narratives of infection since the 1880s (Laukötter 2021, 51). Contemporary definitions of prostitutes were still negotiated and could include any economically independent working women or all unmarried women who had sexual relations (Sauerteig 2001, 77). Further statistics cover the numbers of prostitutes being infected with syphilis, the prospects of success in case of "controlling" them, and the "dangers" of secret prostitution practiced by groups like maids or waitresses. Also, the general reasons for prostitution are mentioned, including rather implicit connections between prostitution and syphilis as part of both series.[18]

Even though the slide series' statistics in general introduce characters from all classes, narrate syphilis by looking at both genders, and trace infections of different groups over time, they keep highlighting the role of certain classes and female professions, mainly prostitution. Their presentation was partly adjusted to the changing society and criticism of urban living conditions, merging social problems and ideas about a "loosening" morality with scientific authority and disease.

Establishing an Expert Focus and a New Enemy

The emergence of rather new characters, while retaining old ones, raises the question of how this was connected to further arguments and behavioral rules going beyond controlling prostitutes presented in further depictions. Following the statistics, before the slide series turn to syphilis, depictions of other diseases like gonorrhea are included. Afterwards, the sections on syphilis in both series are introduced by microscopic pictures, similar to Fig. 2.[19] It presents the effect of the anti-syphilis

17 *"Wo holen sich die Männer die geschlechtliche Ansteckung?"* N.d.. DHMD 1999/1609. Interestingly, the widespread allegation of a connection between Jewishness and syphilis (Pietzrak-Franger 2017, 136) is not mentioned in any statistic depiction.

18 *"Die meisten Prostituierten werden syphilitisch."* N.d. DHMD 1999/1611; *"Die Gefahr der geheimen Prostitution. (Nach Erhebungen von Dr. Gans, Karlsruhe."* N.d. DHMD 1999/1613; *"Äußere Ursachen der Prostitution."* N.d. DHDM 1999/1615. In picture series 10, the statistics on prostitution are included at a later stage of the presentation.

19 *"Spirochaeta pallida. (Mitr. Bild eines frischen Präparates bei Dunkelbeleuchtung)."* N.d. DHMD 1999/1628; *"Spirochaeta pallida in einem syphilitischen Anfangsgeschwür (Primäraffekt). Mikroskopisches Bild eines Schnittpräparates. Färbung nach Levaditi."* N.d. DHMD 1999/1011.

drug *Salvarsan* on the pathogens in the blood of an infected chicken. Salvarsan was a treatment option introduced in 1910 but did not always work and often came with side-effects (Sauerteig 2001, 81).[20] The figure provides a rudimentary before-and-after story depicting syphilis' curability. It shows the blood before being treated with the drug and several steps of pathogen reduction, ending with a healthy chicken.

Fig. 2: The effect of Salvarsan on the spirochetes of a chicken / Die Einwirkung von Salvarsan auf die Spirochäten eines Huhns, Deutsches Hygiene-Museum; DHMD 1999/1037

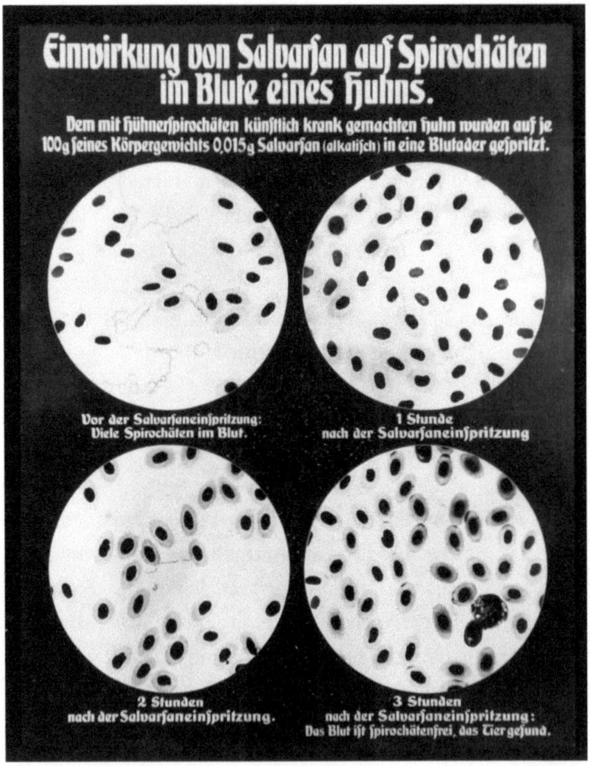

The differences in the four depictions seem obvious, but understanding them was problematic for lay people as this form of representation was not part of their everyday visual consumption (Bethke 2007, 79). However, oral presentations guided audiences through the presented scientific data and ensured "correct" conclusion: a

20 This is the only depiction of the drug, whereas no pictures of the drug itself or the packaging are included.

quick visit to the doctor in case of a possible infection increased healing chances (*Erläuterungen* n.d., 18). This underlined the importance of scientific authority and experts as characters in this campaign against syphilis. Only they were able to properly evaluate the "other" syphilitic blood results which made them a necessary condition for diagnosis, healing and ultimately protecting society from the disease.

At the same time, Fig. 2 gives insights into formerly invisible body parts on a microscopic level. The human body became subsumed under the medical gaze. These changes also impacted the character of the disease enabling a moral-recoding as the discovery of the syphilis pathogen provided a new identifiable enemy, adding an antagonist to the narrative (Gertiser 2015, 59). Alfons Labisch argues that such research results of bacteriology were liberating, as they allowed to present health as a less moral and political goal (1992, 144). The research allowed for a new, non-human actor – the pathogen which could affect the entire society, not merely a subset deemed morally deviant. At the same time, this enemy was presented as curable, thereby largely changing the syphilis narrative. This also created space for new connections between disease and this enemy: For example, series 40's oral presentation guide uses metaphorical language presenting the pathogen as a living creature that would "invade" the body, multiply quickly, and "infiltrate" all parts of it (Galewsky n.d., 10). Simultaneously, the centuries old public idea about syphilis impacting "healthy" blood remained intact. This as well as the idea of the "disease of lust" were two major reasons why research on the disease was intensified and infused with a special moral urgency (Fleck 2021, 102–103). Thus, once again, old moral ideas remained in use and were adapted to a "new enemy." As the statistics and the following sections show, it did not completely replace the role of human antagonists and moral ideas related to them.

Framing Symptoms and Directing the (Emotional) Gaze

Other motives with a prominent role in the series are visible physical symptoms covering almost the entire body. They are communicated through photographs of wax moulages that were created based on human body parts (Fig. 3), photographs of infected people or their body parts, and anatomic drawings of organs.[21]

21 Cf. "*Hirngewichte (Männer) – Gesamthirn und Großhirn, normale und bei Syphilis-Paralyse.*" N.d. DHMD 1999/1052; "*Syphilis der Leber. (Frische und alte – verkäste – Gummiknoten, Lappung infolge Narbenbildung).*" N.d. DHMD 1999/1027. For an introduction to moulages, cf. Schnalke 1995; Eßler 2022; and on the moulages in Dresden Walther, Hahn and Scholz 1993. Only a photograph of a moulage showing a hand that does not allow for the identification of the subject is reprinted here, as photographs of humans and moulages are sensible. Due to lack of documentation, it is unclear whether they were produced voluntarily and authorized for the slide series by the depicted persons. Additionally, they often depict exposed sensible body parts,

Especially moulages like Fig. 3 even enabled the display of male and female genitalia – body parts, that conventionally remained invisible (Laukötter 2021, 156), integrating them into the public depiction of the medical gaze. This gaze was, however, not free from contemporary discourses. For example, visible diseases served as a metaphor for social stigma (Nussbaum 2004, 174). Especially the skin's history is often told as a story of dirt, cleanliness, and disgust (Sarasin 2016, 264). Syphilis's symptoms contradicted a "normal" and "healthy" skin, even though contemporary viewers were likely more used to seeing skin changes than we are today.

Fig.3: Initial ulcer on the finger / Anfangsgeschwür am Finger, Deutsches Hygiene-Museum; DHMD 1999/1638

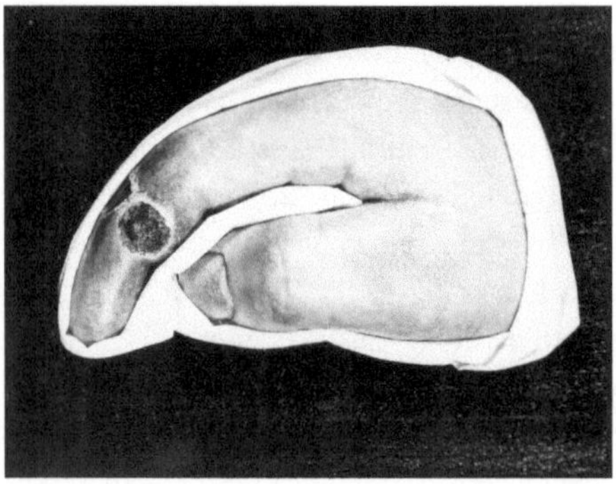

The cultural relevance of skin and the stigmatizations hint at a further function of the depictions: arousing emotions. An additional goal of moulages was to shock viewers and deter them from certain kinds of behavior using confrontation (Sauerteig 1999, 211). Moreover, similar to movies, depictions showing wounds and infected sexual organs were presumably meant to arouse disgust, reminding viewers of the possibility of infection (Laukötter 2015, 311), and triggering the fear of being infected or identified as infected. Emotions could also go in another direction: the description of Fig. 3 adds another layer of information to stimulate the viewers' imagination or even cause empathy with certain groups that were connected to the hand. The explanatory text mentions that the syphilitic "poison" would often have consequences for doctors, nurses, and midwives when they became infected while working (Galewsky n.d., 11). Though images of this kind may induce sympathy, this is only the case under certain narrative conditions – such that allow for a minimum

e.g., genitalia, naked newborns, and faces – potentially allowing to identify the subjects (cf. Schnalke 2020).

of identification with the suffering other.[22] Here, pictures of "innocent" babies or children also have a special role as they were depicted in a terrible situation, but yet remained innocent (Frevert 2020, 111).

An example going beyond the skin is the photograph of a naked male patient who is unable to stand without the help of another man, who, in turn, can be identified as a doctor by his clothes.[23] Here, the naked, dependent patient represents a low masculine status since his inability to participate in society independently and productively contradicted contemporary hegemonic concepts of masculinity.[24] Additionally, several photographs depict naked newborns.[25] The nakedness reflects the contrast of healthy and diseased bodies, as it retraces the search for symptoms and de-individualizes people into bearers of a disease – independent from their age (Bethke 2007, 107–108). Thus, the photographs framed syphilis as an outstanding "abnormality," whereas uninfected "healthy" body parts are often omitted. At the same time, the sufferers are related to society and excluded from it through their disease and nakedness marking them as "unhealthy" and "unable" to fulfil their social duties which was strongly related to social shame. Using the "persuasiveness" of shame also seems to have made sense to the creators of the slide lectures as it is one way groups can establish and enforce their identity (Stearns 2017, 1).

Thus, framing symptoms and directing the audience's gaze went beyond informing on a scientific level. Presenting symptoms through male and female characters of all ages underlined that everyone could be affected by syphilis, turning it into a danger for the entire society, not just for prostitutes. This process was part of moral re-coding which is visually narrated through connections to discourses like masculinity or a healthy youth to ensure a healthy, productive public. These connections are strengthened by various emotions supporting their persuasiveness.

Establishing Infection Routes: Prostitution, Alcohol, and Further "Immoral" Behavior

Another topic widely covered in the series on VDs is various routes of infection. These slides' content is presented in a less scientific manner and offers a larger narrative potential: for example, drawings were often used to illustrate certain "typical" behaviors which usually also implied a moral judgement (Bethke 2007, 75). This

22 Cf. Fritz Breithaupt's ideas on empathy for the development of this emotion through narration (Breithaupt 2020). On the role of media and distant suffering, cf. Boltanski 1999.

23 *"Geh- und Stehunfähigkeit bei einem Mann mit Taboparalyse."* N.d. DHMD 1999/1648.

24 On this concept, cf. Connell and Messerschmidt 2005.

25 Cf. *"Angeborene Syphilis. (Ausschlag bei einem Säugling im Gesicht)."* N.d. DHMD 1999/1034.

judgement created space to refer to old, but also new or re-coded moral positions within the lecture series that were impossible in other kinds of depictions.

The "immoral" behavior as a way of infection mentioned most frequently is prostitution, leading back to Fig.1 showing a man talking to a woman connoted as a prostitute. At the time, prostitution still reflected moral fears of certain groups. For example, conservative and religious groups connected the medical idea of "degeneration" and (changing) sexual behavior (Usborne 1992, 69). Fig. 1 connects prostitution with long-existing discourses related to nightlife, gender questions and social origin outside of public health. These connections are supported by several statistics indicating the high numbers of infections among prostitutes, marking them as a major reason for infections among men. Thus, the moral judgement and connection between prostitution and syphilis remained of use and was "updated" in terms of the current living situation within cities.

In addition, the notes accompanying one statistic for the oral presentation add several layers: each non-marital sexual contact would be dangerous and contact with prostitutes would almost certainly lead to infection. This must be avoided since even a cured disease led to social disadvantages, such as postponed marriage, or a lack of time or ability to work, thus potentially impacting male social status (*Erläuterungen* n.d., 19–20). Here, the responsibility for infection is partly divided: whereas female prostitutes are still claimed as a central source of infection, men are asked to actively participate in not getting infected. By referring to "each non-marital sexual contact," all men are addressed and, even further, also all women. The changing perspective to avoid infection also impacted the perception of prostitutes as antagonists. As not only they, but everyone disregarding preventive behavior could be blamed and ideas about "degeneration" potentially affecting the entire society spread, new antagonists were added, including male guilt into discussions. This had also been the case beyond the lecture series and the German-speaking area since the late 19th century (Spongberg 1997, 162). The possibly underlying idea of "hereditary" syphilis became popular from the 19th century onwards. Even though it was scientifically questioned quickly, the idea was part of public discourses and created room for moral hygienists' ideas and their judgement on certain behaviors to spread (Quétel 1990, 166–168).

The images focusing on prostitution also point out another central characteristic of the discourse on syphilis: it is related to two bodies touching each other in a kiss, whereby the "syphilitic body" deviating from "the norm" possibly communicated the disease through this touch (Pietzrak-Franger 2017, 37). Kissing, in particular, was a typical symbol of infection and immoral behavior that pathologized the behavior of people (Gertiser 2015, 131–132). The slide depicting the kiss is followed by a photograph showing a woman's mouth with symptoms.[26] These depictions build a short sequence about the communication of disease and moral ideas, which once again aimed to evoke an emotional reaction: the disgust at the physical deformation. As Martha Nussbaum describes it: "disgust concerns the borders of the body: it focuses on the prospect that a problematic substance may be incorporated into the self" (2004, 88). The generality of the kiss as dangerous behavior again strengthens the argument that everyone could potentially be infected and infections in case they did not follow the scientifically supported moral guidelines presented in these depictions.

Male characters shown in situations of close physical contact cover various classes, from soldiers and sailors to a man in a suit walking towards his misfortune – represented by a mermaid.[27] Fig. 1 is only included in series 40, but series 10 contains similar depictions referring to prostitution and consumption of alcohol. It is indicated that the consumption of alcohol could lead to losing control which was related to sexual contacts and disease – adding another moral discourse of the time to the syphilis narrative.[28] Again, the manuscript for the oral presentation asks all men to avoid non-marital sexual relations in the same way as it was also expected of women (*Erläuterungen* n.d., 21).

Consequently, syphilis as a disease and the scientific knowledge about it were actively used to support this argumentation, highlighting questions of guilt and potentially judging everyone who did not follow moral norms preventing the spread of a disease presented as avoidable. Men and women from all classes disregarding certain sexual behavioral rules were judged in the drawings. This also impacted the role of prostitutes as infectious antagonists, but it changed only partly as they were still presented more negatively than others.

Establishing Infection Routes: Risks for the Working Class

Not only prostitutes, but also other working-class women were depicted as both, endangered and dangerous. Fig. 4 picks up a common story: the role of the infected mother infecting others (Laukötter 2021, 51). It presents a chain of infections including several female characters, whereas the only male character is among the chil-

26 *"Syphilisübertragung durch Kuß."* N.d. DHMD 2002/2330; *"Syphilitischer Schanker an der Unterlippe."* N.d. DHMD 1999/1634. Like other social situations, this is only included in series 40 on the social conditions of VDs.

27 *"Alkohol – Prostitution – Geschlechtskrankheiten. Nach Untersuchungen von Lomholt aus Kopenhagen."* N.d. DHMD 1999/1653; *"Blind ins Unglück. Nach Untersuchungen von Lomholt aus Kopenhagen."* N.d. DHMD 1999/1654.

28 *"Alkohol und Prostitution."* N.d. DHMD 1999/1046; *"Alkohol und Geschlechtskrankheiten."* N.d. DHMD 1999/1047.

dren. The individual images do not directly refer to disease and only give hints at the women's professions via clothes and symbols, but the caption adds a short narrative including several characters. It starts with a 21-year-old maid who becomes pregnant and infected with syphilis, implying immoral behavior. During childbirth, her midwife is infected through a wound on her finger. At the same time, the child seems healthy, but turns out to be sick two years later. Thus, it has the role of an innocently infected victim, but also turns infectious: its foster mother, a wife with children of her own, is infected. Additionally, three of her children also have the disease, leading to at least seven infected people in total. A supporting visual motif that is included in both series before or after this slide is the drawing of a naked woman's upper body marked by what are supposed to be "abnormalities" on her mouth and breast.[29] A comparable male depiction is not provided. These depictions connect a variety of topics focused on women: moral misbehavior, sexual reproduction, motherhood, social origin, family life, and childcare, and the ever-present potential guilt. All of these offer points of connection to a great number of viewers.

The focus on working class children also seems striking, since during the first decades of the 20th century, their bodies were for instance often perceived as sick and anomalous due to their home and living conditions (Cunningham 2021, 144). Slide presentation 40 visualizes such conditions reinforcing chains of infections: photographs and drawings showing small, crowded apartments, e.g., a room where a woman is nursing a baby, while the father is watching her, one child is taking a bath, and further children spread in the room.[30] The picture's caption points out the housing situation as well as negative moral development.[31] In contrast to such "dangerous" situations, series 10 hints at an option for "saving" the children: fostering sick children in special places (*Erläuterungen* n.d., 13).

In sum, the examples highlight further dimensions of the role of working-class women in the syphilis narrative that were related to motherhood and children. The latter, too, are introduced as potentially infectious or endangered. They are closely linked to the consequences of urbanization and its social discourses through the potential spread of disease. But the extension of "dangerous" characters through such images went even further than just individual groups of characters: public health and ideas of healthy living of this class were at focus as this could potentially impact the entire society. Individuals were not only morally responsible for their own, but also their family's and society's health (Labisch 1992, 169). Here, the narrative of an avoidable disease was crucial.

---

29 *"An welchen Körperteilen erfolgt die Ansteckung mit Syphilis?"* N.d. DHMD 1999/1643.

30 *Wohnungselend und Sittlichkeit (nach einer Radierung von Heinrich Zille)*. N.d. DHMD 1999/1655.

31 Series 10 only contains a statistic on this topic but mentions a similar situation in the text (*Erläuterungen* n.d., 22), cf. *Wohnungselend und sittliche Verwahrlosung*. N.d. DHMD 1999/1048.

Fig.4: Example of a chain of infections with syphilis (according to Professor Werther, Dresden) / Beispiel einer Kette von Ansteckungen mit Syphilis (Nach Professor Werther, Dresden), Deutsches Hygiene-Museum; DHMD 1999/1013

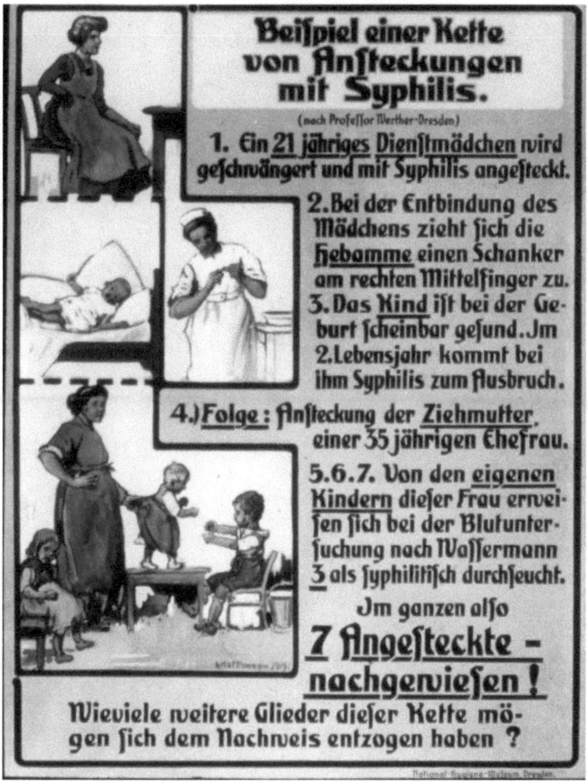
Beiſpiel einer Kette von Anſteckungen mit Syphilis.
(nach Profeſſor Werther-Dresden)
1. Ein 21 jähriges Dienſtmädchen wird geſchwängert und mit Syphilis angeſteckt.
2. Bei der Entbindung des Mädchens zieht ſich die Hebamme einen Schanker am rechten Mittelfinger zu.
3. Das Kind iſt bei der Geburt ſcheinbar geſund. Jm 2. Lebensjahr kommt bei ihm Syphilis zum Ausbruch.
4.) Folge: Anſteckung der Ziehmutter, einer 35 jährigen Ehefrau.
5.6.7. Von den eigenen Kindern dieſer Frau erweiſen ſich bei der Blutunterſuchung nach Waſſermann 3 als ſyphilitiſch durchſeucht.
Jm ganzen alſo
7 Angeſteckte – nachgewieſen!
Wieviele weitere Glieder dieſer Kette mögen ſich dem Nachweis entzogen haben ?

Establishing Infection Routes: How to Protect Your (Bourgeois) Family?

Whereas the visual vocabularies described in the previous section mostly refer to working-class families, series 40 also presents bourgeois settings. Judging from context and clothing, Fig. 5 is a case in point. Here, the experts who created the series actively engage with members of their own class. In the right picture, a father is turned into the protagonist guilty of infecting his family. In the left picture, a "healthy alternative" is given. The depiction probably encouraged this class's imagination, as the model of the nuclear family was considered crucial for bourgeois existence, with children demonstrating the health and capabilities of their parents by mere existence (Winkler 2017, 80–83). It is therefore not surprising that the idea of family was used for the syphilis narrative regarding this and other classes in educational material since the early 20th century (Gertiser 2015, 187).

Fig.5: VDs and marriage / Geschlechtskrankheiten und Ehe, Deutsches Hygiene-Museum; DHMD 1999/1665

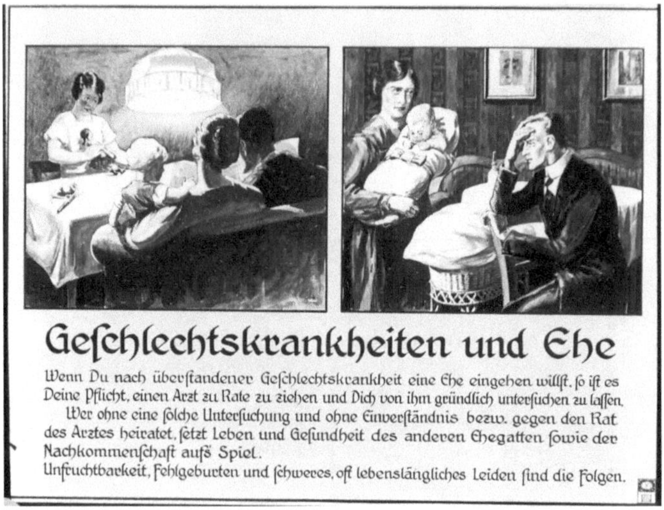
Geschlechtskrankheiten und Ehe
Wenn Du nach überstandener Geschlechtskrankheit eine Ehe eingehen willst, so ist es Deine Pflicht, einen Arzt zu Rate zu ziehen und Dich von ihm gründlich untersuchen zu lassen.
Wer ohne eine solche Untersuchung und ohne Einverständnis bezw. gegen den Rat des Arztes heiratet, setzt Leben und Gesundheit des anderen Ehegatten sowie der Nachkommenschaft aufs Spiel.
Unfruchtbarkeit, Fehlgeburten und schweres, oft lebenslängliches Leiden sind die Folgen.

Whereas the slide's pictures only implicitly refer to immoral behavior and its consequences, the text directly mentions it, revealing the underlying moralistic views on nonmarital sexual behavior and not consulting a doctor. Another slide further underlines this by showing a couple with bandaged eyes standing in front of an abyss – metaphorically representing the danger of VDs.[32] These slides' ideas again possibly also hint at eugenic ideas that became crucial during the 1930s.[33] Monika Pietzrak-Franger points out the "syphilitic child" became an icon of future anxieties in Victorian fiction (2017, 261). In the German context, male guilt of infecting children was raised since the 19th century (Sauerteig 2001, 78–79). Fostering future anxieties was presumably also intended by the series' creators, as series 40's additional text for the oral presentation mentions the "danger" of syphilis being

32 *"'Geh' nicht blind in die Ehe!' (nach einem amerikanischen Flugblatt)."* N.d..DHMD 1999/1669.

33 Discussions whether people infected with VD should be regulated regarding marriage were frequently discussed since the late 19th century, cf. Weindling 1989. On the public development of ideas on "hereditary syphilis," cf. Quétel 1990. On related eugenic ideas, cf. Kaufmann 1998.

"transmitted" to future generations. Notably, this part also talks about a man infecting a woman (Galewsky n.d., 14). Thus, infected people were considered guilty of infecting their children in the series, a belief that was common at the time (König 2016a, 118–119, 137–138). Underlying this was also a dimension of fear for the nation due to the consequences of the spread of VDs. As the previous sections show, this argument of parents being responsible for infection was also crucial for the working class.

The idea of "rescuing" the youth is also present in other slides referring to good parental care, including an example showing parents with their baby and pointing out the universal right of being born healthy, a statistic giving advice to parents about educating their children due to high infection rates among students, two drawings comparing the "wrong" education in the streets to the "right" education at home, and another drawing showing parents educating their children while standing in front of a group of chickens and their offspring.[34] Here, the depictions hint at ideas like the connection between streets and moral danger for children as especially urban childhood was considered a threat around 1900 (Winkler 2017, 103).

Therefore, the bourgeois characters were presented as endangered, but also as being able to change and protect their children which differed from the working class's depictions. The mere addition of the bourgeois family and their connection to nonmarital sexual behavior was part of the process of re-coding the syphilis narrative, spreading it across the entire society. Yet, class boundaries were kept up visually. Syphilis remained strongly connected to lower classes as it was still associated with prostitution, uncleanliness, and the working class's urban living conditions. Even though the bourgeois non-marital contact could include prostitution, the other aspects are mostly visually excluded from their lives in the slide series. Instead, their ability to protect their families and inform their children is highlighted.

Offering Ways of Treatment and Methods of Avoiding Infection

In the series, medical examinations are not only listed as a necessity before marriage to avoid the spread of syphilis,[35] but also visualized. Pictures showing doctors' practices and counselling offices were a common motif (Bethke 2007, 61). For example,

34 *"'Jedes Kind hat das Recht wohlgeboren zu sein. Wollt Ihr Euren Kindern einen gesunden Leib mitgeben und einen guten Eintritt ins Leben sichern?' (nach amerikanischem Flugblatt)."* N.d.. DHMD 1999/1667; *Eltern, sorgt für die Aufklärung eurer Kinder!* N.d.DHMD 1999/1670; *"Wie erhält Dein Kind geschlechtliche Aufklärung?" (nach einem amerikanischen Flugblatt).* N.d. DHMD 1999/1671; *"'Eltern, laßt es Euch nicht entgehen, Euren Kindern das Wunder der Fortpflanzung rein und unbefangen nahe zu bringen!' (Nach einem amerikanischen Flugblattt)."* N.d. DHMD 1999/1672.

35 Their legal requirement was frequently discussed by various groups at the time, cf. Sauerteig 1999.

pictures of an advice center (*Beratungsstelle*) in Dresden depict the institution, not the disease, frequently hinting at the possibility of healing in case of early treatment.[36] As syphilis was long known as not or barely curable before, this marked a change in its narrative.

Fig. 6: Boys, girls! Keep yourselves pure! / Jünglinge, Mädchen! Haltet Euch rein! Deutsches Hygiene-Museum; DHMD 1999/1673

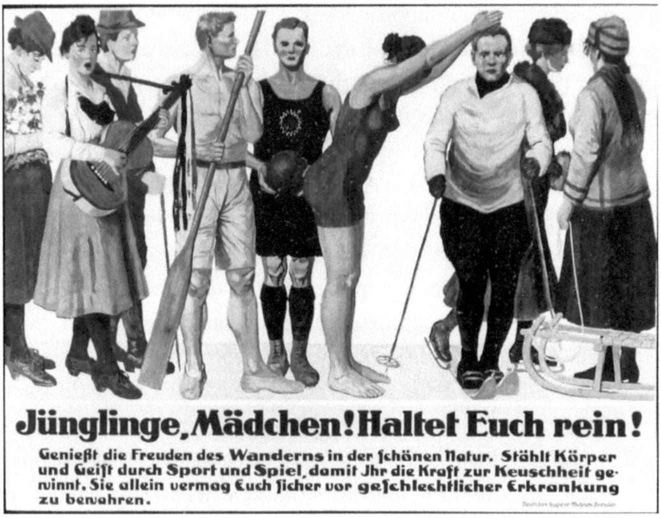
Jünglinge, Mädchen! Haltet Euch rein!
Genießt die Freuden des Wanderns in der schönen Natur. Stählt Körper und Geist durch Sport und Spiel, damit Jhr die Kraft zur Keuschheit gewinnt. Sie allein vermag Euch sicher vor geschlechtlicher Erkrankung zu bewahren.

However, it is also mentioned that chastity outside of marriage would be the safest way to avoid VDs. A concrete suggestion to avoid sexual contacts was movement. The 1920s and 1930s were a time when athletic performance was linked to ideas of cleanliness, rationalization of work, and discipline among other things by some groups (Eichberg 1998, 474). Fig. 6 links such ideas of keeping an abstinent and healthy life by representing various activities as positive examples of alternative behavior to prevent VDs referring to both men and women (Bethke 2007, 76).[37] Similar to the encouragement of medical examinations, this once again linked ways to avoid syphilis or to treat the "curable" disease to moral discourses. By offering alternatives

36 *"Bilder aus der Beratungsstelle Dresden der Sächsischen Landesversicherung."* N.d. DHMD 1999/1051.

37 When thinking about the VD prevention from today's perspective, condoms seem to be an obvious part of it. Even though this contraceptive already existed around 1900, the marketing of condoms was legally restricted and condoms or contraception in general were highly controversial topics at the time (König 2016b, 11, 40).

and informing about their impact, individual moral responsibility to protect oneself and others was strengthened.

Slide Series Building a Narrative Frame

Regarding the general order of slides, it is crucial that both series begin with statistics highlighting the general relevance of VDs for everyone and introducing rather new characters, but also retaining groups that had already previously been considered as endangered and dangerous in the picture. Both series then start the syphilis section with a microscopic depiction of the syphilis pathogen establishing medical authority and the idea of syphilis as being curable by experts, but also introduce a non-human antagonistic character. Still, human antagonists remained crucial.

Series 10 goes on to briefly mention chains of infection and the risks of taking care of children. This is followed by a large, rather scientific part showing symptoms. It ends with another part concerned with social topics such as statistics and pictures on prostitution, alcohol, education of the youth, and exercise as an alternative of mode behavior. In contrast, series 40 contains more depictions, mostly painted ones, on social aspects, like various care institutions for infected people, situations that can lead to infection, and a larger part on family, marriage, and children's education that often seems repetitive – to ensure that viewers will not forget their message. As the title "VDs" for series 10 suggests, it contains fewer images addressing the social conditions of VDs than series 40. However, especially these drawings seem to leave more room for encouraging the viewers' imagination than more scientific depictions such as microscopic pictures. Also, in series 40 especially these drawings are used to engage with classes other than the lower ones.

The depictions' orders differ in both series. Nevertheless, they repeatedly form short narrative sequences. For example, pictures related to oral infection in certain professions, while drinking or kissing, are followed by a photograph showing symptoms on the lips in series 40 – zooming into the possible consequences of this behavior. Another example are several slides forming short narrations concerning chains of infections similar to Fig. 4. In series 40, this is embedded in several other depictions regarding female childcare, infection, and symptoms: the warning of the dangers of taking care of children other than one's own is followed by the moulage of a finger. The infection risk through wet nurses is followed by a moulage showing a female breast. All in all, series 40 uses the narrative technique of visual sequences more intensively, integrating symptom-related visuals into narrative sequences. The same images often stand alone in series 10, even though the manuscript for the oral presentation adds further narrative layers and moralistic arguments.

Depictions often rely on the lectures or additional textual elements within the depictions to be understood "correctly" and contextualized within narratives, indicating a limitation of their narrative potential when they stand for themselves. Here, we must differentiate between performed and written text. Whereas the written text in the captions was limited by space, oral presentations certainly had more space to unfold narratives. Relying on the written proof we have, the possibilities become clear. This is, for example, the case with the depictions of the pathogen. As mentioned, these seemingly neutral representations of science were semantically shaped by metaphors turning the pathogen shown in the depictions into an actively invading enemy.

Conclusion

The two series on VDs by the DHMD are examples of attempts to reshape the public perception of syphilis. Similar to other educational measures like movies, especially series 40 shows a common didactic pattern: syphilis and its consequences are presented along with measures to combat them, often repeating the same contents and messages several times (Laukötter 2021, 146–7). The main measures in the combat against syphilis that everyone was asked to follow, were a celibate life outside of marriage, education on sexual matters, and physical examinations before marriage or in case of infection. Despite moral links such measures indicated, one declared goal of campaigns like the slide series was also to overcome moral implications regarding VDs. However, the previous analysis shows that a de-moralization of syphilis is not applicable to the slide series. Instead, a moral re-coding of existing narratives took place, with one moral stance gradually being supplanted by another or even standing next to each other. This re-coding did not mean that all stereotypes regarding syphilis as a "disease of lust" and prostitutes were suddenly overcome. They were changed slowly and sometimes even utilized to support new or changed moral arguments. This process can be broken down into several factors:

Firstly, a crucial basis for the re-coding in the slides was the depiction of syphilis in a more scientific way including its pathogen as an antagonist. This had two effects: On one hand, it was the base for re-framing syphilis as a (newly) curable disease. On the other hand, the pathogen re-shaped the relationship between humans and the disease by enabling a less moralistic perspective. This made it possible to include all classes and genders. The entire society was added to the visual narrative of syphilis, strengthening a new variant of a "national body" (*Volkskörper*). These arguments were supported by the increasing medical expertise and the subsumption of the human body under the objectifying medical gaze. In parallel, medical experts were presented as heroic and ascribed authority. Microscopic depictions and statistics are two ways of putting this into visual practice.

Secondly, many depictions in the slide series merge scientific appearance with moral implications. Here, the general function of these slide series – which I consider similar to that of educational films – must also be taken into account: they had to educate about medical knowledge and at the same time convince of viewers to adopt behavioral changes, which might have encouraged certain modes of presentation (Gertiser 2015, 32). Through "syphilitic" symptoms on human bodies, oftentimes linked to specific behaviors, people were marked as "sick" and "abnormal." This implied consequences that partly differed from older ones and were intertwined with the changing characters: in the slides, each male or female body is presented as potentially syphilitic and as a metaphor for decline. However, certain bodies, for example those of the urban working class, were presented as more endangered than others. In contrast to them, the potentially endangered bourgeois couple was assigned more capability for self-protection. Here, the suggestion to get medically tested before marriage played a central role. If the couple did not follow such instructions, the consequences would negatively affect their duty towards their family and in the long term potentially the entire nation. Especially the increasing extent by which men were asked to avoid guilt of infecting women and children was an addition to the narrative. To create a more convincing re-shaped syphilis narrative and allow viewers to connect to the characters, various emotional layers were added, for example: fear of being infected or infectious, shame, guilt of endangering future generations, responsibility, disgust, but potentially also empathy.[38]

Thirdly, the fact that the former focus on prostitutes and urban lower classes was kept alive shows that supplementing one moral stance by another was a gradual process leading to coexisting moral stances. Especially the role of the prostitute remained clearly distinct from that of the caring and educating (bourgeois) mother. In general, female groups with a low social status were depicted more frequently and in more negative positions than other women, keeping gender and class boundaries at least partly intact. We also find changes in the depiction of lower-class characters as they were adjusted to changing knowledge; living conditions and professions like the wet nurse were added to the narratives. In general, depictions often combine various discourses (e.g., urban or sexual morals) with VDs, with syphilis being only implicitly shown in the depictions or added via textual components.

To convince viewers of all classes and gain their trust, creators had to bear in mind common viewing practices and regimes of what could be shown. This might explain why especially series 40 contains many non-scientific drawings and moulages, broadening the range of what could be depicted. On top of this, the

38 As other recent studies have shown, such emotions often played a central role in educating about VDs at the time, for example in movies or exhibitions, cf. Laukötter 2021; Gertiser 2015; König 2014; Nikolow and Brecht 2000. These works also show that the series' depictions reproduce the topics and ideas of other educational measures in many ways and make use of the same or similar depictions, even though their materiality differs due to the nature of the slides.

slides' space and narrative potential were limited which might explain why the depiction of different social groups often followed established stereotypes for easier readability – despite of the existing stigmatizations associated with them.

In sum, the range of people potentially affected by syphilis was "officially" opened in comparison to previous centuries. However, the experience of the disease remained a story related to morality and emotions with conflicting ideas coexisting at the same time and impacting each other. As all parts of society now had to be convincingly included in the syphilis narrative, social and class-specific adjustments to former methods of combatting VDs were required. This led to the necessity of new information campaigns and didactic methods – one of these were the slide lectures. Their syphilis narrative was supported by bacteriological changes in knowledge and treatment options turning syphilis into a curable disease with a combatable pathogen. However, widespread moral ideas were visually kept, added, and adjusted to the changing knowledge about syphilis and its characters.

Bibliography

Bethke, Berit. 2007. "Sichtbare Spuren / Spuren der Sichtbarkeit. Betrachtungen zur hygienischen Volksbelehrung in der Weimarer Republik anhand von Lichtbildreihen des Deutschen Hygienemuseums." Magisterarbeit, University of Leipzig.

Breithaupt, Fritz. 2020. *Kulturen der Empathie*, 6th edition, Suhrkamp.

Boltanski, Luc. 1999. *Distant Suffering. Morality, Media and Politics*, Cambridge UP.

Brecht, Christine/Nikolow, Sybilla. 2000. "Displaying the Invisible: *Volkskrankheiten* on Exhibition in Imperial Germany." *Studies in History and Philosophy of Biology & Biomedical Science*, vol. 31, no. 4, 511–530.

Connell, R.W., and James W. Messerschmidt. 2005. "Hegemonic Masculinity: Rethinking the Concept." *Gender and Society*, vol. 19, no. 6, 829–859.

Cooter, Roger, and Claudia Stein. 2010. "Visual Imagery and Epidemics in the Twentieth Century." *Imagining Illness. Public Health and Visual Culture*, edited by David Serlin, U of Minnesota P, 169–192.

Cunningham, Hugh. 2021. *Children and Childhood in Western Society since 1500*, 3rd edition, Routledge.

Daum, Andreas. 1998. *Wissenschaftspopularisierung im 19. Jahrhundert. Bürgerliche Kultur, naturwissenschaftliche Bildung und die deutsche Öffentlichkeit 1848–1914*, Oldenbourg.

Der hygienische Lehrbedarf. 1926. Edited by Deutsche Hochbildgesellschaft/Deutsches Hygiene-Museum, Dresden/Munich.

Deutsches Hygiene-Museum Dresden (DHMD). N.d. "Collection Online." https://www.dhmd.de/en/collections-research/collection-online.

Die Geschlechtskrankheiten. N.d. Edited by Deutsches Hygiene-Museum/ Lehrmittelinstitut. DHMD 2022/109.

Eichberg, Henning. 1998. "Sport zwischen Ertüchtigung und Selbstbefreiung." *Erfindung des Menschen, Schöpfungsträume und Körperbilder 1500–2000*, edited by Richard van Dülmen, Böhlau, 459–481.

Ellenbrand, Petra. 1999. *Die Volksbewegung und Volksaufklärung gegen Geschlechtskrankheiten in Kaiserreich und Weimarer Republik*, Görich & Weiershäuser.

Erläuterungen zu den Lichtbildreihen des Deutschen Hygiene-Museums. Vortrag 10: Die Geschlechtskrankheiten. N.d. Edited by Aktiengesellschaft für hygienischen Lehrbedarf. DHMD 2002/415.

Eßler, Henrik. 2022. *Krankheit gestalten. Eine Berufsgeschichte zur Moulagenbildnerei*, transcript.

Fleck, Ludwik. 2021. *Entstehung und Entwicklung einer wissenschaftlichen Tatsache. Einführung in die Lehre vom Denkstil und Denkkollektiv*, edited by Lothar Schäfer and Thomas Schelle, 13th edition, Suhrkamp.

Frevert, Ute. 2020. *Mächtige Gefühle. Von A wie Angst bis Z wie Zuneigung. Deutsche Geschichte seit 1900*, 2nd edition, S. Fischer.

Galewsky, Eugen Emmanuel. N.d. *Erläuterungen zu den Lichtbildreihen des Deutschen Hygiene-Museums. Vortrag 40: Soziale Bedingungen der Geschlechtskrankheiten*. Edited by Aktiengesellschaft für hygienischen Lehrbedarf. DHMD 2002/745.

Gertiser, Anita. 2015. *Falsche Scham. Strategien der Überzeugung in Aufklärungsfilmen zur Bekämpfung der Geschlechtskrankheiten (1918–1935)*, V&R Unipress.

Gossmann, Jill. 2022. *Mediziner und die Erziehung der "Massen." Gesundheitspädagogische Diskurse in der Weimarer Republik*, Tectum.

Hall, Stuart. 2006. "Encoding/Decoding." *Media and Cultural Studies. Key Works*, edited by Meenakshi Gigi Durham and Douglas M. Kellner, Blackwell, 163–173.

Hüppauf, Bernd, and Peter Weingart, editors. 2009. *Frosch und Frankenstein. Bilder als Medium in der Popularisierung von Wissenschaft*, transcript.

Kaufmann, Doris. 1998. "Eugenik – Rassenhygiene – Humangenetik. Zur lebenswissenschaftlichen Neuordnung der Wirklichkeit in der ersten Hälfte des 20. Jahrhunderts." *Erfindung des Menschen, Schöpfungsträume und Körperbilder 1500–2000*, edited by Richard van Dülmen, Böhlau, 347–365.

König, Malte. 2014. "Syphilisangst in Deutschland und Frankreich. Hintergrund, Beschwörung und Nutzung einer Gefahr 1880–1940." *Infiziertes Europa. Seuchen im langen 20. Jahrhundert*, edited by Malte Thießen, de Gruyter Oldenbourg, 50–75.

König, Malte. 2016a. *Der Staat als Zuhälter. Die Abschaffung der reglementierten Prostitution in Deutschland, Frankreich und Italien im 20. Jahrhundert*, de Gruyter.

König, Wolfgang. 2016b. *Das Kondom. Zur Geschichte der Sexualität vom Kaiserreich bis in die Gegenwart*, Franz Steiner Verlag.

Labisch, Alfons. 1986: "'Hygiene ist Moral – Moral ist Hygiene' – soziale Disziplinierung und Medizin." *Soziale Sicherheit und soziale Disziplinierung*, edited by Christoph Sachße and Florian Tennstedt, Suhrkamp, 265–285.

Labisch, Alfons. 1992. *Homo Hygienicus. Gesundheit und Medizin in der Neuzeit*, Campus Verlag.

Laukötter, Anja. 2015. "Vom Ekel zur Empathie. Strategien der Wissensvermittlung im Sexualaufklärungsfilm des 20. Jahrhunderts." *Erkenne dich selbst! Strategien der Sichtbarmachung des Körpers im 20. Jahrhundert*, edited by Sybilla Nikolow, Böhlau, 305–319.

Laukötter, Anja. 2021. *Sex – richtig! Körperpolitik und Gefühlserziehung im Kino des 20. Jahrhunderts*, Wallstein.

Lichtbildreihe 10. "Die Geschlechtskrankheiten" (70 LB). N.d. Edited by Deutsches Hygiene-Museum Dresden/Lehrmittelproduktion. DHMD 1999/982–1051.

Lichtbildreihe 40. "Die sozialen Bedingungen der Geschlechtskrankheiten" (58 LB). N.d. Edited by Deutsches Hygiene-Museum Dresden/Lehrmittelproduktion. DHMD 1999/1605–1653.

Matt, Susan J., and Peter N. Stearns, editors. 2014. *Doing Emotions History*, U of Illinois P.

Nikolow, Sybilla, and Lars Bluma. 2009. "Die Zirkulation der Bilder zwischen Wissenschaft und Öffentlichkeit. Ein historigraphischer Essay." *Frosch und Frankenstein. Bilder als Medium der Popularisierung von Wissenschaft*, edited by Bernd Hüppauf and Peter Weingart, transcript, 45–78.

Nikolow, Sybilla. 2006. "Imaginäre Gemeinschaften. Statistische Bilder der Bevölkerung." *Konstruierte Sichtbarkeiten. Wissenschafts- und Technikbilder seit der Frühen Neuzeit*, edited by Martina Heßler, Fink, 263–278.

Nikolow, Sybilla. 2015. "'Wissenschaftliche Stillleben' des Körpers im 20. Jahrhundert." *Erkenne dich selbst! Strategien der Sichtbarmachung des Körpers im 20. Jahrhundert*, edited by Sybilla Nikolow, Böhlau, 11–43.

Nussbaum, Martha. 2004. *Hiding from Humanity. Disgust, Shame, and the Law*. Princeton UP.

Paul, Gerhard. 2014. "Visual History, Version: 3.0." *Docupedia-Zeitgeschichte*, March 3, 2014, http://docupedia.de/zg/paul_visual_history_v3_de_2014.

Pietzrak-Franger, Monika. 2017. *Syphilis in Victorian Literature and Culture. Medicine, Knowledge and the Spectacle of Victorian Invisibility*, Palgrave Macmillan.

Plamper, Jan. 2015. *The History of Emotions. An Introduction*, Oxford UP.

Quétel, Claude. 1990. *History of Syphilis*, translated by Judith Braddock and Brian Pike, Johns Hopkins UP.

Ruchatz, Jens. 2003. *Licht und Wahrheit. Eine Mediumgeschichte der fotografischen Projektion*, Fink.

Sarasin, Philipp. 1997. "Mapping the Body. Körpergeschichte zwischen Konstruktivismus, Politik und 'Erfahrung.'" *Historische Anthropologie*, vol. 7, no. 3, 437–451.

Sarasin, Philipp. 2016. *Reizbare Maschinen. Eine Geschichte des Körpers 1765–1914*, 4th edition, Suhrkamp.

Sauerteig, Lutz. 1999. *Krankheit, Sexualität, Gesellschaft. Geschlechtskrankheiten und Gesundheitspolitik in Deutschland im 19. und frühen 20. Jahrhundert*, Steiner.

Sauerteig, Lutz. 2001. "'The Fatherland is in Danger, Save the Fatherland!': Venereal disease, sexuality and gender in Imperial and Weimar Germany." *Sex, Sin and Suffering. Venereal Disease and European Society*, edited by Roger Davidson and Leslie A. Hall, Routledge, 76–92.

Schnalke, Thomas. 1995. *Diseases in Wax. The History of the Medical Moulage*, translated by Kathy Spatschek, Quintessence Publishing.

Schnalke, Thomas. 2020. "Alles auf Anfang. Einige Nachgedanken zum Umgang mit medizinischen Objekten als historische Quellen." *Virus – Beiträge zur Sozialgeschichte der Medizin*, vol. 19, 229–236.

Scholz, Albrecht. 2009. "Eugen Galewsky und die Bekämpfung der Geschlechtskrankheiten." *Die Geschichte der Urologie in Dresden*, edited by Dirk Schultheiss and Friedrich H. Moll, Springer, 118–123.

Serlin, David, editor. 2010. *Imagining Illness. Public Health and Visual Culture*, U of Minnesota P.

Soziale Bedingungen der Geschlechtskrankheiten. N.d. Edited by Deutsches Hygiene-Museum/Lehrmittelproduktion. DHMD 2002/282.

Spongberg, Mary. 1997. *Feminizing Venereal Disease. The Body of the Prostitute in Nineteenth-Century Medical Discourse*, Macmillan.

Stearns, Peter N. 2017. *Shame. A Brief History*, U of Illinois P.

Steller, Thomas. 2014. *Volksbildungsinstitut und Museumskonzern. Das Deutsche Hygiene-Museum 1912–1930*, Universitätsbibliothek Bielefeld.

Sturken, Marita, and Lisa Cartwright. 2009. *Practices of Looking. An Introduction to Visual Culture*, 2nd edition, Oxford UP.

Usborne, Cornelie. 1992. *The Politics of the Body in Weimar Germany. Women's Reproductive Rights and Duties*, Macmillan.

"Vereinsnachrichten." 1925. *Mitteilungen der Deutschen Gesellschaft zur Bekämpfung der Geschlechtskrankheiten*, vol. 23, 84–85.

Walther, Elfriede/Susanne Hahn and Albrecht Scholz. 1993. *Moulagen. Krankheitsbilder in Wachs*, Deutsches Hygiene-Museum Dresden.

Weindling, Paul. 1989. *Health, Race and German Politics between National Unification and Nazism, 1870–1945*, Cambridge UP.

Weinert, Sebastian. 2017. *Der Körper im Blick. Gesundheitsausstellungen vom späten Kaiserreich bis zum Nationalsozialismus*, de Gruyter.

Winkler, Martina. 2017. *Kindheitsgeschichte. Eine Einführung*, Vandenhoeck & Ruprecht.

Wildt, Michael. 2014. "Volksgemeinschaft." *Docupedia-Zeitgeschichte*, June 3, 2014. https://docupedia.de/zg/Volksgemeinschaft.

Caring or Curing?

Social Practice and Narration of Leprosy Work in Colonial East Africa

Richard Hölzl

In 1946, the American-born writer and foreign correspondent James Negley Farson, who was living in Cape Town at that time, published a review of a medical handbook in the Royal African Society's journal *African Affairs*. The handbook was authored by the South African doctor Michael Gelfand and bore the title *The Sick African*. Farson remarked that, for him as medical layman, the book's "real reward" was "that it will help to ease the sufferings, and save the lives, of an ever-increasing number of his fellow-men":

> I can see the White Fathers, up at Kabgaye in Ruanda-Urundi, studying it eagerly in the evenings, or a Tanganyika doctor referring to it, when he starts to diagnose the symptoms of a Native who looks as if he had malaria – or what? It is that kind of book; a hand-book, destined to lie upon the table *of doctors, nuns, priests, medical-missionaries, colonial administrators*; in fact, *every white man and woman working in Equatorial Africa, who has to treat the sick African*. And it is a book that would be of great value to the average Britisher, if only you could get the people at home to read it; it might *shock* them out of their dangerous indifference about the *obligations of the British Empire.* (Negley Farson 1946, 49; emphasis added)

Farson's remarks put a spotlight on the continued cultural and racial stereotyping of the colonial discourse on public health. Empire is cast as a two-body-problem: "white" men and women on the one hand and "the sick African" on the other, revolving around each other at a distance, but bound by the invisible forces of empire. Colonial public health is presented as an endeavor that assembled "white" experts of all kinds: scientific, religious, and political. In stark contrast, the alleged object of the joint effort remained in the collective singular, "the sick African." Of course, this "African" was a fellow-man, but very distant, almost as if "he" was living on another planet. Even if the medical handbook had originally intended to focus sick Africans as opposed to healthy ones: the journalist's eye did not miss the opportunity for a telling *pars pro toto*. He was quick to conflate "the sick" African individual with Africa as whole. Moreover, Farson wrote, the medical handbook of more than 800 pages in length had some lessons in store for the general British public at home, with the potential to "shock" them out of their "indifference" and remind them of the "obligations" of an Empire (Negley Farson 1946, 49–50). These are Farson's readings. Yet, the medical text yields itself easily to such spin-offs. Patients are always referred to in the colonial collective singular, being "the African," or "the native." The whole book appears as an exercise in cultural boundary work. It continuously employs a comparative gaze, holding a supposedly "white" or "European" experience of disease against an "African" one (Gelfand 1957).

Farson's brief review takes a wide gap in a bold stride. He bridges the divide of the cultural and the scientific with great ease. Farson distilled (or fabricated) a grand narrative from a voluminous medical handbook, projecting racial differentiation between "white" doctors and "native" patients, objectifying Africans as carriers of disease, conjuring up a diverse community of white experts to face health crises. According to Farson, the practical notes on diagnosis, therapy, or prevention addressed colonial practitioners on the ground. The grand narrative of colonial public health targeted at a much broader audience. It addressed the citizens of empire at home and abroad, thereby bridging another big gap, the one between the colonies and the metropole.

This chapter takes up some these implicit propositions. It examines non-fictional accounts of medical doctors, colonial officials, and missionaries in terms of their narration. Beyond and beneath the immediate descriptive and factual claims about colonial health, spatial connections and narrative plots become apparent, as well as the framing techniques with regard to events, actions, or agents. I focus on those textual moments, in which diseases become metaphors or even agents in a story, or in which patients as well as colonial medical practitioners are transformed into characters who play the roles of heroes, victims in distress, and antagonists, or, on the contrary, when crucial social agents transform into flat stock characters.

Factual texts claim to represent reality and truth. They are supposed to be adequate depictions of actual events, social formations, people's actions, or material effects (for example of diseases, microbes, unhealthy environments). Historians ought to take these claims seriously and need to go beyond examining them as pro forma. They will have to ask: what do these factual texts do to alter the social and material event that they claim merely to represent? How – by which means and to what effect – do they recreate and transform such events? To answer these questions a historiographical examination of narrativity will involve engaging with the social and material realities of the narrated events. Yet, these events can only be recreated as history through the analysis of factual representations (written, oral, graphical). Thus, contrasting social reality and its narrative transformation is rather less a clinical operation and more of a thought experiment.

The aim of this chapter is to show how colonial public health is narrativized. Why would this be important for our understanding of historical change? Here, I follow the thinking of Stuart Hall who proposes that modern societies experience social reality mainly encoded as mass media narratives (Hall 1984; 2006). In addition, social and narrative realities are mutually entangled. Social and material events are constantly processed (encoded and decoded, as Hall put it) into stories and received as such in society. These broadly distributed narratives provide the basis of very material decision-making in society, for instance about who is allocated funds, who has the right to move across borders, who is to be cured or cared for, and in which way.

The leprosy eradication campaign of the 1920s through the 1940s is a suitable historical case to study narration in the field of colonial public health (Worboys 2000). The colonial medical experts who engaged in the campaign believed that they had found an effective cure for this archetypical infectious disease: regular (intravenous, intramuscular, or subcutaneous) injections of an oily substance derived from the Indian chaulmoogra plant (*hydnocarpus wightianus*). The *British Empire Leprose Relief Association* (BELRA) campaigned among colonial administrations, the British public and existing anti-leprosy initiatives to take up the new curative treatment. BELRA put forward the idea of eradicating the disease through drug therapy, rather than containing it by isolating and providing care for the infected. Most of the existing initiatives were rooted in Christian missionary work. BELRA offered them funding to build infrastructure and treatment with chaulmoogra oil preparations. By the mid-1930s, it became increasingly doubtful whether the chaulmoogra oil injections were actually effective enough to end leprosy. As a consequence, the eradication campaigning petered out in the following decade. More effective multi-drug-therapies against the disease became available only in the 1960s and 1970s and were adopted by the World Health Organization (WHO) in 1981 (Riha 2004). Currently, the WHO registers leprosy as a *Neglected Tropical Disease* and has issued a global strategy to eradicate leprosy by 2030 (WHO 2017).

As a case study, this chapter concentrates on leprosy work in Southern Tanzania between the World Wars, and analyzes health reports assembled by BELRA medical experts, Catholic mission doctors, as well as missionary priests and nuns. The narratives in these texts are put into relation with the social realities within and around a Catholic mission's leprosy settlements including the active participation, negotiating, and resistance of African patients. It is through these relations that the social productivity of narration becomes tangible.

The argument of this chapter develops in four steps. The first is a brief reconstruction of leprosy work in Southern Tanganyika during the 1920s through the 1940s. The second addresses the grand narrative(s) of colonial public health in a spatial sense as exercises in *connecting* and *scaling*. This step, as well as the following, will afford comparing religious and secular variants of narrating colonial public health. This distinction is not always clear-cut: Marcel Dreier provides an instructive account on the difficulties of medical doctors attempting to fit into existing missions and their outlooks on conversions and care work in East Africa (Dreier 2015, 179–224; on medical missions, cf. Ratschiller 2023; Ratschiller/Weichlein 2016; Grundmann 2014; Hölzl 2011). Thirdly, I will discuss the impact of the *materiality of leprosy* on narration in an attempt to open the circle of possible authors and characters to include the *Mycobacterium leprae*. Fourthly, I focus on a particular group of agents within the network of leprosy work who shaped leprosy policies in local settings and were frequently the topic of reports but had hardly any access to the reporting process: African leprosy patients.

Negotiating Leprosy in Colonial Settings: A Mission's Leprosy Settlements

In the years before the First World War, the German colonial government in East Africa, as well as in other German colonies, initiated health inquiries and rudimentary treatment programs. The aim was to prevent the spreading of infectious diseases to Europeans in the colonies, to ensure the sufficient availability of a colonized workforce and to demonstrate the ability to govern colonial societies efficiently. Leprosy, however, rarely burdened Europeans, since infection happened only after close and long-term contact in poor and unhygienic living conditions. The colonial system made sure that such circumstances, in all likelihood, did not affect Europeans. Still, leprosy infection endangered the ready availability of the workforce, and German colonizers intended to compete with other colonial powers in every field of the colonial health sector. While leprosy was – unlike sleeping sickness, malaria, or syphilis – not a priority, the scope of the disease was regarded as a serious enough threat to German colonial objectives. German authorities briefly believed that the drug Nastin developed by Georg Deycke could possibly present a cure for leprosy and allowed tests in leprosy institutions in the colonies. They turned out to be disappointing (Eckart 1997, 319–340; on German colonial health policies cf. Bauche 2017; Ehlers 2019; Walther 2015).

Most governmental leprosy institutions in the German colony East Africa operated in the more populated coastal areas or near larger government posts. They also became testing grounds for new therapies (Eckert 1997, 336–340). After 1900, colonial authorities began to monitor the leprosy situation in their territories regularly. They found leprosy endemic in remoter places, where Christian missions were often the only colonial institutions. These missions readily established leprosy settlements as part of their efforts of evangelization. Thus, governments and missions became "public private partners" in yet another field of colonial rule (Eckart 1997, 329–336; Larson 2021, 10–14).

In Southern Tanzania, the Catholic Missionary Benedictines established several leprosy settlements after 1909 near their mission centers at Peramiho, Kwiro,

Madibira, and Ndanda. Leprosy work, in concert with other medical services, resulted in a long-term engagement of the Catholic Church in the health sector of the region. While Kwiro parish, for instance, still operates a local health center, the Catholic hospitals at Peramiho and Ndanda have become important parts of the area's medical infrastructure (Bruchhausen 2006, 353–357). In 1887, Benedictine monks and nuns entered coastal Tanzania and extended their reach to Southern Tanzania during the 1890s (Napachihi 1998). After the major colonial war of 1905–06, the so-called Maji Maji Rising, education and health policies became door openers for evangelization and state building (Hölzl 2016).

The mission's leprosy work added to the general trend of expanding colonial public health, but it also answered to the local conditions. Medical work had hardly been professional during the German colonial period. Priests and nuns with a few weeks of training as nurses, at best, were dispensing medicine, tending to wounds, and administering the last rites (Bruchhausen 2006, 299–314; for a biographical example, cf. Brockmeyer 2021, 104–112, 163–178; on the prevalence of social care rather than therapy, cf. Eckart 1997, 328). Leprosy became a starting point to establish a more lasting and professional medical infrastructure. From the 1920s, the missions at Ndanda and Peramiho also employed medical doctors, e.g., Sister Dr. Mary Thekla Stinnesbeck. She headed Ndanda Hospital, including the leprosy settlement, from 1927 to 1958, advanced new therapies, built up lab capacities, and made the institution a training site for African health workers (Stinnesbeck 1935; Hertlein 2017; Bruchhausen 2006; Dreier 2015; Iliffe 1998, 42).

The leprosy settlements in Southern Tanzania in the 1920s through the 1940s were quite large villages, housing several hundreds, sometimes more than a thousand patients, who dwelled in and around a treatment center and a church or prayer house.[1] Mobile patients would build their own small homes in the local style and tend to their own fields and gardens. Those who were unable to fend for themselves lived in huts near the center of the village (Anon. 1921, 60–65). Increasingly, during the 1930s and 1940s, the improvised structures gave way to larger residential, therapeutic, and liturgical brick buildings. BELRA, for instance, funded modern treatment buildings for the settlements at Peramiho and Ndanda; both places, in turn, became testing grounds for BELRA's chaulmoogra injections.[2]

1 For the description of the social life in these leprosy settlements I rely on my earlier study on the Morogoro settlement at Peramiho Mission (Songea), Larson's recent article on the Tabora settlement at Kwiro Mission (Mahenge), and Dreier's account on the same institution in the 1930s to 1970s (Larson 2021; Dreier 2015, 185–192, Hölzl 2015).

2 As Dreier reports for the Mahenge leprosy settlement (Tabora village), injection treatment was phased out in the late 1930s. With the end of curative treatment options, medical services as a whole seemed to have suffered and the situation of leprosy care was in steep decline. The mission reinvigorated leprosy work when new drugs became available in the 1950s; cf. Dreier 2015, 190–192.

Patients were not interned in these institutions, but were able to move independently and did so, sometimes moving back to or visiting their places of origin, sometimes choosing to live further away from the settlement's center. They were largely free to interact with their families if the symptoms allowed it. A large part of the patient population grew their own agricultural produce, ate their own food. They received regular medical treatment, education (with a bias towards religious subjects), and other benefits (garments, special food items, tools, medals, prayer objects). Treatment was voluntary but connected to the livelihood of patients who had settled on mission land. Conversion and adherence to the Catholic Church was expected and most benefits were tied to some form of openness to evangelization, if not medical therapy: for instance, significant gifts were handed out during the Christmas festivities (Weber 1923; Gilg 1932). Missionary sources do report conflicts with patients' families, as well as baptisms without the consent of families or patients themselves (Morrissey 1936). However, coercion seems not to have been the rule. Non-leprous patients and their families resisted involuntary baptisms in the hour of death, for instance, by removing patients who were about to die from the hospital grounds. This left Ndanda hospital with a very low mortality rate, as the resident doctor remarked (Stinnesbeck 1933, 178).

When the mission introduced regular treatment with chaulmoogra oil in the late 1920s, African health workers administered the weekly injections under the supervision of European nurses and doctors (Stinnesbeck 1936). These relied on African agents for practical treatment, heavy labor, language translation and socio-cultural expertise. Gradually, the education and expertise of African personnel changed. In the early decades of mission work, African intermediaries primarily relied on their language and cultural skills. During the 1930's, health workers were becoming professionals who had received several years of specialized training and completed government examinations (Groß 1937, 33–35; Bruchhausen 2006).

Both European and African personnel had to rely on patients' cooperation. As Megan Vaughan put it: "Even the most ardent medical missionaries, who had at times tried to make leprosy sufferers into blank pages, in which to inscribe their ideas about new African identities, had generally found themselves reinventing village life and African 'traditional' structures of control in their leper colonies" (Vaughan 1991, 88). This concerned the immediate treatment by at times painful injections and regular appearances at the treatment center, but also the social order of the quite large settlements, the upkeep of buildings and infrastructure, and the subsistence of most of the inhabitants of the settlements. Force could hardly have achieved this level of cooperation. The German medical officer Richard Wolf had attempted the internment of over 400 leprosy patients in a camp in Southeast Tanzania (Kionga) in 1910, threatening punishment if the inmates did not contribute to their sustenance by providing agricultural labor. The patients resisted, demanded assistance, and walked out of the camp after a few weeks (Eckart 1997, 325).

Similarly, missionaries needed cooperation in the field of evangelization. They would visit the village regularly for mass, prayer, or baptism. African mission teachers, however, were the backbone of the evangelical work, giving daily instructions, fending off other evangelists, and watching over the continuous observance of the creed (Hölzl 2016). Yet the mission's medical and educational staff did not live in the settlements. Hence patients largely organized social life themselves, under the supervision of a government appointed chief (Sr. Konstantia 1929, 199–200). Missionaries and doctors, however, controlled goods, which gave them power to ensure compliance: some were economic (nutrition, tools, paid jobs), some religious (the Christian rituals and the "goods of salvation," to quote Max Weber), some medical (access to treatment) (Weber 1986, 247–248).

To sum up: the life in the leprosy settlements was structured by a variety of interactions of cultures, material interests, and social groups. Patients had various social roles, as members of families, as participants in local economies, as practitioners of religious creeds and cultural traditions and as subjects of colonial administrative rule. Doctors, nurses and missionaries had to adapt therapies and policies to these interactions and could only do so because they were relying on a number of African intermediaries such as nurses and teachers. The following paragraphs examine how these social realities turned into narratives.

Local Stories and Grand Narratives: Connecting and Scaling

Advocates of colonial anti-leprosy work proposed "to rid the empire of leprosy" (Anonymous 1928, Cover). This was the motto of a prominent medical advocacy group, the British Empire Leprosy Relief Association (BELRA). It constitutes a kind of narration *in nuce* because it plots medical interventions along a grand utopian trajectory. Local and particular narratives link up with such longer, more elaborate narratives about colonial leprosy work.

From a spatial point of view, narrating leprosy was as an exercise in *scaling* and *connecting*. BELRA's journal *Leprosy Notes* (later: *Leprosy Review*) provides ample evidence of this. The mission statement of BELRA, for instance, connected local medical efforts and individual casework with the grand medical trajectory of this organization and its vision of empire:

> The British Empire Leprosy Relief Association … has as its object the *ridding of the Empire of leprosy*. The Committee of the Association believes that if this object is to be achieved it needs the *co-operation of Government in India and the Colonies and Protectorates, the Missionary bodies carrying on work in those territories, the commercial community and the natives of the various countries*. In order to secure such co-operation the Association, which is a voluntary body, has done all that is possible to se-

> cure the formation of branches of the Association in each part of the Empire where lepers are to be found. Each branch of the Association is responsible for the work in its own area, but the Association seeks to aid in every way possible. (Anonymous 1928a, 2; emphasis added)

This short paragraph establishes at least three important connections: of the metropole and its various peripheries (1), of local colonial agents and the umbrella organization (2), of government, civil organizations and colonized populations (3). Imperial society is portrayed as a tightly woven network of agents of various "classes," respective social groupings which work together in harmony for the greater good. In this greater framework, leprosy and the fight to "eradicate the disease altogether" (Anonymous 1928a, 2) acquired a metaphorical quality. If BELRA had not gotten rid of leprosy yet, it had at least put together a vision of imperial society, in which anything was possible if cooperation at all levels and between all classes was assured.

In 1940, the medical secretary of BELRA and widely acknowledged leprosy expert Ernest Muir published a sweeping survey on *The Leprosy Problem in Africa*. Muir had toured the British colonies in West and East Africa to assess the state of leprosy treatment and facilities on invitation by the British Colonial Office. In his survey, he presented the Uzuakoli Settlement in Nigeria as a specific and localized model institution. The site was run by the Church Missionary Society and received grants by BELRA:

> The Uzuakoli Settlement is thus much more than a well-organized center for segregation and treatment of lepers. It is rather the hub of a wheel which is gradually radiating in the village life of the people. It is a center of training of leprosy patients, who are found to be the most enthusiastic and efficient apostles of anti-leprosy methods. Its sanitary village planning is gradually "taking on" with the people. What astonishes one most is the modest cost at which all this is managed, though doubtless with more resources it could be more rapidly extended and more effectively done. To return to the two different points of view regarding the control of leprosy referred to above, we find in the Uzuakoli and similar institutions that instead of waiting till sanitation and other general improvements bring about the disappearance of leprosy, the disease itself is used as a key with which to open the door to general educational, sanitary and agricultural reform, this being done with the aid of voluntary societies at a minimum of expense to Government. In any case it may be said that the solution of the leprosy problem will be closely bound up with the future progress of Africa. (Muir 1940, 142)

The leprosy settlement becomes quite effectively a metaphor for empire: A "centre ... gradually radiating" to its peripheries, "well-organized", "sanitary" with "most enthusiastic" subjects who become the best advocates of good governance, and all this at a surprisingly "modest cost." To "rid" an "empire" of a widespread infectious disease equals making whole the empire itself.

Denominational missions would not subscribe to this secular and political narrative in the same way or degree. As Megan Vaughan wrote about English protestant missions: "Each sick person was a potential convert, each had a 'soul' as well as a body to be attended to … Healing, for medical missionaries was part of a programme of social and moral engineering through which 'Africa' could be saved." In this respect, "the mission hospital" was a place where the "individual patient was 'created'" (Vaughan 1991, 74). There are some structural similarities with regard to narrative *scaling* and *connecting*: much as in BELRA's narrative, leprosy work for missions was a means to an end. This end was imperial in a transcendental sense: it was supposed to do two things – (1) to open up a site for practicing faith and sacrifice to Christians in Europe (as donors) as well as in the mission field (as medical and care workers), and (2) to function as a door-opener for the evangelization. Leprosy work, again, connected the European metropole with the colonial mission fields, the Church's old constituencies with new ones and worldly efforts with divine redemption. It connected the local, daily struggle for converts with the global Church and God's empire.

A concise rendering of the local, global, and transcendental framing of leprosy work can be found, for instance, in a travel account by Norbert Weber published under the title *Children of Sorrow* around 1923 (Weber 1923, cf. Larson 2021). The Benedictine Arch Abbot was based in Germany but had travelled the mission fields in Africa and Asia. Weber described a "walk" through three of the leprosy settlements operated by the Benedictines in East Africa (at Peramiho, Madibira, and Kwiro). Several chapters are devoted to portraying social life in the settlements, judging the moral character of the patients (their contentment and gratitude), as well as praising the nurses' sacrifice. Frequently, Weber's account also featured direct interactions and conversations with patients. Further chapters narrate critical moments in the religious life of the village, the celebration of Christmas (when grateful patients receive gracious gifts sponsored by European Christians) as well as a baptism ceremony. The finale of the pamphlet recounts, in the style of a sermon, Jesus Christ's encounter with the ten lepers (whom he healed and of whom only one returned to express his gratitude). Weber reminded his European readers of Europe's own history of leprosy and ended with an appeal to repay God's grace by donating to African lepers: "We so favoured by His love and benefits could find no better form of expressing our gratitude than by sharing with others less fortunate the benefits we have received in such an abundance." Weber pointed out that donations and assistance to missionary endeavors were not merely altruistic gestures: the transaction of goods only seemingly went directly from the European donors to the African lepers, but "the work of saving the souls of others is in reality the surest guaranty for our own predestination" (Weber 1923, 49).

Melania Vollmer, a leading figure of the Missionary Benedictines Sisters, published a short travel account in 1925. Travelling across Southern Tanzania, Vollmer perceived a huge demand for medical care. In particular, she noted the competition of Anglican missionaries, who had been offering professional medical treatment at several stations in the area since the turn of the 20th century (Bruchhausen 2006, 296–298). To retain the Catholic influence, Vollmer urged more emphasis on the material welfare of the people: "mission doctors – men and women – willing to give sacrifice" were in urgent demand. "From the very beginning the expansion of Christianity rested on acts of compassion" (Vollmer 1925, 121). The true aim of missionary medical work was not merely pioneering medical discoveries or curing the sick, but to provide the foundation for evangelization. The competitive tone was characteristic and added to the imperialist character of the mission's leprosy narrative.

A third aspect of the leprosy work and other medical efforts of missions emerges in a travel account by Thomas Ohm. Ohm was a professor of religious studies and member of the Missionary Benedictine congregation. He visited East Africa in the 1930s. The account I am referring to here focuses, however, on a journey to South Africa. Ohm underlined that missionary medicine was primarily a service to God and a door opener for mission work. Yet, more importantly the mission's new capacities of professional Western medicine could effectively "destroy the basis and the core of heathendom as well as its strongholds," because Western medicine was "destroying traditional, heathen concepts of disease and … healing." Consequently, it undermined traditional society ("heathendom"). Ohm stated that it was possible to "annihilate the bulwark" and "stronghold" of traditional societies, the "witch doctors" (Ohm 1934, 14–17). In this martial narrative as in other medical missionary writings (Vaughan 1991, ch. 3; Hölzl 2011; Bruchhausen 2006, 317), local ritual and healing experts transformed into the prime antagonists in the fundamental and existential struggle of expanding God's empire.

These three missionary travel accounts highlight how worldly and religious characteristics intersected in missionary narratives of colonial public health: the service primarily rendered to God and the instrumental character of health initiatives in relation to evangelism, often not only directed towards conversion, but in a belligerent tone against European and African competitors in the field.

"Superstition" was also a frequent trope in the narratives on leprosy work in Africa disseminated by BELRA, not least because missionaries published in the association's journal and propagated the infamous figure of the "witch doctor" (Murray 1931; Wallace 1932; Robertson 1932; Langauer 1940). BELRA's leprosy experts identified similar obstacles from a medical perspective. For instance, Ernest Muir:

> How does the native African regard leprosy? He has, of course, *superstitious ideas* connected with the breaking of taboos. … Leprosy is supposed to be the result of

> vengeance of the gods for something done to provoke them, either by the victim himself or by his ancestors. (Muir 1940, 137; emphasis added)

The figure of the ignorant and superstitious "native African" was hardly a strong antagonist to the cause of eradicating leprosy. The colonized were sketched as immature, yet intelligent and ready to develop sounder and healthier ideas on leprosy and diseases more broadly:

> There is a very definite responsibility on the shoulders of the British public, which they cannot shift on to the back of Government. We who claim to be a democratic nation have deliberately taken over or adopted a number of countries peopled by backward races. Anyone who adopts a child holds himself responsible for its education and well-being, and above all for its health. We are proud of these colonies and few would be willing to give them up. Surely then it is our duty to see that everything possible is done to free them from the living death of leprosy and the ignorance, superstition and insanitary conditions which breed leprosy. (Anonymous 1938, 53)

Muir concluded: "In controlling leprosy it is therefore necessary to study the ideas of the natives, and after sympathetically separating out useful knowledge and customs from harmful and useless superstition, to help them to put their correct ideas into practice" (Muir 1940, 138–139).

Creating Leprosy Plots: Conversion and Self-Transformation

Texts about leprosy in the colonial public health context frequently employed *conversion* to structure narrative plots. The comparative perspective on religious and secular contexts highlights several characteristics: for one, conversion was hardly an exclusively religious concept, but was also present in secular texts – as a "conversion to modernity," modernity understood here as a colonial category (van der Veer 1995; Cooper 2004). Secondly, conversion of "others" involved transformation of one's own self; much like missionaries only completely fulfilled their role when they achieved conversion, medical experts truly became worthy imperial agents when they achieved cure of bodies and minds of patients. Thirdly, these conversions of the colonized and self-transformations of the colonizing individuals metaphorically linked up with the secular and religious empires as grander collective subjects.

In the Benedictine mission care work for lepers was relegated to nuns and male African medical workers for theological reasons. Male priests were – in theory – to concentrate exclusively on the primary aim of evangelism. Close encounters with the physical body supposedly presented a worldly distraction. As Lorne Larson underlines for the period before 1914, leprosy work provided Benedictine nuns with an attractive field of agency beyond the ancillary position of organizing the kitchens, washhouses and farmsteads of the larger mission stations. This significant transformation and expansion of professional activities of female Catholic missionaries continued in the 1920 to 1940s. Although baptisms were the prerogative of male priests, nuns exercised this key rite frequently on patients, claiming emergencies. Already in 1910, the mission's leader, Bishop Thomas Spreiter, warned missionaries and explicitly lay brothers and sisters of turning the mission's health institutions into "factories for baptisms."[3]

In the narratives presented to their home audiences in Germany, nuns developed this transformation of their role and pushed gender boundaries. They transgressed the narrow paths laid out for women in mission theology and canon law: they reported not only conversions of patients, but also repeatedly the baptisms that they had themselves performed. A nun's first baptism resembled a rite of initiation not only for the baptized but for herself. A great number of baptisms were considered as a stroke of luck. The mission journal of the Missionary Benedictine nuns, for instance, featured following characterization of Sister Cosma in 1936: bringing the "poor lepers to god ... and even baptizing them herself" was her "special joy." She had been "lucky very often", the journal stated: nine people had died at the leper settlement at Peramiho that year, "eight of which were baptized in their hour of death" (Anonymous 1936, 11–12).

The same journal published a travel account – another "walk" to a "leper settlement" – by Sister Bilhild Groß who was a newcomer at Peramiho mission station. The other sisters had done her the favor of sending her to the leprosy settlement to tend to a mother with a newborn and several other children. The woman was infected with leprosy and apparently very sick. Sister Bilhild Groß rejoiced. According to her account, overpowering religious emotions accompanied her journey:

> [The women] sat at the fire with her youngest child, a three-month-old boy. How her eyes shone in her completely disfigured and consumed face, when I told her, that I came to baptize her. After the necessary questioning I exercised the great, eternal act that opens the gates of heaven. I gave the baptized the name Theresia, Josepha, Emma. *I felt very peculiar, almost not of this world.* We prayed together, the new Christian received a little picture and a medal. Eight days after, the women died. *I was really lucky. Some sisters are here for years without having the chance to baptize.* O dear black Theresia, Josepha, Emma pray for me at God's throne. May he give his blessing to my mission work among your fellow countrymen and women! (Groß, 1930, 224; emphasis added)

3 Circular Letter, Bishop Spreiter, 15 Jan 1910, Archive St. Ottilien, Z. 1. 01.

The nun put forward a powerful narrative about Catholic women's claim to colonial agency. The baptized Theresia – her original name now erased by ritual and narrative – is presented as a willing object to the sister's powerful acts. The name Theresia is no coincidence here. It likely refers to Saint Thérèse of Lisieux, a nun who died in young years of tuberculosis 1897. Her autobiography *The Story of a Soul* was published shortly after her death and became a bestseller all over Catholic Europe. Thérèse of Lisieux (known in English as "little flower of Jesus") constituted a role model for Catholic nuns in the early 20th century, especially after she was elevated to sainthood in 1923. Thérèse expressed the wish to become a missionary and a soldier to expand God's empire. She lamented that as a woman she could not and had to resort to the so-called little ways of faith (Thérèse 1996).

Once women missionaries acquired medical degrees, they were able to expand their roles further, wielding expert authority in the missions' increasingly important health sector. Often this involved setting themselves off against indigenous women by combining religious and secular tropes of Christian and Western superiority. Anna Dengel (1892–1980), who practiced as a mission doctor in Rawalpindi (Punjab), published an appeal to female German doctors and medical students to join the missionary cause in 1925. Dengel was one of the first female German Catholic mission doctors. In her account, she characterized Hindu women as good mothers, who wished to acquire the best health care for their children. At the same time, Dengel portrays them as ignorant, filthy, superstitious, and "like children." Muslim women appear as members of a wealthy upper class, rich but confined to their home without "nurture for body and brain" (Dengel 1925, 20). European missionary women, much to the contrary, are presented as faithful, hard-working, physically agile, and fearless professionals:

> In a country were climate, lack of hygiene, epidemics, ignorance, superstition, flies and filth all come together, there is a lot misery to ease. Where two million children under the age of two die annually, there is ample opportunity to baptize. … A new beautiful, blessed, but hard profession is now open to girls: To set out to hot or cold uncivilized or barely civilized, dangerous or less dangerous countries as mission doctors, nurses, or apothecaries, in order to contribute to the propagation of faith and do good according to talent and grace. (Dengel 1925, 20)

Religious motivations are in the foreground of Dengel's narrative. Yet, the undercurrent of a medical civilizing mission, which enabled European Catholic women to transcend conventional gender roles, is clearly distinguishable.

The prominent role of female medical doctors in missions is somewhat exceptional in the colonial health care sector. The medical experts of BELRA were men and they conceptualized colonial medicine primarily as a white, masculine sphere. When the organization's medical adviser, Ernest Muir, arrived at the Benedictine leprosy settlement at Peramiho in 1938, he perceived a site that "has grown to proportions which are far beyond the control of the present staff." He wrote: "I consider that the Sister-in-Charge and the African Superintendent are both exceptionally devoted and able workers. ... but to conduct this Settlement with full efficiency there should be *a fulltime medical man*" (Muir 1939, 67–8, emphasis added). This imperial masculinity was not only acquired by racial identification, birth or education. It demanded full engagement for the medical civilizing mission. Ridding the empire of leprosy meant saving the empire from dysfunctionality. Curing leprosy and having the colonized population voluntarily subscribe to treatment signified not only the colonized populations' acceptance of colonial rule but their willingness cooperation. This made the empire whole, analogous to the human organism.

The positioning of the "medical man" in relation to other roles (European women, African health workers, patients) in the *mise-en-scène* of colonial leprosy becomes apparent in another one of Muir's accounts. As mentioned, the Uzuakoli settlement (Nigeria) served Muir as a kind of model institution, or lab in Helen Tilley's metaphorical use (Tilley 2011), for a well-functioning empire:

> The *doctor in charge* is a Methodist missionary; a second doctor is being sent out by the Leprosy Association, and the Association also supplies two layworkers. The doctor's wife and another honorary lady assistant help with the women and children, and there are four nonleper African workers. The rest of the work is done by the patients themselves. There are eleven hundred patients housed in neat rows of sanitary huts, arranged in villages within the settlement. The site is healthy and suitable for agriculture. *From the doctor's bungalow one gets a fine view over miles of undulating woodland country.* The hospital, treatment centre and other administrative buildings and the European staff quarters are of a permanent type, and have been erected chiefly with the labour of patients. The treatment arrangements are excellent, including occupation therapy in all its forms and communal physical exercises. (Muir 1940, 140; emphasis added)

The "doctor in charge" is not only in the center of the narrative's *dramatis personae*, but also put in an extraordinary geographical position. The elevated location of the doctor's residence, which allows for a mile-wide view of the country below, reminds of Marie Louise Pratt's ingenious observation of the "promontory scene" in colonial travel narratives. Such a viewpoint renders the observer the "monarch of all I survey" (Pratt 1995, 197, 217). Of course, the quote also steers us to Foucault's prison wardens and their panoptical gaze (Foucault 1977). Although the perspective of choice of the leprosy expert should perhaps be a microscopic one, Muir emphasizes the big picture, the macroscopic view on the colonial landscape. The protagonist is more like a general on a battle hill than a scientist behind a desk, examining samples under a microscope.

In this narrative, patients are cured physically and become socially productive members of the institution, while the medical expert is transformed into a civilizing missionary and key agent of empire. On the structural level, this is remarkably similar to the conversion narrative of missionaries that render patients faithful members of the Christian community, while transforming themselves into true agents of God's empire.

Narration and Materialities

Asking how leprosy narratives were assembled and what they did, a further actor (or agent) comes into play: the disease in its material aspects and the ways by which it communicates or reacts to treatment, its symptoms and trajectories (on why materiality matters: Latour 1999 and 2004). If communication is perceived as comparatively slow and affecting a specific portion of society, as was the case with leprosy in the colonial context of the 1920s and 1930s, a disease may more readily be categorized as a disease of *others* (Muir 1938, 12–14).[4] This, in turn, enables close inspection and care. The disease becomes connected to a different set of emotions, i.e., compassion rather than fear. Paradoxically, the very "otherness" of leprosy, as a disease of the colonized poor, explains the illusion of intimacy and tilted emotional relation that the above-cited missionary narratives transported to European publics. In this respect, leprosy resembled, for instance, hookworm disease or yaws. However, these were less relatable to the biblical and European historical traditions. Leprosy differed from highly infectious diseases which were communicated over a greater distance (e.g., via insect vectors) and thus were not confined to a particular social stratum. The "colonial other" infected with malaria or sleeping sickness was conceived of and narrated less as a patient to be cured or even commiserated, but as a dangerous carrier of a disease, a threat to be controlled, separated, and confined.[5]

How material ways of communication have affected narratives becomes obvious when looking at sexually transmitted diseases such as syphilis. During the long 19th century patients were often branded as immoral, as adulterers or prostitutes. The disease served as a signifier of sin. Around the time of the First World War, secular doctors and public health administrations in Europe tried to change this

4 Conversely, African societies were accused of cruelty and superstition, because they feared and ostracized members infected with leprosy (cf. Dow 1945, 57–63).

5 See the variety of contributions in Bashford and Hooker 2014. It was, of course, possible that general considerations of racial segregation and "purity" in a settler society led to very different interpretations, e.g., in 19th century Australia. The Australian government introduced racialized policies of "isolation, separation, and containment" against leprosy patients, much in line with general health policies (Bashford/Nugent 2014).

narrative. Moralizing the disease seemed to block efficient prevention and treatment, as the infected tended to hide the disease out of shame and fear of stigmatization (Sauerteig 2001; Morick 2026). Christian activists, however, often adhered to the older narrative much longer (Ratschiller 2023; Hölzl 2024). Leprosy, in comparison, was recounted as a disease of social outsiders, but generally did not come with the same degree of moral deviation and subsequent ostracization. Megan Vaughan, however, points to cases of patients suffering from both diseases, and moral connections that were drawn between them (Vaughan 1991, 82).

The relations of material contexts and narratives are also historically volatile: if, for instance, curative treatment is believed to become available, the narrative of a disease changes. Curability alters roles, hierarchies of characters and plots. Stories of compassion, of self-sacrificing care, or of moral outrage may then turn into martial narratives of heroic conquest and eradication campaigns. The figure of the self-sacrificing female care worker gives way to the pioneering male medical expert. For instance, Victor G. Heiser, one-time director of a leprosy isolation colony on the Philippines (Culion Colony on Cebu), as well as health director of the US colonial administration of the country, and then a director of the International Board of Health (Rockefeller Foundation):

> The real gains have been due […] to the disinterested cooperation of physicians and sanitarians who have shared knowledge and experience, and helped governments and institutions to organize systematic measures of isolation and treatment. Their aim has been not merely to relieve the afflicted but to protect whole populations. These *modern crusaders* will not be content until leprosy has been banished from the world. (Heiser 1925, 688; emphasis added)

Changing the narrative on leprosy, however, was a gradual, non-linear, and not necessarily teleological process. The leprosy campaign of the 1920s and 1930s and its narratives are exemplary of this volatility. The perceived efficacy of the chaulmoogra oil injections initiated and motivated campaigning for leprosy eradication. The disease featured as a simple and conquerable entity in this campaign. Although the pathogen (*Mycobacterium leprae*) was known at the time und used for diagnosis, it hardly appeared in the narratives. Leprosy's long history served to highlight the spectacular novelty of 20th century pharmaceutical cures. While the use of substances derived from the chaulmoogra plant was old and historically located in Indian medicine, medical experts (such as Heiser, Rogers or Muir) from various countries introduced new methods of extraction and marketability (as powder, concreted liquid) as well as various injection techniques. They attempted to improve the viscosity as well as tolerability of the medication and to reduce the cost of production and shipment (Rogers 1934).

In answer to this, Leonard Rogers, a prominent physician and colonial medical expert, explicitly called for a paradigmatic shift regarding leprosy – from caring to curing:

> The organisation of the great humanitarian work of *caring* for the leper, which is so largely in the hands of Christian missions of various denominations, requires to be remodelled in the light of the new situation, for it is evident that a far greater service is rendered by *curing* the leper in the early stages of the disease, than in providing a home for him after the affection has reduced him to a helpless wreck. (Rogers, as cited in: Anonymous 1928a, 3)

Rogers and BELRA counted on chaulmoogra oil, which, they claimed, to have developed into a medication that was efficient, cost-effective, and tolerable for patients. The organization not only distributed the medication and offered advice on treatment. It also distributed the seeds of the Indian chaulmoogra tree to be planted near leprosy hotspots (Rodgers 1928, 6–9).

Yet, by the early 1930s doubt was mounting about the success of the chaulmoogra treatment and the curability of leprosy. With increasing diffusion of the therapy and the substance, more and more negative reports circulated among leprosy experts: They exposed low curing rates and many relapses after treatment had ended, as well as adverse physical reactions to treatment. In 1935, the *Leprosy Review* decided to publish an article by José Rodriguez, a very experienced doctor who headed a children's clinic on the Philippines and whose studies casted further doubt on the "curability" of leprosy. They suggested that not even in early cases and in children was the chaulmoogra treatment very effective. Rodriguez noted that after nine years of treatment, "we are no longer so sure that the chaulmoogra treatment is effective in this very early stage" (Rodriguez 1934, 102).

This met with an emotional response from the BELRA medical community. The journal editors did not deny the findings, but expressed confusion, sadness, even grief, and they signaled hope. Rodriguez positions were "startling" and cause for experts to think "furiously." The editors conceded that the initial expectations for the treatment were very much "diminished." Even though chaulmoogra was the only available drug, it was effective only in a very small group of patients. The editorial ended with a plea that is striking due to the density of emotive and psychopathological references:

> Let us continue the search for better remedies but let us not forget that our most efficient remedies still are the derivatives of hydnocarpus oil, and that these cannot be *put into the limbo* of forgotten things. We would strike this note of *hopefulness* that while our ideas concerning specific treatment *are apparently in the melting pot*, we have never been more *convinced* of the value of leprosy work and the pos-

> sibility of the control of this scourge than we are to-day. We must *keep our vision clear*, not letting our *enthusiasm* for treatment *blur our view* of prevention, or be so *obsessed* by apparently unfavourable reports that we *lose our faith* in the efficacy of all treatment. We plead for a *sane* outlook so that our view of the problem may be complete, and no part of the picture be out of focus because one aspect of the problem is stressed at the expense of another. (Anonymous 1934, 100–101; emphasis added)

This statement is indicative, because it appeals to readers not only as an expert group, but as an *emotional community* bound by the heroic narrative of colonial leprosy eradication (Rosenwein 2010). Critically, this heroic narrative hinged on the curative efficacy of the medical treatment.

In the process, the disease itself acquired a different quality in the eyes of the BELRA experts. Its medical secretary, Robert Cochrane, stated: "One must confess that we have a long way to go in our search for better remedies for the disease. It may be that leprosy does not lend itself to specific treatment and that our greatest advance will be along epidemiological and preventive lines" (Cochrane 1934, 139). In short: back to square one. The *Leprosy Review* editorial speculated about physical dispositions to contract leprosy or not, and whether "the life of the Mycobacterium leprae" ought to be conceived of more like a parasite: "We have felt for some time that the M. leprae in many of its aspects can be looked upon as a cellular parasite, and if this is the case then, as with other parasitic diseases, a symbiosis tends to be set up between the parasite and its host. It is well known that specific therapeutic remedies, in the case of parasitic diseases, are apt to fail" (Anon. 1934, 100).

Unexpectedly resisting treatment, the pathogen acquired a much more central place in the narrative of leprosy. Having previously almost disappeared under the general entity of leprosy, it now became a very particular agent whose character and life story warranted much closer attention. Scientists thus stepped up efforts to isolate the Mycobacterium leprae and reproduce it in vitro under lab conditions (Muir 1938, 105–109).

Missionary health policies never fully embraced the curative narrative and retained a broad focus on care, compassion and evangelism. Missionary doctors navigated between various strands of narrating leprosy, alternately stressing the curative and caritative aspects of their work. A case in point is the Thekla Stinnesbeck, a Benedictine nun with a medical degree who headed a mission hospital. A whole set of articles on her work are available to study – published in *Leprosy Review*, the German medical missionary journal *Katholische Missionsärztliche Fürsorge* and in illustrated mission journals, including the Benedictine women's journal *Missionsecho*. Stinnesbeck's reports for *Leprosy Review* were more matter-of-fact with less emotional emphasis on the curative aspects of leprosy work than most texts of the journal: they reduced leprosy work to statistical results of treatment and infection in the area, accounts of building and therapeutic activities, and to ethnographic descriptions of traditional approaches to leprosy among the societies of the region. Stinnesbeck's portrayal of indigenous attitudes on leprosy are to degree more expressive and indirectly stress an alleged superiority of European biomedicine. Local African societies and patients are described as "cruel," "afraid," and lacking "confidence in European treatment." According to Stinnesbeck, indigenous societies in the area regarded leprosy as "infectious and incurable disease," reacted with separation of varying degrees of severity, and were unable to detect early cases. Yet, they had herbal medicine that could stall the development of disease for some time (Stinnesbeck 1936, 1936a).

In comparison, Stinnesbeck's articles for mission journals were quite different. These also contained statistics of treatments and expenses, accounts of medical procedures and descriptions of the built environment of the settlement. Yet this information was framed by an emotionally dense appeal to the readership. It presented leprosy patients as worthy and in need of assistance as well as compassion. Between 1933 and 1936 Stinnesbeck published the very same text in three different mission journals. The publications – all involving the "walk to the lepers" – differed in their aspects: the *Leprosy Review* had featured several photographs, one of Stinnesbeck performing an operation on a gangrenous foot, one of an African nurse (possibly Vincent, the mission's leprosy worker) dressing a wound (Stinnesbeck 1936). The article in *Katholische Missionsärztliche Fürsorge* came without any illustrations (Stinnesbeck 1934). The journal of the Benedictine Fathers of St. Ottilien (*Missionsblätter*) featured an orderly photograph showing Dr. Stinnesbeck teaching four rows of male African student nurses in a small lecture theater (Stinnesbeck 1933). The journal of the Benedictine Sisters (*Missionsecho*) had two photographs depicting Stinnesbeck in a caring role: one surrounded by an Indian patient's family on the doorsteps of Ndanda hospital and the other among joyfully dancing female leprosy patients at the settlement (Stinnesbeck 1934a). The curative aspects of leprosy work had become part of the missionary narratives. Yet they were never as central to the narrative as they were in a more secular colonial health context, where the practical failure to cure had significant impact on narration.

Framing Patients' Agency

Leprosy patients not only navigated the conditions of colonial health policies but also shaped them to a considerable extent. As laid out above, leprosy settlements in Southern Tanganyika between the World Wars were large, open, and underfunded institutions. Many of the patients led rather self-sufficient lives, but received some assistance, care, medical treatment and evangelical education from teachers, nuns, health workers, and doctors. While these had some powerful assets to bring to table, the whole idea of evangelical leprosy work relied on the cooperation of patients, who in the end had to attend regular treatment and education for years. Of course, agency depended on the severity of the symptoms a patient experienced. Abandoning the settlements was less of an option for patients with more severe symptoms that ostracized them from communities and immobilized them.

Coercive models of leprosy work were difficult to uphold. Largely failing German attempts at internment in Southern Tanzania during 1910s are mentioned above. The American colonial health administration on the Philippines (Anderson 2006) centralized internment at Culion leper colony (est. 1906 on Cebu) under the administration of the US occupational government and health experts of the Rockefeller Foundation. BELRA perceived it to be a failure brought on by the resistance of the involuntarily interned patients and the refusal of the population to hand over the infected to the government for distant internment. BELRA took the inability of the full force of the US colonial military administration and medical expertise to force treatment on people as a hint and put forward alternative approaches, which were also considerably less costly (Muir 1938; Rogers 1929; Anonymous 1928a). Suggesting outpatient clinics and open leprosy settlements, where patients could organize their economic and social life themselves, BELRA was actually selling the status quo in the mission institutions as an innovative anti-leprosy strategy. Ingeniously, even the subsistence farming of the infected inhabitants of the leprosy villages was remodeled as "occupation therapy" of special "therapeutic and economic value" (Rogers 1929a; cf. Wilson 1930 and Kerr 1938).

As mentioned above, injecting patients with plant-based substances every week for years in open facilities depended on high levels of cooperation. Patients' reaction to treatment forced pharmaceutical researchers to look beyond the therapeutic impact of drugs on the disease and cost-effectiveness. Side effects (the "leprosy reaction") had to be minimized and the level of pain caused by injections reduced (Rogers 1934). This also spurred the professionalization of African health workers, who were responsible for administering the hardly trivial procedure.

The realization that drug therapy promised only moderate success in the immediate future plus the fact that patients in many colonial contexts would not be forcibly concentrated and isolated also pushed preventive concepts such as decentralized "propaganda work" directed at the colonial villages, households and families (Lowe 1934, 40–44). BELRA advocated an integrated approach here under the headline of "Propaganda Treatment Survey Centres." In villages, and in cooperation with local authorities, surveys, information events, and treatment in small clinics (dispensaries) were to go hand in hand:

> First of all, the information available from the decennial census returns is collected. This information, though not accurate, as it has been collected by enumerators who have no special knowledge of leprosy, is useful as a starting-off

> ground. Villages are visited, and with the aid of the Union Presidents and Village Watchmen known cases of leprosy are looked up and members of their families are examined for early signs of leprosy. By conversation, demonstration of charts and lantern lectures, the villagers are taught about leprosy--how it is contracted, how it may be prevented and how remedied. An out-patient clinic is opened at the headquarters of the thana [local administrative unit] and patients are treated there once or twice a week, while on the remaining days of the week other villages are visited. Alongside of treatment and propaganda the survey proceeds. With the help of grateful and willing patients more and more cases of leprosy are found.... In this way much useful information is collected which again is used in propaganda work. The sufferers from leprosy are generally found to be' eager for treatment. Within three or four weeks of starting such a centre as many as two or three hundred patients have been found to attend for treatment. Villagers are taught to isolate infectious cases in huts outside the village, and to discern the earliest signs of disease and bring their patients in the first stage in which leprosy is so remediable. (Muir 1928, 5)

This text is quoted here at some length because it demonstrates how experts folded patients' considerable agency back into the powerful narrative of colonial public health: by employing refined social engineering and propaganda techniques patients would be happily convinced of the superiority of the colonial biomedical approach to disease.

Extensive propaganda work in tune with local socio-cultural settings was the key to missionary success. For evangelization, just as for medical treatment, missionaries needed a high level of cooperation among the local population since missions expected adherence to Church law and a restrictive set of moral prerequisites. For their evangelical work the Benedictines in East Africa relied heavily on the cultural expertise of African mission workers (catechists, teachers, nurses). These translated and negotiated Christian faith in a wider cultural sense for the various societies in the region. This included education and health policies, which were increasingly bundled up with evangelism during the 20th century. Even if missionaries emphasized the instrumental character of schools and hospitals to European audiences, education and health care were closely tied to religion and vice versa in the mission field, not least because the services were in high demand among potential converts.

Mission teachers were often presented to European audiences as key to local evangelism; sometimes medical workers featured in such a role as well. In the grander scheme of things, however, these key agents were objectified as examples of missionary success. In addition, the colonial social hierarchy was steep: "[t]rustworthy" African mission activists lead local African parishes but deferred to European superiors. In contrast, the Benedictine mission's leprosy patients appeared as malleable, good-natured, happy, but unfortunate stock characters. In the highly individualized conversion stories of female Catholic missionaries, leprosy patients appeared as largely empty canvasses to be inscribed with powerful projections of female European imperial agency.

The variable ways in which patients made homes in leprosy settlements and negotiated the offers of missions were reconfigured in missionary narratives as proof of worthiness and convertibility. Missions appealed to European Christians as intermediate, yet powerful agents of God's empire. This becomes tangible in Norbert Weber's 1923 account of his travels to the leprosy settlements in Southern Tanzania:

> These poor afflicted people in their anxiety and eagerness even went so far as to declare themselves willing to cultivate sufficient land to meet the requirements of the entire leper community comprising a large number whose infirmities had disabled them from all manual labour. [We] promised to supply two dozen of the required implements [hoes]... The distribution had taken place amidst hushed silence, but now it was over, a great demonstration of joy followed, manifesting itself in a mighty shout of "asanti" "thank you." ... The "stupid" negroes are so often denied both heart and feeling and accused to be strangers to all sensations of gratitude, that after witnessing so striking an exhibition of all these qualities I feel bound to stand the advocate of this much maligned and misunderstood people. (Weber 1923, 15–16, 21)

The abbot's narrative exposes communication strategies of missions for the home constituencies. Weber portrayed Africans as poor, sick and in urgent need of help, at the same time eager, grateful and able to express joy and happiness, if given assistance. European Christian readers were expected to be compassionate and giving in emotional communion with the newly converted – a common trope among missionaries of various denominations (Haggis/Allen 2008). Weber evoked the desired *emotional regime* (Reddy 2001) with authority: "The retrospect on the sufferings of our fellow men *pierces one's inmost soul*, and through the keen *sympathy* with which our *hearts are filled* at the sight of *anguish*, there comes forth a soothing song of *peace and love*, which to the poor sufferer is almost akin to the voice of angels" (Weber 1923, 3, emphasis added). Both, secular and missionary narratives were able to reconfigure and almost extinguish the vital agency of Africans, not by actually removing them from the story, but by objectifying them as part of the syndrome of leprosy, as obstacles to be overcome by social engineering efforts, or as worthy objects of European Christians emotional (and material) engagement.

Conclusion

There were significant differences between religious and secular narratives of leprosy in the colonial context of the 1920s through the 1940s, for instance, in the way religious narratives tended to foreground *care* or the triangular and transcendental connection of European Christians, African patients, and God's grace. Medical experts put the work for the secular empire center stage, an empire to be saved and ridded of disease. The *curative* aspect was a prime mover for these secular narratives of leprosy and for the emotional bonds that formed the community of leprosy experts in the 1920s and 1930s.

However, both strands of colonial leprosy narratives had similar structural features: the *scaling* and *connecting* effects that bound together local stories and grand narratives of secular and religious empires; the way conversion and self-transformation stories allowed for narrative plots; the impact of patients on programs and policies; and the disease's structuring effect on leprosy narratives. Religious and secular reports presented distinctly different, yet not fundamentally diverging versions of colonial public health. The colonial mode of narrating pandemics came in different guises but remained with a colonial framework.

The leprosy narratives examined in this chapter have proven to be volatile and multifaceted, so much so that they do not submit themselves to summaries, such as a "story of hope" (Vaughan 1991, 84) or "confidence trick" (Iliffe 1987, 225) played on African patients by European doctors and missionaries. On the contrary, these narratives were impressionable with regard to the physical aspects of the disease as well as the terms and conditions under which African leprosy patients chose to undergo caring or curing treatments. These patients used institutions to carve out space for survival under very dire conditions. However, the impact became manifest on an intermediate and practical level. The grander framework of colonial public health narration remained surprisingly intact.

Perhaps, there was a "confidence trick" to the narration of leprosy after all. If that was at all the case, it worked on the medical and religious experts and their European audiences. Leprosy narratives, secular and religious, had a way of thoroughly masking the profound impact of the material disease and patients' agency alike. Presenting these agents as passive obstacles to be overcome by European ingenuity (in the case of medical experts), or self-sacrificing care and the Lord's grace (in the case of missionaries) allowed the overarching paradigm of the European civilizing mission, and superiority, to largely stay intact. A case of self-deception, as the decades of decolonization were going to prove.

Bibliography

Anderson, Warwick. 2006. *Colonial Pathologies. American Tropical Medicine, Race, and Hygiene in the Philippines*, Duke UP.

Anonymous. 1921. *Passionsblumen und Pfingstblüten in dem Wirken der Missionsbenediktinerinnen von Tutzing*, Mission Press.

Anonymous. 1928. "Annual Meeting of the Association." *Leprosy Notes*, vol. 1, no. 1, 4–5.

Anonymous. 1928. "Cover." *Leprosy Notes*, vol. 1, no. 2, sine pag.

Anonymous. 1928a. "The Work of the Association." *Leprosy Notes*, vol. 1, no. 1, 2–3.

Anonymous. 1934. "Editorial." *Leprosy Review*, vol. 5, no. 3, 100–101.

Anonymous. 1936. "Aus der Mission Peramiho." *Missionsecho*, vol. 5, no. 1 (January), 11–12.

Anonymous. 1938. "Editorial." *Leprosy Review*, vol. 8, no. 2, 52–54.

Bashford, Alison, and Claire Hooker, editors. 2014. *Contagion*, Routledge.

Bashford, Alison, and Maria Nugent. 2014. "Leprosy and the management of race, sexuality and nation in tropical Australia." *Contagion*, edited by Alison Bashford and Claire Hooker, Routledge, 106–128.

Bauche, Manuela. 2017. *Medizin und Herrschaft. Malariabekämpfung in Kamerun, Ostafrika und Ostfriesland (1890–1919)*, Campus.

Brockmeyer, Bettina. 2021. *Geteilte Geschichte, geraubte Geschichte. Koloniale Biografien in Ostafrika (1880–1950)*, Campus.

Bruchhausen, Walter. 2006. *Medizin zwischen den Welten: Geschichte und Gegenwart des medizinischen Pluralismus im südöstlichen Tansania*, V&R Unipress.

Cochrane, Robert. 1933. "The Treatment of Leprosy. A Paper read at the Calcutta Leprosy Conference on 27th March, 1933." *Leprosy Review*, vol. 5, no. 3, 135–139.

Cooper, Frederick. 2004. "Development, Modernization, and the Social Sciences in the Era of Decolonization: the Examples of British and French Africa." *Revue d'Histoire des Sciences Humaines*, vol. 10, no. 1, 9–38.

Dengel, Anna. 1925. "Als Missionsärztin unter indischen Frauen." *Katholische Missionsärztliche Fürsorge*, vol. 2, 20–24.

Dow, Donald. 1945. "Occupational Therapy in Leprosy Institutions." *Leprosy Review*, vol. 16, no. 2, 57–63.

Dreier, Marcel. 2015. *Health, Welfare and Development in Rural Africa. Catholic Medical Mission and the Configuration of Development in Ulanga/Tanzania, 1920–1970*. Ph.D. University of Basel. https://edoc.unibas.ch/72455/1/Dreier_Diss_Health_Welfare_Development_Africa_Mission_Medicine_Ulanga_Tanzania.pdf.

Eckart, Wolfgang U. 1997. *Medizin und Kolonialimperialismus, Deutschland 1880–1945*, Schöningh.

Ehlers, Sarah. 2019. *Europa und die Schlafkrankheit. Koloniale Seuchenbekämpfung, europäische Identitäten und moderne Medizin 1890–1950*, Vandenhoeck & Ruprecht.

Foucault, Michel. 1977. *Discipline and Punish: The Birth of the Prison*, Random House.

Gelfand, Michael. 1957. *The Sick African. A Clinical Study*, 3rd edition, Juta & Co.

Gilg, Alois. 1932. "Weihnachten bei den Aussätzigen." *Missionsblätter*, vol. 36, no. 1 (January), 7–9.

Groß, Bilhild Sr. 1930. "Mein erster Täufling." *Missionsecho*, vol. 9, no. 8, 224.

Grundmann, Christoffer. 2014. *Sent to heal! – Emergence and Development of Medical Missions*, 2nd edition, Centre for Contemporary Christianity.

Haggis, Jane, and Margaret Allen. 2008. "Imperial Emotions: Affective Communites of Mission in British Protestant Women's Missionary Publications c1880–1920." *Journal of Social History*, vol. 41, no. 3, 691–716.

Hall, Stuart. 1984. "The narrative construction of reality: an interview with Stuart Hall. – Reprinted from a transcript of an interview by John O'Hara on the ABC programme 'Double Take.' 5 May 1983." *Southern Review* (Adelaide), vol. 17, no. 1, 3–17.

Hall, Stuart. 2006. "Encoding/Decoding." *Media and Cultural Studies. Key Works*, edited by Meenakshi Gigi Durham and Douglas M. Kellner, Blackwell, 163–173.

Heiser, Victor G. 1925. "The Future of Leprosy." *The North American Review*, vol. 221, no. 827, 680–688.

Hertlein, Siegfried. 2017. *Ndanda Abbey. Part III: From Mission to Local Church*, EOS.

Hölzl, Richard. 2011. "Der Körper des Heiden als moderne Heterotopie. Katholische Missionsmedizin in der Zwischenkriegszeit." *Historische Anthropologie*, vol. 19, no. 1, 54–81.

Hölzl, Richard. 2015. "Lepra als entangled disease. Leidende afrikanische Körper in Medien und Praxis der katholischen Mission in Ostafrika, 1911–1945." *Der afrikanische Körper als Missionsgebiet. Medizin, Ethnologie und Theologie in Afrika und Europa, 1880–1960*, edited by Linda Ratschiller and Siegfried Weichlein, Böhlau, 95–121.

Hölzl, Richard. 2016. "Educating Missions. Teachers and Catechists in Southern Tanganyika, 1890s to 1940s." *Itinerario* vol. 40 no. 3, 405–428.

Hölzl, Richard. 2024. "Missionary Anxieties, Psychopathology, and Decolonization: A Biographical Approach." *Psychiatric Contours: New African Histories of Madness*, edited by Nancy Rose Hunt and Hubertus Büschel, Duke UP, 68–92.

Iliffe, John. 1987. *The African Poor: a History*, Cambridge UP.

Iliffe, John. 1998. *East African Doctors. A History of a Modern Profession*, Cambridge UP.

Kerr, George. 1938. "The Organization of Occupational Therapy." *Leprosy Review*, vol. 8, no. 2, 64–69.

Langauer, L. "Leprosy in the Benin and Warri Provinces of Nigeria." *Leprosy Review*, vol. 11, no. 2, 96–99.

Larson, Lorne. 2021. "Disease, Science and Religiosity: A Case Study of Leprosy in German East Africa." *Zamani*, vol. 13, no. 1, 1–43. https://journals.udsm.ac.tz/index.php/tz/article/view/4618.

Latour, Bruno. 1999. *Pandora's Hope. Essays on the Reality of Science Studies*, Harvard UP.

Latour, Bruno. 2004. "Why Has Critique Run out of Steam? From Matters of Fact to Matters of Concern." *Critical Inquiry*, vol. 30, no. 2, 225–248.

Lowe, John. 1934. "The Leprosy Clinic and the Control of Leprosy." *Leprosy Review*, vol. 5, no. 1, 40–44.

Morick, Victoria. 2026. "Visually Narrating Disease? Syphilis in the German Public Sphere During the Early 20th Century," *Narrating Pandemics*, edited by Silke Schicktanz, Andrew S. Gross, Richard Hölzl, transcript.
Morrissey, Ermenlinde. 1936. "Glück im Leid." *Missionsecho*, vol. 15, 215–218.
Muir, Ernest. 1928. "The Campaign Against Leprosy." *Leprosy Notes*, vol. 2, no. 2, 2–7.
Muir, Ernest. 1938. "The International Congress of Leprosy." *Leprosy Review*, vol. 9, no. 3, 105–109.
Muir, Ernest. 1938. *Leprosy. Diagnosis, Treatment and Prevention*, 6th edition, BELRA.
Muir, Ernest. 1939. "Tanganyika Territory." *Leprosy Review*, vol. 10, no. 1, 58–80.
Muir, Ernest. 1940. "The Leprosy Situation in Africa." *Journal of the Royal African Society*, vol. 39, no. 155,134-142.
Murray, Janet. 1931. "Work Among Tanganyika's Lepers." *Leprosy Review*, vol. 2, no. 1, 15–17.
Napachihi, Sebastian W. 1998. *The Relationship Between the German Missionaries of the Congregation of St. Benedict from St Ottilien and the German Colonial Authorities in Tanzania, 1887–1907*, Mission Press.
Negley Farson, James S. 1946. "Review of: The Sick African, by Michael Gelfand." *African Affairs*, vol. 45, no. 178 (January), 49–50.
Pratt, Marie Luise. 2005. *Imperial Eyes. Travel Writing and Transculturation*, 2nd edition, Routledge.
Ratschiller Nasim, Linda Maria. 2023. *Medical Missionaries and Colonial Knowledge in West Africa and Europe, 1885–1914: Purity, Health and Cleanliness*, Palgrave Macmillan/Springer International.
Ratschiller, Linda, and Siegfried Weichlein, editors. 2016. *Der schwarze Körper als Missionsgebiet. Medizin, Ethnologie, Theologie in Afrika und Europa 1880–1960*, Böhlau.
Reddy, William M. 2001. *The Navigation of Feeling. A Framework for the History of Emotions*, Cambridge UP.
Riha, Ortrun. 2004. *Aussatz. Geschichte und Gegenwart einer sozialen Krankheit*, Hirzel.
Robertson, Russel L. 1940. "Garkida Agricultural-Industrial Leprosy Colony." *Leprosy Review*, vol. 3, 1932, 2, 50–58.
Rodriguez, José. 1934. "Results of the Chaulmoogra Treatment in Very Early Cases of Leprosy." *Leprosy Review*, vol. 5, no. 3, 102–107.
Rogers, Leonard. 1928. "Report of the Hon. Medical Secretary." *Leprosy Notes*, vol. 1, no. 1, 6–9.
Rogers, Leonard. 1929. "Voluntary Leper Colonies and Clinics. In Place of Compulsory Segregation." *Leprosy Notes*, vol. 4, no. 2, 10–12.
Rogers, Leonard. 1929a. "The Therapeutic and Economic Value of Work for Lepers." *Leprosy Notes*, vol. 7, no. 3, 16–17.
Rogers, Leonard. 1934. "History of the Foundation and the First Decade's Work of the British Empire Leprosy Relief Association." *Leprosy Review*, vol. 5, no. 2, 54–58.

Rosenwein, Barbara. 2010. "Problems and Methods in the History of Emotions." *Passions in Context*, vol. 1, no. 1, 1–32.

Sauerteig, Lutz. 2001. "'The Fatherland is in Danger! Save the Fatherland!' Venereal disease, sexuality, and gender in Imperial and Weimar Germany." *Sex, Sin, and Suffering. Venereal Disease and European Society since 1870*, edited by R. Davidson and L. A. Hall, Routledge, 76–92.

Sr. Konstantia. 1929. "Ein Gerichtsverhör im Aussätzigenheim in Kwiro." *Missionsecho*, vol. 8, no. 9, 199–200.

Stinnesbeck, Thekla. 1933. "Bei den Aussätzigen in Ndanda." *Missionsblätter*, vol. 37, no. 10, 307–309.

Stinnesbeck, Thekla. 1933. "Das Missionshospital in Ndanda (Ostafrika) in seinen ersten fünf Jahren." *Katholische Missionsärztliche Fürsorge*, vol. 10, 174–180.

Stinnesbeck, Thekla. 1934. "Bei den Aussätzigen in Ndanda." *Katholische Missionsärztliche Fürsorge*, vol. 11, 147–50.

Stinnesbeck, Thekla. 1934a. "Wanderung zu den Aussätzigen in Ndanda." *Missionsecho*, vol. 13, no. 1, 4–7.

Stinnesbeck, Thekla. 1935. "Letter, 6 August 1934." *Katholische Missionsärztliche Fürsorge*, vol. 12, 108–110.

Stinnesbeck, Thekla. 1936. "How Leprosy was regarded by the African Natives before Europeans came?" *Leprosy Review*, vol. 7, no. 1, 17–18.

Stinnesbeck, Thekla. 1936a. "Ndanda Leper Camp, Tanganyika Territory. Annual Report 1935." *Leprosy Review*, vol. 7, no. 3, 119–121.

Thérèse de Lisieux. 1997. *Story of a Soul: The Autobiography of St. Therese of Lisieux (the Little Flower)*, 3rd edition, ICS Publications.

Tilley, Helen. 2011. *Africa as Living Laboratory: Empire, Development, and the Problem of Scientific Knowledge, 1870–1950*, Chicago UP.

van der Veer, Peter. 1995. "Introduction." *Conversion to Modernities. The Globalisation of Christianity*, edited by Peter van der Veer, Routledge, 1–21.

Vaughan, Megan. 1991. *Curing their Ills. Colonial Power and African Illness*, Polity Press.

Vollmer, Melania. 1925. "Not an katholischen Missionsärzten in Ostafrika." *Katholische Missionsärztliche Fürsorge*, vol. 2, 119–21.

Wallace, C.A. 1932. "Leprosy in Ukuguru District, Tanganyika." *Leprosy Review*, vol. 3, no. 4, 159–161.

Walther, Daniel J. 2015. *Sex and Control. Venereal Disease, Colonial Physicians, and Indigenous Agency in German Colonialism, 1884–1914*, Berghahn Publishers.

Weber, Max. 1986. *Gesammelte Aufsätze zur Religionssoziologie*, vol. 1, 8th edition, Mohr Siebeck.

Weber, Norbert. 1923. *Children of Sorrow. A Walk through the lepper stricken villages of Southern East Africa*, Mission Press.

WHO. 2007. *Towards Zero Leprosy. Global Leprosy (Hansen's disease) Strategy 2021–2030*, World Health Organization, Regional Office for South-East Asia.

Wilson, R.M. 1930. "Industrial Therapy in Leprosy." *Leprosy Review*, vol. 1, no. 1, 25–28.
Worboys, Michael. 2000. "The Colonial World as Mission and Mandate: Leprosy and Empire, 1900–1940." *Osiris* (2nd Series), vol. 15, 207–218.

"But We Were All in the Same Boat Anyway"
How Factory Workers in Austria Narrate the Covid Pandemic

Laura Bäumel

Introduction

Shortly after the COVID-19 pandemic hit Europe in March 2020, a public narrative emerged suggesting an imaginary collective subject ("we") that had to "stick together" in view of the common fate of a pandemic that allegedly was affecting everyone equally. In fact, this was not the case: people under precarious material circumstances were in many ways more affected by the pandemic than those with more capital (Nolan 2021, 102). In order to "fight the virus together," this discourse suggested there was a simple distribution of roles between people working in essential occupations on-site on the one hand and people working remotely from home on the other. Large parts of the working population were omitted in that discourse, however: people working as tilers, painters or factory workers, for example, had to continue working, in many countries, risking their lives, regardless of the fact that their services were not necessary for the maintenance of the critical infrastructure. Thus, one might assume that factory workers perceived the pandemic and its management as unjust. However, interviews with women, especially mothers, working in factories at the time of the pandemic show that the outbreak of the disease was *not* perceived and narrated as an exceptional crisis by many within this part of the population.

In this chapter, I will show that working class women in Austria recount the pandemic as an event that did not significantly affect their daily lives: at home, they had to pursue their reproductive work – and in the factory, their productive, i.e., salaried, work. The pandemic is not so much narrated as an exceptional state, but rather as a moment in which the needs of workers are in accordance with those of the companies and employers. The working mothers in my case study talk about the fact that they were relieved to be able to continue to work and found the protective measures in the factory annoying, but they also perceived them as a necessary concession towards their employers. In that sense, I argue that the hegemonic discourse regarding the need for strong cohesion within society was taken up by these workers in a relatively direct manner.

The Hegemonic COVID-19 Pandemic Discourse: Narratives of an Exceptional Crisis

In the following, I attempt to shed light on the prevailing discourse at the onset of the COVID-19 pandemic that was characterized by narratives suggesting a predicament in which all people found themselves together. Setting the tone at this time were political leaders and their advisors on virological issues. For example, Christian Drosten, who became somewhat of a cult figure in the German-speaking world (Kupferschmidt 2020). "We're all in this together" can be understood as the "linguistic hallmark," as described by linguists Piotr Blumczynski and Steven Wilson (2023, 1), through which the first phase of the pandemic was characterized across national borders. During these months clear social roles were drawn by governments, experts and public figures: either one stayed at home and thus saved lives and one maintained critical infrastructure and therefore left one's house for work only. Each person, the narrative suggests, had a clear role in which they would become a hero, provided one followed the rules set for that particular situation in which they found themselves.

Celebrities took up those narratives and addressed their fans and followers with glimpses of their own lives in quarantine. They acted as role models in that they depicted a creative approach to the situation in which they found themselves. Many celebrities encouraged their followers to show civic engagement by donating money or volunteering (Lookadoo et. al. 2021, 412) and frequently called for the measures to be followed. They also appealed to social cohesion (ibid., 413–415). UN Secretary-General António Guterres released a video teaser via Twitter for his report "COVID-19 and Human Rights. We are all in this together." Although the report addresses the socio-demographic differences in the consequences for individuals, and actual and potential human rights violations during the pandemic, the discursive slogan also made it onto the title and teaser graphic of the report (UN 2020).

This discourse functioned as the backdrop of Austria's political and discursive crisis management as well. The COVID-19 virus was first registered in Austria at the end of February 2020. On Friday, March 13, three days before the start of the first lockdown in the country, President Alexander Van der Bellen sent a nearly six-minute video announcement from the Hofburg Palace in Vienna, which was broadcasted by the Austrian Broadcasting Corporation (ORF):

> Ladies and gentlemen, you all know and see it every hour on the news. The corona crisis has reached our country. It is a serious challenge for us, for our families, for our society, for our economy, for our cohesion in general. [...] Well ladies and gentlemen, I stand here today to tell you, yes, we are in a serious situation. The Corona crisis affects us all and it cuts deeply into our everyday lives. And we can all do something. [...] Ladies and gentlemen, we all have practical concerns now as well. Who will look after my child when there are no more classes? [...] What will happen to my business, my job? How will I even make ends meet? We humans have the quality and the gift to adapt quickly to sudden changes. This characteristic will also help us now and hopefully lead us out of this crisis in the shortest possible way. But it will be a big challenge for all of us, for all of us (emphasized). [...] Thank you, ladies and gentlemen who live in Austria, thank you for helping. Ladies and gentlemen, we have to go through this situation together now. And the more we stand together now, the better we work together now, the faster we will master this situation together. I am confident that we will manage this too, as we have already managed so many things together in our country. So, please take care of yourselves and together we will take care of our Austria.[1]

Van der Bellen stressed the collective "we" and emphasized that "we all have worries now" and that it "will be a great challenge for all of us." He pleaded to stick together to get out of this crisis as quickly as possible. The (then) Chancellor, Sebastian Kurz, announced the "Emergency Mode in Austria" [*Notbetrieb in Österreich*] on Sunday, March 15, 2020. In a speech, he thanked "all of Austria's parties" who helped making the "Emergency Mode" possible and finally addressed a few professional groups to express his gratitude:

> Dear Ladies and Gentlemen, dear Austrians. We are living in a time of challenges, in a time of crisis, in a time when it is necessary to stand together. [...] We have to shut down Austria to "emergency mode" starting tomorrow. That means classes at schools will no longer take place, care will of course be provided. Businesses will remain closed, with the exception of grocery stores, pharmacies and other necessities. Events will no longer take place and mobility will also have to be restricted. This means: stay at home unless you have to go to work, run necessary errands or help other people who are in urgent need of assistance. [...] I would especially like to thank all the people who are going above and beyond in our country right now. Who are doing great things, whether in the health care system, in the police force, or all those who do their duty every day in the supermarket, in the pharmacies, or in food production.[2]

---

1 Emphasis by the author (https://tvthek.orf.at/history/Politischer-Rueckblick/13557947/Erster-Appell-des-Bundespraesidenten/14047789).

2 Emphasis by the author (https://tvthek.orf.at/history/Politischer-Rueckblick/13557947/Kanzler-Kurz-verkuendet-Notbetrieb-in-Oesterreich/14047788).

The two social groups that Kurz named in this announcement would dominate the discourse in the first weeks and months of the pandemic: those who stay at home and those who have to work in essential occupations at their workplaces. The group of workers he addresses in the speech are in sectors that are obviously necessary to maintain the critical infrastructure. The word "production" is only used in connection with food production. It seems implausible that groups whose professions are not relevant to maintain the critical infrastructure, such as those in automobile production, were simply forgotten here, given their numbers and economic importance – it seems more likely that they were deliberately not being addressed. One can only speculate about possible intentions for this omission. Presumably, however, including these groups and thereby making the concession that not only *systemrelevant* groups had to risk their health and lives by working, would have contributed, or initiated, a broad debate or even dissent.[3]

The regulations regarding the "interim measures to prevent the spread of COVID-19" issued on the 15th of March 2020 by the Federal Minister of Social Affairs, Health, Care and Consumer Protection concerned "entering the customer area of business premises of trade and service companies as well as of leisure and sports facilities for the purpose of purchasing goods or using services or leisure and sports facilities"[4] – accordingly, the restrictions do not affect the industrial sector.

The nationwide (first) lockdown in Austria began on Monday, March 16, 2020, and applied with gradual relaxations until May 1 of the same year. Both narratives – the one about "us" who had to pull together as well as the second narrative that emerged from this, suggesting everyone was either working for the maintenance of the critical infrastructure or staying at home – were taken up and transmitted by the media. For people working at home, there were tips on ergonomics and how to deal with the fact that one's own four walls now must function as workplace. For example, the left-liberal magazine *Der Standard* headlined "Tips for the home office in times of coronavirus. How to communicate effectively with the company from home." It explained legal principles, gave tips for suitable office communication software and how to protect oneself against distraction and procrastination.[5] The pub-

---

3 Inquiries to the Federal Ministry of Justice, the Chancellor's Office and the Federal Ministry of Social Affairs, Health, Care and Consumer Protection have not shed light on the dichotomous representation and omission of those workers who did not contribute to the maintenance of the critical infrastructure. The Chancellor's Office and the Federal Ministry of Justice each pointed out that they were not responsible for specific decisions and therefore could not provide any information. The Federal Ministry of Social Affairs, Health, Care and Consumer Protection had not responded to the author's inquiry by the time of publication.

4 https://www.ris.bka.gv.at/Dokumente/BgblAuth/BGBLA_2020_II_96/BGBLA_2020_II_96.pdfsig.

5 https://www.derstandard.at/story/2000115573498/tipps-fuers-home-office-in-corona-zeiten.

lic television station ORF aired a fifty-minute program *Am Schauplatz* on March 27, 2020, which focused on those who ensure "that vital areas of the country continue to function." Here, too, the population is depicted as divided into those who work in a system-relevant area (warehouse workers, truckdrivers for supermarket chains, supermarket workers, doctors) and those who by staying at home or in their allotment gardens take care of each other and contribute to saving lives.[6]

It can thus be stated that the political and media discourse represented a clear social dichotomy: either one is at home strictly adhering to the exit restrictions, working remotely (if gainfully employed), or one is working in an industry that contributes to the maintenance of critical infrastructure, and thus counts as a "frontline worker." In terms of public representation, the situation of factory workers was different from that of nurses and other care workers, and in general those who were now perceived as "essential workers" who suddenly became subject of intense appreciation, like when people were clapping form their balconiesfor healthcare workers.[7] Due to their essential role in the crisis moment of the pandemic, workers of certain precarious and scarcely visible professional sectors became heroes of the everyday life (cf. Cook et al 2020, 75).[8]

The sociologists Antonia Kupfer and Constanze Stutz point out that while personal services were being closed on the grounds that people come into direct physical contact, governments still "refrained from lockdowns of large corporations and companies in the production sector, despite these being locations of contact" (2022, 14). People who were obliged to work and risk their lives, without being "relevant to the system" and without the attention of media,[9] politicians, and applauding people on balconies, mostly belonged to the low-income groups and precarious class (Autor*innenkollektiv Governance, Demokratie, Solidarität 2023, 13). They were therefore often more vulnerable to the virus (Meisterhans 2022, 81), for example due to cramped living conditions. The risk of infection and the chance of survival were therefore unequally distributed in society from the beginning (Lessenich 2020, 225). But what seems particularly problematic from a public health and safety perspective is that people continued to work in factories, even if they did not have to risk their lives for essential goods (such as food production).

6 https://tvthek.orf.at/history/Der-Alltag-mit-Corona/13557955/Ein-Land-in-Quarantaene/14047159.

7 And there have been the subsequent discussions about how this kind of symbolic tribute was something of a mockery if it was not accompanied by improvements in working conditions and wage increases (cf. Hürtgen 2022).

8 However, this is not to negate the fact that despite the temporary (mostly discursive) recognition, no significant structural improvements in working conditions have been achieved in this sector (cf. Kreimer et al. 2023, 91–112).

9 With the exception of the meat industry in Germany, where mass infections in meatpacking plants prompted a public debate (cf. Birke 2022, 249–292).

And yet, although they were not valued or even represented in the discourse, the hegemonic narrative of "We're in this together" also had a pacifying impact on them. on how the pandemic is perceived and told by the interviewees, as I will show in the following.

Mothers as Factory Workers Before and During the Pandemic

First, however, a short overview about the specifics of the research field in general. In my research, I am concerned with the question of how mothers who work in factories as temporary workers reconcile the productive and reproductive sphere in times of neoliberalism.[10] They belong to what I call, following Andreas Reckwitz, the "precarious class" (2019, 72), that is, they have little overall capital in Bourdieu's sense, insecure employment and poor wages. The local context of my research is the Austrian state Styria (*Steiermark*) where, the automobile industry, together with the timber industry, has long been the economic backbone (Kühberger 2011, 10). I became interested in this research field because I worked in a factory that manufactures side mirrors for cars during my first years of university. The people who worked on the assembly lines of that factory were mostly women who had very similar biographies: they had learned other professions, such as hairdresser, painter, cook/waitress, and had acquired professional certifications in these fields. When these women became mothers, a rupture occurred in their professional careers – and instead of working in the fields they had spent years being educated for, they went into the factory. This happened because jobs in the professions they had learned no longer suited their new circumstances. The most significant reasons for this were a) that the salary from working in a factory is higher than in their learned (mostly low-waged) occupation; b) that in the factory, working hours are clearly defined (shift work makes it possible to always get home on time); and c) that it is possible to work night shifts, which many of the women choose to do, especially while their children are still very young. The children are put to bed, their mothers go to work, when the child gets up, they are back home and can take care of the children and the household. This is what one of my interviewees described as "just the normal everyday life."[11] However, working in a factory comes with many disadvantages that are accepted for the advantages mentioned above; there are two reciprocal factors for the precarious position of mothers who decided to work in factories. To be employed as an unskilled worker in a factory is in most cases only possible through a temporary employment agency, which

10 At the time of publication, the empirical data material consists of 19 qualitative, guided, interviews (duration between 1.5 and 3.5 hours) and a two-week research phase in a factory. The data collection phase lasted from December 2020 to August 2022.

11 Hilde Schwarnhofer, 01/21.

means less financial and job security. In general, there would be the possibility of being taken on by the company as a direct employee at some point, but this is often limited by a range of factors, such as the responsibilities tied to reproductive work.

Being a temporary worker means not to be employed directly by the company for which you work, but by an employment agency such as Randstad or Manpower. Nevertheless, as a temporary worker, one often performs the same work as workers who are contracted directly by the company that operates the factory. As a result of this classification, workers are sitting next to each other on the assembly line, performing the same manual steps, while the difference is only the contract that is underlying their work – and, therefore, the pay and job security. Most direct employees in the factory had previously been temporary workers, especially amongst the younger employees. If laborers do a good job from management's perspective, work full-time and have little sick leave, there is a chance to be taken on by the company itself. That usually means having a more secure job. The advantages and disadvantages of temporary employment vary depending on the legal basis and the actual practice in the company. Austria is noteworthy in that many rights for temporary workers have been fought for by the production trade union (*Produktionsgewerkschaft, PROGE*) over the past decades (Mendel et. al 2017).

The difference between the two forms of employment, which, as I mentioned above, usually does not equate differences in the actual everyday work, became clear at the very beginning of the pandemic. Most factories continued to produce uninterruptedly in Austria, however, in many cases the workforce was reduced through different means.[12] Many direct employees were signed up for "short-time work" (*Kurzarbeit*), i.e., replacement payments from the government, while many temporary workers were laid off (even if many of them were taken back on after some weeks). Thus, the immediate consequence was a serious difference in income: being registered for short-term work usually meant receiving up to 90% of the former salary and staying on the contract. Temporary workers who were laid off had to register as unemployed and were only entitled to receive unemployment benefit, which in Austria is 55% of the salary for the first 20 weeks and decreases after this short period of time. This highlights an underlying problematic and conflict that came to a head in the pandemic: being a temporary worker increases the degree of precarity.

Motherhood plays a great role within this precarious situation, as it restricts social mobility. Regarding the type of employment, being a mother is decisive, insofar as mothers are less likely to work full time. Hence, they are less likely to become contracted by the factory itself. If they somehow manage to become direct employees, this status can still be lost if they continue to work part-time for too long after the

12 It should be noted at this point that a frequent reason for the workforce reduction was supply shortages, not interest in infection control (cf. Kupfer, Stutz 2022, 14–15).

birth of their children.[13] The (non-)availability of childcare is a crucial context when analyzing the intersection of production and reproduction: in Styria, only 31% of the childcare facilities offer services that are suitable for parents working full-time jobs. The others offer less than 10 hours of care per day (Statistik Austria 2022, 10). The situation is worse in the less densely populated rural areas, where most of my interviewees live, as opposed to Graz, the state's capital. Volatile support structures enabled the mothers' pre-pandemic daily waged work – neighbors, grandparents, friends who looked after the children in times when formal care was not available, especially in afternoons and during vacation season.

This structure was shaken with the outbreak of the pandemic, as options to send children to school and kindergarten were severely limited. Suddenly, parents had to home-school their children or had to deal with teenagers they could not motivate to study or could not help them properly with their homework tasks. Informal forms of care fell away due to imposed restrictions on personal contact outside the own household.

Inequalities, based on androcratic structures, that already existed before the pandemic, intensified. Mothers in general took on most of the unpaid care work during the pandemic, as several studies show. For Austria, a study documents that mothers were more likely to "voluntarily" reduce their working hours due to the repeated lockdowns (Derndorfer et. al 2021, 4) than fathers. In the terminology of feminist Marxist theory, the spheres of production and reproduction had to be renegotiated on several levels during the pandemic (cf. Federici 2020, 24). A differentiated analysis shows that the pandemic-induced changes in the relationship between reproductive and productive labor also have a class-specific component: Women with a high level of education and higher income are more likely to report that they performed more unpaid housework because of the COVID crisis. The reason for this is that activities could not be outsourced to cleaners, babysitters, and similar workers (Mader 2020). Outsourcing reproductive activities, especially within one's own household, is significantly less common (and possible) among mothers in the precarious class. This means that the pandemic-related changes were less drastic.

To summarize: being a temporary worker increases the degree of precarity in general and motherhood plays a great role within this precarious situation as it re-

13 Employees in Austria have, with minor restrictions, a legal entitlement to part-time employment at the longest until the child's 7th birthday (or any later start of school) (https://www.oesterreich.gv.at/themen/arbeit_und_pension/elternkarenz_und_elternteilzeit/Seite.3590004.html). In many cases, mothers who wish to remain employed part-time at the factory for longer than this time allowed by the law, are being dismissed with the option of being hired as part-time workers through a temporary agency (while performing the same work as they used to but having a more insecure form of employment).

inforces the degree of immobility within the "social space" (Bourdieu 1998, 15–23). In that sense, the mothers interviewed are confronted with a complex structure of injustice that was exacerbated during the pandemic. Accordingly, it might be assumed that those affected talk about the pandemic as a situation in which the unjust structures they have already found themselves in in pre-pandemic times aggravated. In the interviews I conducted, I first assumed that the interviewees would complain about difficulties like these, and I accordingly began to pose my questions.

(Non-)Narrations of Injustice

In the following, I try to analyze how mothers working in factories (most of them as temporary workers) during the pandemic speak about that time. The analysis is based on the ethnological method of narrative analysis of qualitative interviews. Cultural anthropologist Ove Sutter describes the specifics of a culturally oriented narrative analysis as one in which *speaking* is viewed as an *everyday action* and the socio-cultural background and the performance of speaking and the functions associated with it are included in the analysis (Sutter 2013, 83). Following Bourdieu, Sutter argues that the social location in which a speech act is performed, i.e., the capital resources the speaker has, as well as the habitual dispositions, must be considered in the analysis (ibid., 100–101). Following this model of narrative analysis, I ask what is (and what is not) represented and narrated by the interviewees and how it is represented. I will formulate interpretations on the question of the meanings of the narrative forms and narrative modes in the respective passages and thus attempt to "look at them across hegemonic discourses" (Meyer 2014, 249).

"Having Work": Maintenance of Normality

G **We were happy. [...] Yes, it is, life actually went on normally for us, for us actually normally, really.** We didn't, except we went shopping or what, you know. But otherwise [...] They have actually taken care, there, protection. [...] Such plastic walls between the people have been installed [...] You could talk, but you didn't spit on each other or so, you know, and that, they have actually taken care. They just made sure that we kept working. That's why it went so well. // L: Ok, yes. // so they actually took care.

L And you were glad, because you said //

G //**and normality was there too.**[14]

14 Gerlinde Payer, 08/22.

This is an excerpt from a three-and-a-half hour conversation with Gerlinde Payer[15] in August 2022. When Gerlinde (54) was 18, she completed an apprenticeship as a hairdresser and worked in this profession for several years. When her children were in their teens, she started working in a fish packing factory, a job she had to give up for health reasons. Afterwards she worked in a supermarket for a short period of time as a semi-skilled worker. For about ten years now, she has been working in a parquet flooring factory. Gerlinde told me that at the beginning of the COVID-pandemic, she was neither laid off nor put on short-time work. She continued to work without interruption, which she found pleasant because life "actually went on normally,"[16] as she put it. When I asked directly what having to continue producing during the pandemic was like for her, even though they were not actually part of any "critical" infrastructure, she did not address what I was implying, but rather talked about how she was worried that the demand situation at her workplace would weaken. Rather surprised, Gerlinde then reported that the order situation remained stable due to the fact that many private individuals laid new floors in their homes, during the first phase of the pandemic. Gerlinde's answer, which is representative of other similar answers here, surprised me to a certain extent, since I had assumed that the interviewees would express dissatisfaction or even complain about the situation in some way. This, however, is not Gerlinde's focus: she is mainly concerned about having and keeping this job. The next interview sequence from an interview with Jana Gross is similar to Gerlinde's:

L [...] Was that an issue then, so that you have to produce during the pandemic, for example, although actually cars could be dispensed?
J No, was not an issue.
L Was not at all?
J No.
L Were people rather happy//
J //**Yes, that they have a job. Well, that wasn't a topic at all. I just never thought about that before** *laughs*. Yes, I mean, there was short-time work in the meantime. Some were laid off for one or two months and then rehired. [...] There was short time work once, but that didn't really affect us part-timers anyway, it was only for the full-time employees. [...] **But otherwise, actually, no, I was glad that I could go to work, yes.**[17]

Jana graduated from high school in 2015 and went on to study at a university. She dropped out of her studies and started a training as a massage therapist. Until her

15 The names of all interviewees are pseudonyms to maintain their anonymity.
16 Ibid.
17 Jana Gross, 08/22.

pregnancy, she worked in a hotel as a masseuse. She had her first child a few months before the pandemic and started working during the night shift in a car parts plant eleven months after giving birth. The reason for her relatively early return to work was that she and her partner took out a loan to build a house and one of the bank's conditions for obtaining the loan was that Jana had an income. She described the household income at the time of the interview in August 2022 as just about sufficient for their everyday life and that they are already far away from "saving something away." After an hour and a half of talking, I asked Jana what working during the pandemic was like for her. She first described that it was exhausting to work with the mouth-nose-protection mask and how the measures at the workplace were not very useful. I then asked if they had discussed within the staff that they had to produce during the pandemic. She answered that it was not an issue at all for her and her colleagues and that she had never thought about this matter. While she found the measures in the factory annoying, the most important aspect of her narrative regarding working during the pandemic, as for Gerlinde, seems to be that she *had* work.

These passages indicate that workers perceived the fact that they could continue to go to work as positive. Instead of complaining about having to continue to produce during a pandemic in which large parts of the population did not have to risk their health through working, as I was expecting, they expressed their satisfaction about being able to be continuing working and thus experienced a certain maintenance of "normality." Accordingly, the hegemonic discourse is not contradicted, rather it is taken up and adapted to one's own reality. It manifests the attitude towards gainful employment, which can be understood as shaped by hegemonic structures, as part of a *common sense [Alltagsverstand]*, as Sutter, following Antonio Gramsci, describes it (2016, 55–57). An incorporated interest in maintaining work can be identified, as this is a way of maintaining "normality," i.e., the everyday life.

Reporting Reproductive and Care Work

L This first phase, at home, with school care, how was that?
J Yes, they were at home then anyway.
L That's when you had to look after everything.
J Mhm.
L What was that like?
J Exhausting, looking after everything (nochischaun), they did quite a lot online anyway. She [daughter] is well behaved, actually. But the little one [son], always wants to go to her [when she was studying]. And well, keeping him busy.
L So keep him busy?

J Exactly, exactly. You almost can't go out, then she wants to go out too. That's tough.[18]

As described above, childcare had to be reorganized during the pandemic. Especially at the beginning, when public care was massively restricted, it was even more difficult for many workers to juggle gainful employment with reproductive and care work. However, when I asked Judith Moser how she experienced the time of home schooling with her children during the pandemic, she simply answered: "Well, they were at home then." I asked if she then had to look after everything (*nochischauen*) she only answered "Mhm." I asked her again "What was that like?" and only then she very briefly described how she experienced the beginning of the pandemic in terms of childcare. Neither having to work during the pandemic nor having to handle school chaperoning for their children seems to be perceived as an exceptional challenge.

When asking my interviewees about the role of the fathers of their joint children was, I felt like they found my question somewhat odd. When, for example, I asked Lena Schwaiger about the role of her ex-husband, she answered: "Pff... that doesn't concern him at all."[19] She then explained that she has asked her ex-husband if he could take care for their two children for one more day per week during the first lockdown because of the difficult situation she was in (normally he sees them every second weekend for two days). But he just said that Lena also did not care how he struggles during this crisis. Due to the challenging time of repeated lockdowns, their conflicts came to a head and even ended in a lawsuit about alimony payments. This, of course, also meant that she again had to deal with an additional mental load during this time.

Judith and Lena responded to my question about childcare during the first lockdown by answering briefly. Clearly, the interviewees could have told me more about the multiple forms of stress. It took several inquiries on my part to hear how the initial period of the pandemic was organized and what role their partners played in it. This does not correspond to their way of speaking in the entire interview: both narrate in a detailed fashion in other passages.

According to Silke Meyer, meanings can be deduced from non-narratives such as these (2014, 249). In the sections presented above, they resort to "reporting" rather than "narrating," i.e., they summarize their experience in a condensed and abstracted form (Lehmann 1983, 34). This mode of speaking thus indicates the implicitness with which these working mothers look at the challenges between gainful employment and childcare. The omissions in their narrations about the pandemic, one could argue, point to the fact that they did not actually perceive the pandemic

18 Judith Moser, 08/22.

19 Lena Schwaiger, 04/22.

as an exceptional crisis. Lena even reported that she had felt "locked in" before the pandemic: "I just went to work and was at home."[20]

To conclude and state it in a somewhat exaggerated manner: since the interviewees already experienced a life before the pandemic that was so strongly characterized by the pressures of productive and reproductive work, they seem to have felt like little had changed in their everyday lives. While the daily life of the interviewees was in some ways marked by the measures "from above," the crisis was not perceived as exceptional. Also, this pandemic crisis seemed to affect many of the interviewees less than other crises that have determined their biographies. Such statements about everyday life during the pandemic as *not* particularly extraordinary point to a more general problematic that Anne Seeck has discussed – for many people, the experience of being restricted from participating in public life is not an exception:

> They are used to sitting isolated in their apartments and being excluded from social life. For them, going outside has always meant having to spend money they do not have. Many of the things that middle-class people sorely miss in Corona times are not possible for the income-poor in their normal, everyday lives, such as travel, visits to restaurants, expensive concerts and sports classes. (Seeck 2020, 86; author's translation)[21]

In the case of the field studied in this article, it can be added that a decisive factor for being isolated is the overall workload in terms of time between gainful employment and reproductive work. The perception of restrictions on everyday life due to the pandemic seems to be dependent on the class structure and the gendered division of labor.

"It has happened to everyone the same way"

The narrative modes used by the interviewees point to the fact that the additional burdens such as health risks or home schooling during the pandemic are often not seen as exceptional. The fact that they had to work during the pandemic seems to be perceived more as damage or threat (losing one's own job) averted than as an expression of structural inequality, or a manifest contradiction to the hegemonic discourse (home office vs systems-relevant jobs). I contend that my interview partners primarily took up the framings of "being in it together" from hegemonic discourse,

---

20 Lena Schwaiger, 04/22.

21 Stephan Lessenich refers to the same circumstance, focusing on the global context: "What have always been self-evident privations for four-fifths of the world's population [...] became real with corona, at least for a brief historical moment, also for the top fifth of the world's social structure" (Lessenich 2020, 218);author's translation).

thereby taking a non-oppositional and even anti-oppositional stance, especially towards their employers.

When, for example, I asked Judith what having to go to work was like for her when, after all, the production of auto parts was not essential to maintaining critical infrastructure, she expresses her satisfaction with the handling during the early phase of the pandemic:

> "**Well, I don't know, but I must say, it suited me quite well.** Because school and that then started again anyway and then it is okay anyway. But otherwise [...] if I'm afraid of it [the Covid virus], then it's something else, then I have to look anyway, but everyone get's it anyway. [...] **No, that's fine the way it was.**"[22]

Judith Moser works in a car parts factory, part-time on the night shift. Her partner and her father, both craftsmen, had to work throughout the pandemic and had more work than before because people at home had started to renovate their homes. When I asked what she thought of the fact that her family members and herself had to continue working, she, like other interviewees dismissed my question and did not elaborate on it. She did not answer my question about health risk and (as I saw it) the non-necessity to produce cars during the pandemic and answered, "Well, I don't know [...] it suited me quite well." She followed up with reflections that revolved around childcare and concluded her answer similarly to how she began, "No, that's fine the way it was." Similar forms of not complaining during the pandemic are used by many interviewees.

L What was working like then during the pandemic?

A **Well, we continued to produce as before, thank God**. Ah, just, of course, you had to wear a mask. Ah, you had to test yourself. [...] Then you had a certificate, ah, on your cell phone. **So, you may enter, you may go to work.** [...] **And, so, attention was paid somehow.**[23]

Anna Gruber, a full-time temporary worker at an automotive supplier, expresses gratitude that she was able to continue working and emphasizes that "attention was paid somehow" (*also da wurde schon geschaut*) to ensure that certain safety measures were followed. This can be read as a favorable remark that the factory had done something right during the pandemic. In a similar way, Jana first explained that the measures at her workplace did not offer any reliable protection, but stated quickly afterwards that those responsible could not have done more to protect the workers.

---

22 Judith Moser, 08/22.

23 Anna Gruber, 07/22.

L Did you feel well protected in general?

J [...] **That in the company, that was stupid,** because when we chatted, we just leaned forward in such a way that we talked past the security glass, because otherwise you didn't understand anything anyway, and at the seat you just don't have it [mask], where you sit next to each other for eight hours, and in the aisle, where I pass by I have to put it on. **It is not logical, it was actually moronic. Well protected, no** [...]. It was definitely, they, just the usual things. Disinfect hands, wash hands often, put on the mask as well as possible [...] **They did what they were told to do, and I don't see what else you could have done more.**[24]

The statements like "attention was paid," "I don't know what you could have done more," "[w]ell, that's fine the way it was" indicate a shoulder-to-shoulder relationship between employers and employees during the pandemic that is worth paying attention to. The passages presented can be interpreted as a non- and even anti-oppositional stance towards the employers or "those up there": the interviewees look approvingly at the factory's pandemic management, which gives them work and to a certain extent "normalizes" the global state of emergency. The anti-oppositional stance is accompanied by the frequent use of deictic forms, such as the pronoun "they" which partly leaves unclear who exactly is meant in the passages.

This conciliatory view of the employment relationship seems to have been influenced specifically by the pandemic and the ways in which it was made sense of discursively. While in other parts of the interviews, employers or "those up there" are clearly categorized as "others" who are generally not viewed favorably, the pandemic narrations are dominated by an imagery of employees and employers standing shoulder to shoulder. The discourse of "we're all in this together" is to some extent shared or even echoed by the interviewees. Quite clearly, for example, Jana explains that it was tedious for her to work with a mask, but at the same time, she emphasizes that it was probably the same for everyone:

> "[...] **It was just annoying with the mask.** It's really annoying, it's so stuffy inside, in the hall, and then you have to it out somewhere all the time, when you just quickly go over, carry a box over. That really bothered me. **But it was the same for everyone anyway**, I don't think there was almost anywhere where they didn't have them."[25]

The narrated satisfaction, or the non-, i.e., anti-oppositional stance, seems to be related to the hegemonic discourse suggesting that "everyone" had concerns about

24 Jana Gross, 08/22.

25 Jana Gross, 08/22.

work and childcare (including related financial issues) during this time. The employers, large production companies, also made use of the narrative of being in this crisis "together," for which the political and media discourse had paved a way. For example, an international company with several production locations in Styria reports on the website about the good pandemic management from 2020 as well as currently completed measures with the title "COVID-19 measures: Together, Safe & Healthy." Under one article of the regional newspaper *Kleine Zeitung*, which reports the temporary productional stop due to COVID-19 of a local car factory, there was a debate among readers in the comments column discussing employees' rights due to factory closures. One comment of a worker of the factory the article was about first describes the potential labor rights violations that might occur – but concludes the comment with "[b]ut in times like these, we just have to show solidarity." In this case, showing solidarity meant not causing the employer any trouble regarding labor law violations or making any kind of demands.

Conclusion

The article was an attempt to show how factory workers in Austria narrate the COVID-19 pandemic. Although they had to work during the pandemic and were thus exposed to a high health risk, they did not perceive the pandemic as reinforcing their (precarious) pre-pandemic situation. There was rather gratitude that the factories mostly remained open and only in some cases a complete production stop was imposed. Often, the discourse of "togetherness" was taken up and the issues of potential labor rights violations and health risks tended to be left aside – what seemed to be more important was the preservation of the fragile system in which the workers find themselves in. Since this system was not significantly shaken, i.e., the interviewees could still make ends meet and childcare was somehow mastered despite the difficult circumstances, the COVID crisis has apparently not been perceived and therefore narrated as an extraordinary crisis. The interview passages and media material presented indicate that the discourse following the "we're all in this together" paradigm has influenced perceptions and corresponding narratives about the pandemic. Solidarity with the employer was expressed, rather than discontent about the pandemic management. Potential labor rights violations were seen as lower priority. Questions about vaccination were not addressed in the interviews (this presumably would have elicited other narratives). However, the focus on the productive and reproductive sphere seems to expose interesting aspects from the precarious class that often remain unconsidered, as the COVID-19 pandemic was perceived and narrated as a non-exceptional crisis.

Bibliography

Autor*innenkollektiv Governance, Demokratie, Solidarität. 2023. "Pandemische politische Ökonomie. Zur kapitalistischen Verarbeitung der Corona-Krise." https://www.soz.univie.ac.at/ueber-uns/rising-scholars/ifs-working-papers/10.25365/phaidra.391.

Birke, Peter. 2022. *Grenzen aus Glas. Arbeit, Rassismus und Kämpfe der Migration in Deutschland*, Mandelbaum.

Blumczynski, Piotr, and Steven Wilson. 2022. "Are We All in This Together?" *The Languages of COVID-19, Translational and Multilingual Perspectives of Global Healthcare*, edited by Piotr Blumczynski and Steven Wilson, Routledge, 1–11.

Bourdieu, Pierre. 1998. *Praktische Vernunft. Zur Theorie des Handelns*, Suhrkamp.

Cook, Maria Lorena, Madhumita Dutta, Alexander Gallas, Jörg Nowak, and Ben Scully. 2020. "Global Labour Studies in the Pandemic. Notes from an Emerging Agenda." *Global Labour Journal*, May, 74–88.

Derndorfer, Judith, Franziska Disslbacher, Vanessa Lechinger, and Katharina Mader. 2021. "Home, sweet home? The impact of working from home on the division of unpaid work during the COVID-19 lockdown." *PLoS ONE*, November, 1–26.

Federici, Silvia. 2020. *Aufstand aus der Küche. Reproduktionsarbeit im globalen Kapitalismus und die unvollendete feministische Revolution*, edition assemblage.

Hürtgen, Stefanie. 2020. "Gesellschaftliche Arbeit und soziale Demokratie: Der alltagspolitische Diskurs zu 'Systemrelevanz' als Auseinandersetzung um eine sozialökologische Politik der Arbeit." *PROKLA. Zeitschrift für kritische Sozialwissenschaft*, 97–115.

Kühberger, Leo. 2011. "Car(e) Workers. Große Krise und (noch) kleine Kämpfe in der Steiermark." *grundrisse. zeitschrift für linke theorie & debatte*, 10–13.

Kreimer, Margareta, Hanna Hof, and Simone Liesnig. 2023. "Strukturelle Geschlechterunterschiede in den Arbeitsbedingungen. Eine beispielhafte Analyse der sozioökonomischen Folgen der Coronakrise im systemrelevanten Care-Bereich." *Sozialer Zusammenhalt in der Krise. Interdisziplinäre Perspektiven auf Heterogenität und Kohäsion moderner Gesellschaften*, edited by Barbara Ratzenböck, Katharina Scherke, Annette Sprung, and Werner Suppanz, transcript, 91–112.

Kupfer, Antonia, and Constanze Stutz. 2022. "Continuity, not Change: The unequal Catastrophe of the Covid-19 Pandemic: An Introduction." *Covid, Crisis, Care and Change? International Gender Perspektives on Re/Production, State and Feminist Transitions*, edited by Antonia Kupfer and Constanze Stutz, Verlag Barbara Budrich, 7–27.

Kupferschmid, Kai. 2020. "The coronavirus czar: The COVID-19 pandemic has made German virologist Christian Drosten an unlikely cult figure." *Science*, 462–465.

Lehmann, Albrecht. 1983. *Erzählstruktur und Lebenslauf. Autobiographische Untersuchungen*, Campus.

Lessenich, Stephan. 2020. "Soziologie – Corona – Kritik." *Berliner Journal für Soziologie*, 215–230.

Lookadoo, Kathryn, Caleb Hubbard, Gwendelyn Nisbett, and Norman Wong. 2021. "We're all in this together. Celebrity influencer disclosures about COVID-19." *Atlantic Journal of Communication*, 397–418.

Mader, Katharina. 2020. *Zeitverwendung von Paarhaushalten während Covid-19. Blog 1: Genderspezifische Effekte von Covid-19*. https://www.wu.ac.at/economics/mitarbeiter-innen/mader-k/genderspezifscheeffektevoncovid-19/1blog/.

Meisterhans, Nadja. 2022. "Das große Versagen in der Pandemie: Macht- und herrschaftskritische Anmerkungen zu den intersektionalen Dimensionen einer politisch gemachten Katastrophe." *Momentum Quarterly. Journal for Societal Progress*, 79–93.

Mendel, Marliese, Martina Schneller, and Peter Schissler. 2017. *15 Jahre Kollektivvertrag für das Gewerbe der Arbeitskraftüberlassung*. PROGE.

Nolan, Ryan. 2021. "'We are all in this together!' Covid-19 and the lie of solidarity." *Irish Journal of Sociology*, 102–106.

Reckwitz, Andreas. 2019. *Das Ende der Illusionen. Politik, Ökonomie und Kultur in der Spätmoderne*, Suhrkamp.

Seeck, Anne. 2020. "Von Umverteilung ist kaum etwas zu hören. Isoliert und vom gesellschaftlichen Leben ausgeschlossen sein – das kennen einkommensarme Menschen auch ohne Corona-Ausnahmezustand." *Solidarisch gegen Klassismus. Organisieren, intervenieren, umverteilen*, edited by Francis Seeck and Brigitte Theißl, Unrast, 86–94.

Statistik Austria. 2022. "Kindertagesheimstatistik 2021/2022," edited by Statistik Austria. https://www.statistik.at/fileadmin/publications/Kindertagesheimstatistik_2021-22.pdf

Sutter, Ove. 2016. "Alltagsverstand. Zu einem hegemonietheoretischen Verständnis alltäglicher Sichweisen und Deutungen." *Österreichische Zeitschrift für Volkskunde*, 41–70.

Sutter, Ove. 2013. *Erzählte Prekarität. Autobiographische Verhandlungen von Arbeit und Leben im Postfordismus*, Campus.

United Nations. 2020. "COVID-19 and Human Rights. We are all in this together." https://www.un.org/sites/un2.un.org/files/2020/04/un_policy_brief_on_human_rights_and_covid_23_april_2020.pdf.

The Jailbreaker
Exploring the Role of Social Figures in Pandemic Storytelling

Annerose Böhrer, Marie-Kristin Döbler, Larissa Pfaller

Introduction

In spring 2020, Mitterteich, a small town of about 7,000 residents in the southern German state of Bavaria, became one of the first German hotspots of the COVID-19 pandemic, just a few weeks after the first COVID case in Germany had been detected.[1] The epidemic situation in Germany was still unclear when the city hosted the local beer festival at the beginning of March 2020, which the organizers advertised as an "oral vaccination against Corona" (Amtmann and Kettenbach 2020). A little later, an increasing number of infections were registered in the Mitterteich district and eventually a state of emergency was declared in Bavaria.[2] Mitterteich became the focus of nationwide political and media attention. Finally, on the 18th of March, the lives of the town's inhabitants changed from one day to the next, not primarily due to the infections but rather due to the control measures including hitherto unprecedented acts such as a comprehensive curfew. People were allowed to leave their own house only for a "legitimate reason."

Additionally, the entire city was "locked up": guarded roadblocks were set up, the streets were filled with police, firefighters and ambulances, and maps showing the city limits were distributed to citizens. At the same time, numerous journalists made their way to the town, filming its empty streets and interviewing the few people they encountered. While curfews became a commonplace throughout Germany and entered everyday language as "lockdowns" in later stages of the pandemic, the Mitterteich case remained unique regarding the extent of the emergency measures

---

1 The first infection with Corona virus was reported in Germany on January 27th, 2020 (Bayerisches Staatsministerium für Gesundheit und Pflege 2020).

2 In Germany, infection control is regulated at the level of the federal states. When the numbers of people infected with the Corona virus increased in the state of Bavaria, the Bavarian government decided to declare a state of emergency for this administrative district. https://www.bayern.de/corona-pandemie-bayern-ruft-den-katastrophenfall-aus-veranstaltungsverbote-und-betriebsuntersagungen/.

in Germany. Against the backdrop of the beer festival,[3] a specific dynamic of dealing with the spread of infectious diseases quickly emerged: the search for culprits and, with it, multiple moral and often (highly) emotional assessments of the situation. The idea that the citizens of Mitterteich were rightly confined to their homes and city emerged as a recurring motif in these discourses. Various media reported, e.g., "the city in Corona custody" (Herda 2020), blamed "Bavaria's fatal love of beer" (Lill 2020) and, last but not least, Bavarian Prime Minister Markus Söder "threatened" that measures like these could also affect everyone else if they did not behave accordingly (*Die Welt* 2020). The discourse on the pandemic had soon adopted a rhetoric of crime and punishment.

In this chapter, we focus on a specific incident that happened on the very first day of the curfew: the case of a young man who broke the newly established rules by leaving his place of residence without permission in order to attend a party outside of the city's borders. His escape was noticed by neighbors, reported to the police and widely discussed on social media. To analyze how this case appears as a typical form of pandemic storytelling, we first introduce the sociological concept of *social figure – narrative figures, which are an important part of public discourse and processing of new situations*.

After further defining our material (online posts in a local news ticker) and methods (content analysis), we discuss the *social figure* of "the jailbreaker" as a key to understand how the pandemic and healthcare countermeasures were perceived as a manifestation of state violence and incarceration. We explore how narratives of (in)justice emerge in the online discussions about "the jailbreaker" and how this figure became a significant factor in structuring the moral landscapes of the German public discourse at the beginning of the pandemic. In addition, we will discuss how the conceptual metaphor of imprisonment plays a significant role in the creation of this figure and the narratives connected to it. Finally, we discuss the practical consequences of this framing in public communication: working together to combat the spread of the virus often became less a question of acting according to medical findings than of legitimacy and (in)justice.

Theorizing Pandemic Storytelling with Social Figures

"Pandemic" storytelling has already been identified as an important field for understanding how pandemics are socially perceived and processed (cf. Charteris-Black

3 There is a long tradition of annual beer festivals in the town of Mitterteich and the surrounding region. The so-called "Starkbierfest" ("Starkbier" translates to "strong beer"), which is always celebrated at the beginning of March, also took place in March 2020 in a local event hall.

2021; Davis and Lohm 2020; Lee 2014). We learn about an epidemic or pandemic outbreak, Davis and Lohm (2020) note, mostly through stories: news stories, conversations with friends, Facebook, Twitter, emails from employers, etc. – narratives that are widely circulated and modified. Pandemics are therefore also multifaceted narrative phenomena disseminated by a broad variety of media. Especially in the early stages, "pandemic narratives help us to understand contagion, identify its possible ramifications, and take positions and actions, individually and collectively, on the implied threat to life" (ibid., 1). A central element of this negotiation are *social figures* (cf. Moser and Schlechtriemen 2018; 2019; 2020) that carry traces of events and histories. In most cases, these figures are used to delimit and contain the phenomenon and/or articulate how things are supposed to be (or not to be). They are narrative figures that structure the moral worlds of experiences and enable the narrators to position themselves.

The concept of *social figures* has a long history in sociology (cf. le Grand 2019). It has been further developed and elaborated by the German sociologists Sebastian Moser and Tobias Schlechtriemen (2018; 2019; 2020). *Social figures* are, as the authors state, "a suitable means of pursuing the questions that people in present-day society are itching to answer but for which there are no clear or even institutionalized answers so far" (Moser and Schlechtriemen 2019, 5). They do not only function as a sociological form of reflection, but are also produced outside of academia and, thus, form patterns of interpretation that circulate far beyond scholarly debates. This feature makes them connectable, relatable and comprehensible for many people. *Social figures* emerge especially in contexts of crisis or social change whose (potential) effects have not yet been clearly clarified and institutionalized (cf. Moser and Schlechtriemen 2018, 164–165): "They can thus facilitate the explorative investigation of crises-laden social developments" (Moser and Schlechtriemen 2019, 5). The COVID-19 pandemic produced, as Moser and Schlechtriemen (2020) state, a whole firework of *social figures:* in the beginning, there is *the hoarder* leaving the supermarket with significant amounts of toilet paper, ready to isolate for an indefinite period of time. In the course of the pandemic, the German public became acquainted with the names of *virologists* who had been largely unknown before and now became embodiments of the social figure of *scientific experts*. At the same time, names such as those of the Bavarian company Webasto, the Austrian ski resort Ischgl, or the Huanan market in Wuhan gain sad notoriety as the (alleged) places of appearance of the respective *Patient* 0 – a figure that is not only sick, but also contagious, and, for that very reason, provokes questions about the right behavior, about guilt and responsibility (Moser and Schlechtriemen 2020). Questions of a similar nature, especially about irresponsibility and antisocial behavior, were personified in the figure of the *mask refuser* (cf. Müller 2020) or later the *anti-vaxxer*.

The concept of *social figures* is suitable for detecting and defining socially relevant problems, such as those that arise from a pandemic, developments of medical technologies or scientific findings that call central cultural categories and habits into question. On the one hand, they claim to describe social realities, and on the other, they give rise to social self-understanding and ethical-moral positioning (cf. Moser and Schlechtriemen 2018, 168). They can challenge emotional reactions and irritations: one admires them, or one is outraged by them. However, how to deal with them socially has not yet been determined (ibid., 169).

How a *social figure* emerges and solidifies can probably not be traced in all its details. They mark breaking points and describe the fragility of previous interpretations of the world (cf. Moser and Schlechtriemen 2018, 171), but are of only conditional permanence, often appearing temporarily and in the context of specific discourses. This is what Moser and Schlechtriemen refer to as social figures' "special time index," which "sets them apart from theoretical concepts and their claim to universal validity" (ibid., 12). They are "in between time" (ibid); although they may lose their popularity over time, they can always be reactivated (cf. ibid). Thus, they are not simply historical persons in the strict sense, but rather part of social processes and public discourses: they enable communication and shared, intersubjective understanding of events or occurrences collectively experienced.

As "embodied" figures (or at least possessing an imaginary and imaginable body), they enable to imagine an individual and "real" persons and things done by or happening to them (such as getting arrested). *Social figures* enable ethical positioning by representing a role model for how one could behave towards a socially virulent problem. They figure ways of dealing with a social problem or challenge and thus sketch the picture of a possible future in which society is populated by that concrete *social figure* and its associated consequences (cf. Moser and Schlechtriemen 2018, 172; Moser and Schlechtriemen 2019, 13). In their capacity as ethical/moral points of reference, they also have a political function and play an important role in cultural negotiations about (a)moral behavior.

In the following section, we will introduce a case of our empirical data that we call *the jailbreaker* for now. Although the news report that we take as a starting point for the analysis initially does mention a real person, the way in which he is reported on and discussed makes him a "case," a *social figure* that is negotiated in an exemplary way and beyond the individual person. The *jailbreaker case* of Mitterteich thus refers to a broader discourse that took place in the pandemic that war-games not only the medical but also the social challenges of the pandemic.

The Jailbreaker Case: Material and Methods

For presenting the *jailbreaker case* we draw on empirical data of the research project *Spring in Mitterteich* (funded by Volkswagen-Stiftung).[4] Designed as a locally and temporally focused case study the project develops a differentiated understanding of doubt and critique, which are expressed and expressible in the face of political measures during a biomedical emergency. For this article we decided to focus on online discussions[5] for two reasons: these discussions provide a particular form of material with a special epistemic potential for our case study of Mitterteich in general and of (in)justice in the face of a biomedical emergency in particular. They are – unlike interviews which necessarily have a retrospective character – field material generated "in real time." The social media posts represent what people wrote, thought and knew in the beginning of the pandemic. They document the process and the making of the discourse in the face of the knowledge available in spring 2020 and make the dynamic patterns of interpretation traceable.

In the following, we present our findings of the analysis of the *Mitterteich jailbreaker case* – one particular thread of these social media groups initiated on 21st March 2020 by a local news feed. Already existing prior to the pandemic, this news ticker has given short (police) reports about events, and transmitted important local news, for instance, about festivities, road closures or accidents. With the advent of SARS-CoV-2 the ticker also functioned as a medium for communicating "health news," new regulations/rules and general developments regarding the COVID situation in Mitterteich.

Among the first "pandemic posts" is one about the aforementioned young man, who was caught by the police attending a party in a neighboring town. More than 1000 comments from various users were received in a short time as reaction to the report and the discussion soon started to develop its own dynamic. To understand this better, let us briefly look at the unfolding of posts: first, the ticker reports in a comparatively matter-of-fact way that a party had been held in a town close to Mitterteich and that one of the guests was a Mitterteich resident (in the following called

4 The project is funded by Volkswagen Stiftung from Mai 2021 to April 2023a, project number A134525.

5 United by their reference to Mitterteich and their temporal focus on the first curfew, different sorts of data have been collected: (a) We conducted, transcribed and anonymized *narrative, thematically focused interviews* with (so far, as in August 2022) nine inhabitants of Mitterteich, and(b) gathered *official documents* (policy papers, public statements etc. published in the period between March to May 2020) reporting about "a virus," later "the virus, " presenting it as biomedical threat and communicating political measures. Further, we collected *publicly available statements* of different actors made via various media. Thus, there are (c) a set of 107 *newspaper articles* about the pandemic in Mitterteich published between March and May 2020 as well as (d) transcripts of *posts in three Mitterteich related* social media groups.

Max). By attending the party, it was said, he had violated the newly installed *Infection Protection Act* (German: *Infektionsschutzgesetz*) and would therefore be prosecuted. The majority of posted reactions to the "party newsflash" shared an affirmative position regarding the biomedical policy or a condemnatory and pejorative attitude towards the rule-breaking partygoer.

Thus, subsequent posts questioned the knowledgeability of the wrongdoer and called for "considerable," "right," or "just" sanctions. Others struck a more educational tone presuming that only "real" and "true" punishment (e.g., flogging, shooting, denial of medical care etc.) could combat such "foolishness." The few voices, which raised criticism about the authorities' sense and logic, e.g., by pointing to the ambivalence of being allowed to go to work but not to private meetings, became targets of derogatory and condemning comments themselves. The respective users were quickly inundated with accusations of stupidity and lacking solidarity. Additionally, their status as informed citizens and their capacity for rationality was questioned.

In the analysis, we present the online reactions to the illicit attendance of a party by Max. For this purpose, we first sighted the discussion in terms of a qualitative content analysis (Mayring 2014). Posts and thematic strands identified as central were then heuristically analyzed, following the documentary method (Bohnsack 2010), discourse (Keller 2005) and metaphor (Schmitt 2005) analysis.

Due to the ambiguous, semi-public status of social media posts (Merunkova and Slerka 2019, 271) and because we could not ask all (of the more than 1000) group members for their consent, we refrain from making direct quotes or naming groups and group members. This is also important in order to protect the users' anonymity and to avoid their traceability, especially in context of the subsequently presented example, which circles around the misconduct of a concrete person and gave rise to highly emotional debates, violating statements and personal insult.

Analysis: The Narrative Function of *The Jailbreaker*

The ensuing flood of comments on Max's behavior can be summarized in two main strands: much of the commentary is concerned with his cognitive abilities: he is said to be stupid and obstinate, and uncomprehending. A second tendency concerns his social skills: he is said to be selfish and lacking solidarity.

Regardless of whether stupidity or selfishness is suspected as the driving force behind the man's behavior, demands are made for punishment to atone for the crime. These demands can be divided into two categories: monetary and physical. On the monetary side it is, e.g., demanded that he should face a maximum penalty rate and should have to pay an amount of money, varying from 5,000 up to 50,000 Euro. One person demands that the penalty should be so high that it still affects him financially in 5 years. Some participants call for the penalty to be extended to all others involved in the event (e.g., all should pay 10,000 Euro each). Further, although the news ticker post did not mention a name, *the jailbreaker* himself apparently was easily identified. Thus, some particularly resourceful participants found out that Max has a soft spot for cars. Accordingly, they demand that his car and driver's license should be confiscated.

Even more troubling than the demands for monetary reparations are the collective fantasies about corporal punishment. An obvious idea for atoning for a crime seems to be imprisonment. However, some participants are getting even more creative: Max should, e.g., be sent "to [the hotspots in] Italy"[6] without protective clothing or locked in with infected people. Flogging and shooting are also considered, he (optionally also his family) should be denied medical care, he should be forced to stab asparagus.[7] Others demand to send him to a labor camp in Siberia (imagining he would pound stones there), he should be used as a test subject for new vaccines, he should be locked inside his house (or "the barn"[8]) and is encouraged to commit suicide. In a more innocuous variation, participants fantasize about locking him up without TV, internet and toilet paper and little food. Some of these penalties are again expanded to the other participants of the party.

The calls for punishment are essentially legitimized by two arguments that clarify the way in which one feels affected by his action as a community. One side understands his action in terms of the virus and its physical effects: He puts everyone on risk to fall ill with coronavirus disease. Another current thinks of the consequences of his actions exclusively in a legal sense, as it would ensure that the curfew is being prolonged for everyone.

Although the short news post does not mention his age or name, *the jailbreaker* is immediately presumed to be a "young" man. By people who apparently know him or his family, his private online profile is tagged several times in the comments. At some point, he takes part in the discussion and frames his action as a political act of resistance. He says he "will not let them imprison me," and if others let this happen to themselves, it is "their problem, not mine." In this mindset, the pandemic seems to be mainly a political measure (less than a threat of contagious lung disease). "Politics," Max stresses, is not an authority that has to dictate to him and participating in parties would be "a personal decision," which is why he announces that he will

6 At the beginning of 2020, reports on the infectious situation in Italy were very present. In discussions about COVID-19 and the measures associated with the pandemic, "Italy" often functions as a counter-figure to "Corona is just the flu."

7 Asparagus staking is widely known as poorly paid very hard, physical labor that is often outsourced to workers from abroad.

8 The small town is located in a rural area.

continue to do so. Even a state executive in the form of the police cannot harm him; "his lawyer" will take care of this.

In the further course of the discussion, the focus shifts from Max as an individual towards a negotiation of the social figure of *the jailbreaker*. It is, as Moser and Schlechtriemen (2019, 11) as well as Eßbach (2014, 19) state, that the discussion itself turns an individual into a social experience.

So, what can we see by considering *the jailbreaker* as a *social figure*? In the following we are going through the case alongside four "features" of social figures described by Moser and Schlechtriemen which are going to shed light on how they help to articulate social experiences, how they are configured in the discourse, their aesthetic and somatic aspects and their role in ethical positioning.

Articulation of Social Experiences: Negotiating New Rules

Beyond the individual case, the underlying topic of the discussion is the reasonableness and the legitimacy of the infection control measures, which at this point are a new experience and challenge for most people. The fact that one single person "escaped" the metaphorical prison of the curfew and disregarded the rules has an emotionalizing effect, as we can see in the extensive and sometimes violent punishment fantasies. Understanding *the jailbreaker* as an "expression of latent societal tendencies on which contemporaries have not (yet) succeeded in finding a clear stance" (Moser and Schlechtriemen 2019, 11), it may also hint to a subversive potential. The *jailbreaker* discussion appears in a moment of transition when Mitterteich gives everyone else a perspective on their near future events: the rules that got implemented there were soon to be applied – in a modified form – to the whole country as the pandemic continued to spread. In that sense, figures like *the jailbreaker* as a kind of antifigure and antagonist to the political measures have an important function, as they are an essential part of negotiating how to deal with the unknown situation (ibid.).

Moreover, this discussion already reveals what will later become apparent in organized protests all over the country: the role of state and medical institutions, their sovereignty of interpretation and their areas of competence are questioned.

Configuration: Rise and Fall of the Jailbreaker

As indicated above, a social figure like *the jailbreaker* is a highly dynamic affair, a kind of briefly solidified sample:

> As soon as a society has succeeded in elaborating new normative behavioral standards to reflect the changing times, the social figure, as well as the pronounced

> interest in it, disappears. It becomes unattractive and is forgotten, because there is currently no demand for a figurative focus of self-understanding. The process by which social figures fall into disuse may therefore be termed "defiguration:" The key point for all three [(configuration, refiguration, and defiguration] is that they describe constant changes [...]. Hence, social figures represent the (provisional) result of a process of figuration that passes through several stages [...]. (Moser and Schlechtriemen 2019, 12)

As a phenomenon of the early stage of the pandemic, *the jailbreaker* will later be replaced by other characters (such as *the anti-vaxxer*). Configured (Moser and Schlechtriemen 2019, 12) by an urge to negotiate a situation when sickness is not considered a private matter anymore and in which the state reacts with unusual power, *the jailbreaker* increasingly lost his discursive function when people became more accustomed to the pandemic and finally all curfews were lifted. As a breaker of rules, he got modified with each rule and could be refigured (ibid.) when needed. The particular time index (ibid.) of this figure is also related to the highly dynamic perceptions of temporality over the course of the pandemic. Numerous contributions to the discussion reveal how, in this initial phase in 2020, measures are assumed to last no more than 14 days. This perception of time is contrasted in a morally judgmental way with a hedonistic need to meet friends or go to parties. A more general need for social contact would be morally upgraded later in the wider public discourse against the backdrop of longer-lasting contact blocks – a development from which Max cannot yet benefit here.

Aesthetic-Somatic Aspects: Embodiment of Norm-Control and Punishment

Following Moser's and Schlechtriemen's (2019) take on Elias' figurational sociology, one can say the body of the jailbreaker plays an important part in this negotiation about individual practices and risk management. "Social figures are concrete precisely because they 'embody' norm-controlled role-bearers and are therefore observable" (ibid., 13). However, the body of the figure of the escapee is also relevant in another respect. Not only does he make tangible what breaking rules should look like, but through his embodiment he also enables a fictional discussion about what consequences should be drawn from this. Since in this case it is one individual (and not, e.g., an institution or a building), fictional punishments are carried out on his body, among other things, to illustrate how much his behavior is considered wrong. Also infecting the jailbreaker with the (back then) new disease would apparently appear as "fair" to many posters. His body is not one to worry about; rather it is one to suffer illness and punishment. Instead of following a medical ethos that wishes for as few infections as possible, at least a part of the discussants does not seem too averse to the idea that those characters, who do not give in to the community, should get intentionally infected. With such a personification of the right or wrong one can easily get into a fictional dialogue and position oneself near or far from that figure. The negotiation of situations on a figure that embodies (as in this case) the transgression of new rules functions here similarly to a fable and conveys moral messages.

Ethical Positioning: Structuring Moral Fields alongside the Jailbreaker

The last and maybe most important aspect concerns the structuring of the moral field, as "[s]ocial figures constitute a figurative suggestion on how one might behave in the face of a virulent problem in society" (Moser and Schlechtriemen 2019, 13). *The jailbreaker*'s way of dealing with the situation makes people imagine a possible future where all citizens behave like him. The perspective of those who criticize his behavior is pessimistic: many people would get infected with SARS-CoV-2 or the disobedience of the few would lead to an extraordinarily extended curfew for everyone. While the escapee sees himself as a kind of freedom fighter, he obviously represents a moral counter-horizon for the majority; favor a different kind of behavior.

"Argumentative exaggeration" (ibid.) such as demanding draconic punishments is a typical rhetorical device of this kind of discussion. What might appear as an emotionally overloaded social media conversation about a local incident, can thus also be understood as a universal ethical debate beyond the individual case of a person breaking the rules: the question of how to deal with the new and exceptional situation as a society is negotiated. An "ongoing change of social conditions" gets cast into a "human figure and thus making it tangible to the senses" (ibid., 13–14). The fact that *the jailbreaker* is a transgressive figure in several senses triggers the participants in this virtual space to make judgments about him and his actions.

Nonetheless, there is more than one (judgmental) perspective on this incident. While Max himself argues from a position of an unjustified prisoner, the number of his advocates remains relatively small in this imaginary online "court room." Yet there are voices that contest the fierceness of his "verdict" and the intensity of public alertness that "going to a party" receives. The figure we have referred to here as *the jailbreaker* can also be understood as a precursor to a later, broader social discourse. As the pandemic progresses and questions about the appropriateness of political measures are repeatedly raised, other subversive figures emerge. Discursive events around so-called "*Querdenker*" (literally: "lateral thinkers") and "#Covidiots" will shape the further course of public discourse.

Discussion: Narrating (In)justice through Conceptual Metaphors

In public media, the COVID-19 pandemic has often been described as a "silent catastrophe" whose triggers and effects remained very abstract for most people, especially at the beginning. In contrast to flood disasters, earthquakes or other natural events, direct consequences were neither obvious nor evident in public life.[9] What, however, quickly became noticeable and visible were measures taken by policymakers. The pandemic reached the population initially and primarily in the form of laws, rules, prohibitions, and restrictions, combined with moral appeals. In this sense, it is hardly surprising that "the pandemic" as a social phenomenon has repeatedly been perceived primarily as a political issue and discussed accordingly in public. As with other political decisions, questions of (in)justice were raised by the public and a formerly "medical problem" has been translated into a language of law, crime and punishment.

Even beyond the *jailbreaker case*, the idea of having been "imprisoned" is found repeatedly in our empirical data and mostly linked to critical evaluations of this type of infection control measure. Be it, when one year later a member of a social media group posted a reminder to the day when "we got locked in" or interviewees describing the first day of curfew in similar words. *Social figures*, as our example shows, are thus also closely linked to the possibilities of translating new and challenging situations into language in the first place and may rise from conceptual metaphors (Lakoff and Johnson 1980) emerging from practices that appear in the process.

With regard to questions of (in)justice, the conceptual metaphor of imprisoning seems to be especially significant – for both, the overall structure of the respective narratives and the attributions to social figures. In the case of the *jailbreaker*, we can see how the framing of the figure bases the action of the person on normative and moral premises: the mere idea of "jailbreaking" refers to a moral framework of legality, state power, and justice. Demands for "punishment" and "incarceration" or other physical punishments are consequently raised as consequences. It is precisely this idea of being imprisoned or even punished instead of being protected, that is often found in the mind-set of a later developing protest movement. A metaphorical framing of processes of the pandemic with words like "lockdown," "closures," "shutting" etc., coupled with a high public presence of state executives have fueled this. The specificity of this framing becomes even more obvious in comparison to alternative interpretations of the situation. A more protective framing, for example,

9 When the disaster situation was declared in Bavaria in 2020, people only knew this political measure from disasters, which could also be transmitted in clear images (e.g., of destroyed houses). "Corona" as a threat thus seemed rather abstract in comparison and was initially felt primarily through the restrictions on public life.

would have possibly led to the emergence of a different social figure, e.g., *the naïve fool*, taking the warnings not seriously enough.

The *jailbreaker*, thus, resembles other social figures, e.g., Cohen's *folk devil* (le Grand 2019, 416; Cohen 2002) and Tyler's *abject figure* (le Grand 2019, 418; Tyler 2008). "Like the folk devil, the abject figure is a stigmatised scapegoat who emerges during periods of social anxiety and becomes the object of repressive forms of governance and control, although they may also resist such stigmatisation and repression" (le Grand 2019, 418–419). This is an important aspect of the social processing of the pandemic because it does not place the emerging social figures solely in the realm of the fictional. Social figures are not only metaphorical solidifications but are applied to real persons. Along with all attributions and stigmatizations that can have serious repercussions: for example, Max and his family experience hostility in real life. Moreover, our cases study points out to the challenges and complexities of translating medical research into social practices and public narratives.

To summarize this, the analysis of the *jailbreaker case* shows how metaphorical concepts that are used to describe the new and frightening situation of the COVID-outbreak reveal what we can call the moral order of the pandemic. Not only in the local newspapers headlined that Mitterteich was seen as "A Town in Corona custody." Instead, the social figure of the jailbreaker was part of a discursive framing of the counter-epidemic measures as a form of "imprisonment" that helped to articulate and negotiate the new social experience of curfew. The characteristics and re-configurations of the jailbreaker shed light not only on the narrative structure of the pandemic but also its normative and moral premises. It reveals lines of conflict, processes of stigmatization and blaming against the backdrop of a biomedical crisis.

Conclusion: What to Learn from the Jailbreaker Case

In this chapter, we analyzed the *Mitterteich jailbreaker case* as an example of pandemic storytelling. For this, we employed the concept of the social figure as a key to reconstruct the structure of a specific narration and its underlying normative and moral premises. In doing so, we found the character of the *jailbreaker* to be a significant component of the overreaching conceptual metaphor of imprisoning – a concept with far-reaching implications to behavior and meaning-making in the pandemic. We further empirically and exemplarily depicted that using social figures as an analytical concept can help to reveal the social dynamics in the wake of COVID-19 and thus the moral economy of the pandemic. In this vein, the social media group members' attention on the reporting on Max's wrongdoing is not only to interpreted as an interest in local news and the practicability of lockdown regulations. Their various outraged comments mainly convey moral judgments. They document how people at a certain point in time experience the COVID situation and interpret their personal fate. Our analysis of the Mitterteich case reveals that "in empirical reality" implemented measures are understood less in terms of protection than – against the backdrop of a morally evaluative media discourse – as a punishment. In conclusion, compliance to health policy measures seems in praxis often tied to an estimation of (in)justice, rather than to an idea of medical rationality. This ultimately leads not only to questions of dealing with injustice as a task of society, but also to questions of balanced reporting and successful health communication.

Bibliography

Amtmann, Katarina, and Max Kettenbach. 2020. "Weiterhin Ausgangssperre in Mitterteich: Corona-Verbreitung beim Starkbierfest? Brauerei tief betroffen." *Merkur.de*, February 29, 2023. https://www.merkur.de/deutschland/mitterteich-coronavirus-bayern-markus-soeder-starkbierfest-regierungserklaerung-corona-zr-13605704.html

Bayerisches Staatsministerium für Gesundheit und Pflege (Bavarian State Ministry for Health and Care). 2020. "Pressemitteilung. Bestätigter Coronavirus-Fall in Bayern – Infektionsschutzmaßnahmen laufen." https://www.stmgp.bayern.de/presse/bestaetigter-coronavirus-fall-in-bayern-infektionsschutzmassnahmen-laufen/.

Bohnsack, Ralf. 2010. "Documentary Method and Group Discussions." *Qualitative Analysis and Documentary Method in International Education* Research, edited by Barbara Budrich, Verlag Barbara Budrich, 99–124. https://nbn-resolving.org/urn:nbn:de:0168-ssoar-317253.

Charteris-Black, Jonathan. 2021. *Metaphors of Coronavirus Invisible Enemy or Zombie Apocalypse?*, Palgrave Macmillan. http://doi.org/10.1007/978-3-030-85106-4.

Cohen, Stanley. 2002 [1972]. *Folk Devils and Moral Panics: The Creation of the Mods and Rockers*, Routledge.

Davis, Mark and Davina Lohm. 2020. *Pandemics, Publics and Narrative*, Oxford UP.

Die Welt. 2020. *MITTERTEICH: Erster Ort in Bayern mit Ausgangssperre wegen dem Coronavirus*, July 27, 2022. https://www.youtube.com/watch?v=AxXe7udOhMY&t=3s

Eßbach, Wolfgang. 2014. *Religionssoziologie, Vol. 1: Glaubenskrieg und Revolution als Wiege neuer Religionen*, Wilhelm Fink.

Herda, Jürgen. 2020. "Mitterteich im Ausnahmezustand: Eine Stadt in Coronahaft." *Onetz*. https://www.onetz.de/deutschland-welt/mitterteich/mitterteich-ausnahmezustand-stadt-coronahaft-id2997291.html.

Keller, Reiner. 2005. "Analysing Discourse. An Approach from the Sociology of Knowledge." *Forum Qualitative Sozialforschung / Forum: Qualitative Social Research*, vol. 6, no. 3 (September 2005). http://nbn-resolving.de/urn:nbn:de:0114-fqs0503327.

Lakoff, George and Mark Johnson. 1980. *Metaphors We Live By*, U of Chicago P.

Langenohl, Andreas. 2011. "Öffentliche Reaktionen auf das Schweizer Referendum über Minarettbau und auf ‚Deutschland schafft sich ab.'" *Gießener Universitätsblätter*, vol. 44, Gießener Hochschulgesellschaft, 83–94. http://doi.org/10.22029/jlupub-5564.

Lee, Jon D. 2014. *An Epidemic of Rumors. How Stories Shape Our Perceptions of Disease*, UP of Colorado.

le Grand, Elias. 2019. "Conceptualising Social Types and Figures: From Social Forms to Classificatory Struggles." *Cultural Sociology*, vol. 13, no. 4 (September 2019), 411–427. http://doi/10.1177/1749975519859962.

Lill, Tobias. 2020. "Bayerns fatale Liebe zum Starkbier." *Spiegel Online*. https://www.spiegel.de/panorama/gesellschaft/corona-krise-in-bayern-die-fatale-liebe-zum-starkbier-a-b400b534-3f22-4de9-8549-1f657f502e97.

Mayring, Philipp. 2014. *Qualitative content analysis: theoretical foundation, basic procedures and software solution*, Beltz.

Merunkova, Lucie, and Josef Slerka. 2019. "Goffman's theory as a framework for analysis of self-presentation on online social networks." *Masaryk University Journal of Law and Technology*, vol. 13, no. 2, 243–276. https://journals.muni.cz/mujlt/article/view/11836.

Moser, Sebastian J., and Tobias Schlechtriemen. 2018. "Sozialfiguren – zwischen gesellschaftlicher Erfahrung und soziologischer Diagnose. Social Figures – Between Societal Experience and Sociological Diagnosis." *Zeitschrift für Soziologie*, vol. 47, no. 3, 164–180. http://doi.org/10.1515/zfsoz-2018-1011.

Moser, Sebastian J., and Tobias Schlechtriemen. 2019. "Social Figures – Between societal experience and sociological diagnosis." *Fondation Maison des sciences de l'homme*. https://halshs.archives-ouvertes.fr/halshs-01972078/document.

Moser, Sebastian J., and Tobias Schlechtriemen. 2020. "Sozialfiguren der Corona-Pandemie – ein Aufschlag." *Sozialfiguren der Corona-Pandemie*, Kulturwissenschaftlichen Instituts Essen. https://doi.org/10.37189/kwi-blog/20201116-0900.

Müller, Marion. 2020. "Der Maskenverweigerer Die Suche nach einem Schurken in der Pandemie." *Sozialfiguren der Corona-Pandemie*, Kulturwissenschaftlichen Instituts Essen. http://doi.org/10.37189/kwi-blog/20201116-0900.

Schmitt, Rudolf. 2005. "Systematic Metaphor Analysis as a Method of Qualitative Research." *The Qualitative Report*, vol. 10, no. 2, 358–394. http://doi.org/10.46743/2160-3715/2005.1854

Sontag, Susan. 2002. *Illness as Metaphor & Aids and its Metaphors*, Penguin.

Tyler, Imogen. 2008. "Chav mum chav scum. Class disgust in contemporary Britain." *Feminist Media Studies*, vol. 8, no. 1 (March 2008), 17–34. http://doi/abs/10.1080/14680770701824779.

Narratives and Morality

Don't Judge Me!
Anti-Judgementalism and Anti-Moralism in the Corona Pandemic

Moritz Ege, Julian Schmitzberger

Introduction

During the COVID-19 pandemic, the routines of everyday life were disrupted and re-arranged. This crisis was accompanied by reflections and debates on the (un)ethical character of practical decisions concerning one's own personal actions as well as those of others – reflections that were seen to have direct or indirect life-or-death consequences.[1] Governments, public health officials and many others communicated in strongly moral terms.[2] As people maneuvered through these unprecedented circumstances, a sense of moral urgency gained prominence. On the other hand, being confronted with a series of moral demands, many people took the view that it is wrong – or even unjust – to judge others for their behavior, and that, consequently, they – and others – should not be judged.

In the following, we take up the principle foundational to this attitude which we term *anti-judgmentalism*: a felt and/or argued opposition to others' moral judgments in which implied demands are rejected not primarily for their inherent right- or wrongness but rather for being illegitimate in a more categorical sense. Anti-judgmentalism can be seen as a general critique of a propensity for making moral judgments that are seen as overreaching, excessive, inadequate, underinformed, or hypocritical. In consequence, apodictic anti-judgmental statements – such as "don't

1 This is reminiscent to what cultural anthropologist Jarret Zigon terms "moral breakdown" (2007).

2 Moralized (which in this case means focused on others' interests) public health communication was recommended for example, by Luttrell and Petty (2021), based on a psychological study. At the same time, this study also found that people who did not see public health as a strongly moral issue in general were also much less responsive to moral communication.

judge me!" – imply a reference to common-sense understandings of the "right" and the "wrong" place of moral judgments and morality in life.[3]

Recently, moral philosophers have addressed the problem of overreaching or hypocritical moral judgments as core aspects of moralism (Neuhäuser and Seidel 2020; Mieth and Rosenthal 2020). Anti-judgmentalism in the sense in which we are analyzing it here can indeed be seen as a (sub-)form of *anti*-moralism[4]: a generalized rejection of the moral register that is, we argue, rooted in everyday, vernacular culture, and that circulates in popular media as well as in a broader discursive sphere. As researchers of everyday life, we are less interested in developing a general philosophical concept or conducting a straightforwardly normative discussion, but rather in conceptualizing anti-judgmentalism as a "cultural theme" (Lindner 2003) that is embedded in and emerges from everyday narratives. Our goal in this chapter is to explore this theme and its meanings in different arenas; we aim to situate it in its societal contexts and conditions. For this purpose, we use tools from transdisciplinary cultural analysis, combining an analysis of public – including pop-cultural – discourses with a close, ethnographic attention to lifeworld-level dynamics, everyday (linguistic) practices and subjective attitudes and sentiments. Our explication and contextualization of moral (counter-)claims is inspired by (descriptive-analytical) sociological and cultural-anthropological studies of ethics and morality that have shown how social practices establish ethics and morality as seemingly self-evident domains (Thompson 2012; Fassin 2015; Fassin and Lézé 2014; Hinrichsen 2019). This includes work on the "problematization" of morality in relation to shifting forms of subjectivity and subjectivation (Foucault 1992; 1997; Collier and Lakoff 2005; Ege 2022), on public moral panics and moral regulation (Hunt 1999; Hier 2011; 2019), or the morality and politics of humanitarianism (Ticktin 2011; Fassin 2015).

By exploring the sources and the intertextual connections and resonances that define anti-judgmentalism as a cultural theme in the present moment, the chapter will contribute to a phenomenology of "aversive sentiments" in moral interpellations and counter-interpellations, as well as their narrative constitution, and thereby to an analysis of the subjective side of the current conjuncture.[5] Long before the pan-

3 We follow a Gramscian approach to common-sense as historically sedimented, heterogeneous and potentially contradictory (Gramsci 1971: 324; cf. Crehan 2002; Hall and O'Shea 2013; Sutter 2016).

4 See, for example, Coady 2006; Neuhäuser and Seidel 2020 and the contributions to their edited volume, which primarily focuses on moral philosophy and ethics. On anti-moralism, cf. the ongoing research project "Disintegration through morality? Moral argumentation and the moralism charge in public debates," directed by Cord Schmelzle at the research institute on social cohesion.

5 Literary theorist Amlinger and sociologist Nachtwey (2022) have argued that recent protests against COVID regulations exemplify a new political formation of "libertarian authoritarian-

demic, Lawrence Grossberg, Wendy Brown and other critical theorists pointed out that the experiential plane of the present conjuncture is characterized by widespread confusion over the relation and the borders between morality and politics (Brown 2020; 2001; Grossberg 2018).[6] While their diagnoses point to different societal problematics, their basic argument is that there is *dissensus* about these questions, but also widespread (affective) *unclarity*: what is the status of demands for moral or ethical behavior in contemporary public and private lives – when there is so much obvious *systemic* injustice and hypocrisy?[7] What are we to make of demands of morality and moral orientations for the conduct of everyday life that are expressed by authorities of various types that otherwise set demands for people to be ruthlessly competitive? Are "we" demanding moral purity – from ourselves and others – in ways that are unrealistic despite our knowledge that humans and their practices have all sorts of motivations that differ radically from moral self-images and rationalizations? These questions are often experienced as personal and emotional – as our empirical investigation will demonstrate.

Overview

Anti-judgmentalism's roots transcend our present historical moment.[8] To lay the groundwork for an understanding of the rejection of moral claims and judgments during the Coronavirus pandemic, we first need to survey a broader semantic and discursive field and introduce different genealogical strands of the theme. For that purpose, we will first take a closer look at semantics of the German-language equivalences of "to judge" (*urteilen*). Building on the exploratory methodology suggested for the analysis of cross-domain cultural fields by Williams (1977), Lindner (2003), Ehn, Löfgren, and Wilk (2016), and others, we then follow anti-judgmentalism through

---

ism": According to these authors, frustrated demands for autonomy and an "expansion of the zone of narcissistic hurt" (2022, 146–163, dt. *Ausweitung der Kränkungszone*) have given rise to a radically individualistic and resentful formation of protest subjectivities. "Aversive sentiments" are a central aspect in this context.

6 Fassin, Ticktin and other anthropologists have stressed the depoliticizing dangers of humanitarian moralism, while also stressing that the ethical and the political are impossible to disentangle (Fassin 2015; Ticktin 2011).

7 Some commentators in left-leaning Cultural Studies such as Jeremy Gilbert and Alex Williams (2022) come to the political conclusion that "moralism" (which they connect to "liberal identitarianism") should generally be avoided, arguing instead for a politics of solidarity centered around the realization of collectively shared (material) interests. The problem with this position is that definitions of moralism differ widely, as we will see below. It may be more difficult to draw the line between ethical-political positions (in a Gramscian sense of the hyphenated term) and "moralism" than the authors suggest.

8 In the sense of their genealogical *Herkunft*, not their *Ursprung* (Foucault 1978).

very different discursive fields where it has been expressed and shaped – the Bible, pop songs, as well as popular psychology and self-help writings.[9] We then turn to anti-judgmentalism during the rise of the Corona virus to show how people make use of those circulating themes in order to make sense of and navigate through the ethico-political challenges of the pandemic in 2020/2021. We trace anti-judgmentalism through German-language newspaper articles and commentaries which were published during the outbreak of COVID-19. Here, critical reflections on and invectives against "judging" could be found especially in political discussions about the pitfalls of the state's governance of public behavior, and the links between populist and anti-judgmentalist discourse becomes palpable. We then shift registers and draw from Schmitzberger's ethnographic study, which includes extensive and repeated qualitative interviews with partygoers and club culture participants in Germany that took place during the acute phase of the pandemic – i.e., we shift from public narratives to everyday narrations. As putative representatives of a hedonistic fraction of a younger generation, the interviewees provide a particularly interesting case study of the moral experience of life during the COVID crisis.[10] Building on this, we suggest a new typology of two main forms of anti-judgmentalism – and, ultimately, anti-moralism more broadly – which have very different social and political implications.

Verurteilen/judgen: A Note on Semantics

Specific words, expressions and idioms in different languages matter greatly here as they give shape to vaguer sentiments. Our examples are from Germany and German-speaking Switzerland where most people speak of *verurteilen*, one of the two most common translation options for the English word "to judge." "*Verurteilen*" is the main term used in situations in which English-speakers would commonly be speaking of "judging." It refers to negative judgments, primarily to moral condemnation (as in politicians publicly "condemning" acts of other governments), but also to legal judgments.[11] *Verurteilen* not only has the meaning "to judge," and "to condemn," but also "to sentence," as in the activity of judges – or of God.[12] The other German

9 In doing so we draw from an ongoing investigation of popular cultural (anti-)moralisms (Ege 2022, 2024).

10 A few notes on the methodology and contexts of these interviews will be provided below.

11 The role of the "juridical unconscious" and the permutation of trials as models and metaphor will have to remain unexamined here; cf. Felman 2002.

12 Here also is the partly synonymous, more anachronistic German verb "*richten*" – which Martin Luther used in his translation of the gospel of Matthew in the New Testament (Jesus says: "*Richtet nicht, damit ihr nicht gerichtet werdet,*" Matthew 7:1-5).

translation option for "judging" is "*beurteilen.*" It means to judge by merit, aesthetics, or morality in professional contexts (e.g., in the work of teachers or prize juries), but it can also refer to everyday classifications and evaluations, including judgments about attractiveness.[13] *Beurteilen* is also related to a broad spectrum of institutionally embedded social practices.

Most of the sources and data we have surveyed speak of *verurteilen* and *urteilen* where English speakers would only use "to judge." Moreover, the anglicism *judgen* (to judge) has been incorporated into German, especially among younger people. Even the adjective *judgy* appears regularly in some variants of everyday, vernacular language. At first sight, anti-judgmentalism as a cultural theme mostly seems to concern judging in the sense of *verurteilen*. But as we will show, the other semantic elements (including *beurteilen/bewerten*) regularly play into anti-judgmentalist statements as well, and the use of the anglicism can imply further ambiguities. These ambiguities, we argue, are not only crucial for their appeal but have profound consequences on how everyday life – especially in times of the pandemic – is being made sense of and narrated.

Sources of Anti-Judgmentalism

The causes for a generalized desire (and demand) not to be judged to some extent fall into a psychological domain that is difficult to access for cultural researchers. As we are concerned here with anti-judgmentalism as a theme and pattern, we are interested in the sources and the practical logics of common-sense thought, narratives, and arguments, rather than in causal explanations. What, then, are the historically concrete and specific sources of the common-sense "knowledge" that is expressed by an apodictic statement such as "Don't judge me!"?

A provisional sketch of such an inventory can draw from different domains, including religious teachings, popularized secular philosophy, psychology, guidelines for conduct, conventions in vernacular language (sayings, proverbs, quotes) and other popular cultural representations. The Bible contains what are probably the most famous proverbial formulations against judgmentalism: the speck of sawdust in another's eye and the plank in your own; he who is without guilt shall cast the first stone; judge not so that ye be not judged. Judging (*richten*, *verurteilen*) is seen as the domain of God in which mortals with their limited knowledge – and

13 In that sense, *Beurteilung* is close to *Bewertung* and could be translated as "evaluation" as well. It can be argued that judging has taken on specific qualities (and perhaps also a qualitatively different quantity) in the current sociopolitical and technological conjuncture (Fourcade 2016; Groth 2019).

authority – should not interfere.[14] Popular music represents an arena in which normative cultural meanings, including religious ones, have long been activated, translated and recontextualized. This is particularly strong in the – near-globally influential – African American tradition, which famously relies on the Black church, especially in the Gospel/Soul/Disco/House trajectory ("Mother, mother / Everybody thinks we're wrong / But who are they to judge us," Marvin Gaye, "What's Going On," 1971). In popular rap anthems like Tupac Shakur's "Only God Can Judge Me" (1999), theological meanings blend with a form of "hard" sociological naturalism, which represents another discursive thread: In these lyrics, the rapper prototypically claims that "judging" someone like him, a streetwise hustler and gangster in a racist society, should be left to God; those who haven't lived this kind of life ("each and every black male's trapped") and lack the basis for understanding it should not judge it. In newer usages such as FKA Twigs's experimental RnB/rap song "Don't Judge Me" (2021), moral fallibility is also traced back to societal forces and hostile circumstances, whereas judgments are depicted as a form of (internalized) oppression.[15]

There are numerous other discursive threads and arenas that could be considered as sources of contemporary anti-judgmentalism. For present purposes, we confine ourselves to one: In contemporary popular psychology, life coaching and self-help discourse, judging (in the sense of *verurteilen*, but also *beurteilen*) is a particularly prominent theme. These discourses reach a much wider audience than academic philosophy and ethics. Podcasts – a crucial medium of today's popular culture – and life advice blogs are a good starting point for an exploration of this discursive strand. To survey some of the usages and meanings, we performed a (German-language) keyword search for *verurteilen* on Spotify and Apple Podcasts. Aside from entries in the fields of crime/law/jurisdiction and religion/religious ethics, the search led us to podcasts in the intersecting fields of popular psychology, life coaching, self-help and guides for mental health and spiritual mindfulness.[16] Such podcast episodes

---

14 While this is well-known core teaching in Christian and post-Christian contexts, the English term "judging" seems to be more obviously connected to the Biblical interdiction than the German term *verurteilen*, if only because in most Bible translations the word *richten* is used. A more modern English version is "[d]o not judge, or you too will be judged. For in the same way you judge others, you will be judged, and with the measure you use, it will be measured to you. / Why do you look at the speck of sawdust in your brother's eye and pay no attention to your own eye" (NIV).

15 Cf. Ege 2024.

16 We examined five podcasts in-depth in regard to how the word *verurteilen* is used, as well as the argumentative patterns in which such statements are embedded, and the normative beliefs and bodies of knowledge on which those reflections are based. In doing so, we methodologically follow the approach of qualitative content analysis, although our research results are more illustrative in nature rather than claiming to fully represent the popular discourse

have titles like "Life is a walk in the park. How to live a joyful life: Why we judge others," "Love Balance Remembrance: Why it doesn't matter what others think of us – why we evaluate and judge and how we stop our judgment," or "Words don't fail me. Your non-violent communication podcast: 3 reasons why we judge others – and how to transform your judgments."

In most of these texts, judgmental attitudes and judging as a practice are presented as bad habits or as weaknesses to be overcome. Therapeutic writers tend to identify the "subconscious" as the guilty party – the problematic "ethical substance" in the terminology of Foucault's analysis of ethical subjectivity (Foucault 1992). They often propose a plan for better, more efficient self-care: being happier and mentally healthy is the main stated goal. They usually also formulate a related ethical program. This is illustrated by a listicle-style BuzzFeed blog article from 2018.[17] The German version is titled "*10 Tipps für alle Menschen, die gerne mal über andere urteilen*" ("10 pieces of advice for all people who like to judge others"). It includes statements like "[j]udging others doesn't only hurt the people it is directed at. It also very much damages the person who voices the criticism. So be nice to others and show them (and yourself!) some compassion!" The overall goal is to "climb down from your high horse" and become a better, "more loving and caring" person. Coaches recommend therapeutic practices like biographical self-examination, breathing exercises and aromatherapy for relief against judgmental habits. The latter, they believe, are ultimately forms of externalized auto-aggression.

Such snippets from self-help/life-coaching texts offer a glance at the commonsense variant of anti-judgmental, anti-normative discourse. While we based our search on "*verurteilen*," it is remarkable that here and in many other examples, there is no clear distinction being made between *verurteilen*, *beurteilen*, *urteilen*, and *bewerten* – these words are used almost interchangeably. They are presented as "bad" practices, psychologically unhealthy and presumptuous classification, and reproach. In this context, it is important to point out that the objects of everyday judgments are not always of a straightforward "moral" type: the BuzzFeed article, for example, mentions judgments in everyday situations such as not liking the best friend's new boyfriend or judging a colleague for wearing an outfit that one finds unsuitable for a day at the office. Such criticism is directed at the enactment of other forms of normativity, such as evaluations of others' adherence to social conventions, their aesthetic competence, or, to some extent, their chances on the path to a "good life." While morality

on the topic. Our method only yielded empirical data explicitly addressing contemporary understandings of *verurteilen*.

17 The article was partly rewritten and translated into German one year later (Hallett 2018; BuzzFeed 2019) – which illustrates mechanisms of transnational popular cultural circulation and transfer.

and other forms of normativity can be separated analytically, as can the different semantic components of *(ver-)urteilen*, the actual usage of the term "judging" and its equivalents often merges them.

In following these texts, one also learns that those who make judgments about others are per se depicted as problematic subjects. They suggest that this anti-judgmentalist attitude should be common-sense knowledge. While some of the texts also accept judging as a natural human tendency, based on the need to compare oneself to others, they argue that those who judge uninhibitedly are in a sense pathological.[18] They are criticized for projecting their own feelings and needs onto others, and for being unmindful, over-hasty, or superficial – and therefore unjust. But while it is clear, within this logic, that judgmental people are problematic people, the BuzzFeed article also warns of potentially paradoxical effects of thinking through the problematic of judging *in an overly judgmental manner* in reference to one's own self: "Be forgiving to yourself if you have a bad conscience because you judge others. To criticize someone else and then judge yourself for it is a psychic muddle that you don't need!"

While such second-order dilemmas can be seen as amusing, we do not intend to ridicule this discourse here, but to better understand its implications. It has become clear already from this brief overview that the psychological pathologization of "judging" suggests an ego-centered view of human relations and responsibilities: The ability to solve problems relies primarily on one's own capacities and training; it is suggested that it is better to work out problems on your own instead of having arguments with others – or a public debate about them. In that sense, it can be seen a symptom and conveyor not just of a broad sociocultural trend of "therapeutization" (Maasen et al. 2011), but of a neoliberal culture (Hall and O'Shea 2013) that is pervaded by selves that are schooled in reflexive psychological knowledge. The blurring of the lines between judgments of taste and aesthetics, personal and idiosyncratic aversions, and classic tropes of morality, is particularly important in this context. In this logic and in this rhetoric, which is often apodictic, the taboo of judging tends to be understood as a generalized maxim that should be applied to all sorts of circumstances. These texts propagate a generalized ethic of non-normativity and also of non-engagement. This non-engagement and the concomitant abdication of responsibility are the libertarian flipside of an anti-judgmentalism that defends the integrity of the self. As therapeutic vernacular would put it: "you do you!"

---

18 A common, but usually unspoken reference point are psychological concepts from "social comparison theory" (Festinger 1954), which are standard elements of (academic) psychology curricula. According to Festinger, there is a human drive to evaluate each other's abilities and opinions. Comparing oneself to others is a way of determining how individuals fit with certain groups of people and, more broadly speaking, it is a means by which oneself finds a place in the world.

Having sketched these discursive strands and briefly alluded to their political implications, we now turn to anti-judgmentalism during the COVID-19 pandemic, for which these strands provide context and resonance. We will look at German-language newspaper articles, including opinion pieces and more subjective-introspective text genres, during the first year of the pandemic.[19]

The "Don't Judge" Theme in Diagnostics of the Present Moment during the Coronavirus Pandemic

In an opinion piece in the newspapers of the Tamedia group in Switzerland in summer 2021, author Andreas Kurz warned of a coming "*Corona-Apartheid*."[20] The piece is presented as a liberal-conservative take on the pandemic, in line with the country's liberal tradition. Kurz opposes the policy proposals brought forth by the people whom the author calls "the over-cautious," such as requiring vaccination certificates as a prerequisite for using public transportation or entering restaurants and other semi-public spaces. The author goes on to argue that as there are people who have good reasons for not wanting to be vaccinated, there should be no policies that result in disadvantages for the unvaccinated: "These are legitimate opinions which one shouldn't judge (*die man nicht verurteilen sollte*). Firstly, because it is bad form in a democratic society (*weil es sich ... in einer demokratischen Gesellschaft nicht gehört*). And secondly, because it does not work, as the hardening of debates in recent weeks has shown." The presentations of these matters in the anonymous third person is typical here: speakers/authors of such texts often present observations (or speculations) about the ways in which others, mostly nameless "everyday people," perceive unfair judgments – usually without citing empirical evidence that supports their argument.

Why has the author chosen the term "*verurteilen*" that primarily denotes moral condemnation? Implicitly, the argument claims that "the overcautious" propose a direct path from their own moral judgments (about others) to legal rules, but that those moral judgments are spurious and even categorically illegitimate: in a democracy, opinions one disagrees with (at least within a certain corridor) *should not be morally condemned*. This is not a self-evident argument: Many people will feel that some political opinions are indeed morally wrong (as, for example, adhering to them

19 Articles were collected through a search for "Corona" and "verurteilen" (starting in February of 2020) in the LexisNexis newspaper database in September 2021. The sources cited here represent themes collected from this set.

20 Andreas Kurz, *Eine Corona-Apartheid darf es nicht geben*, Kommentar, *Der Tagesanzeiger* (and other Tamedia newspapers), July 24, 2021.

may – like in the Coronavirus case – lead to avoidable deaths). The argument is, however, reminiscent of a prominent strand of writings in German-language political philosophy and theory opposed to "political moralism" (some prominent examples: Gehlen 2004; Koselleck 1979; Lübbe 1985; 2019; Cappenberger Gespräch et al. 1985; Luhmann 2008a) that has been revived in recent years, especially on the political right and among self-described post-left "realists" (Grau 2017; Stegemann 2018; Bolz 2021).[21] In this realm, moral discourses are seen as simplifying complex institutional matters into theology-derived distinctions between good and evil, which necessitate arguments *ad personam* (i.e., from a moralist perspective, good or evil positions are almost inevitably taken by good or evil persons) that are strongly judgmental. Furthermore, from this self-described realist, anti-moralist perspective, moralism is "polemogenous" (Luhmann 2008a), it creates strife because moral absolutism precludes compromise and a sober negotiation of interests.

Whether or not one finds these arguments compelling, it is notable that the author chooses to shift his article onto a (meta-)level reminiscent of that debate in the first place. His argument moves the political debate onto the level of a debate over the legitimacy of moral judgments in general. At the same time, its main thrust concerns government policies, i.e., *legally* binding prescriptions. These can (and, one may add, should) of course be supported by moral arguments, but they are nevertheless different in character, as is the political process of putting them in place. After all, the most pressing political question in that situation could arguably be whether such certificates were in themselves useful and legitimate policy, not whether in calling for such policies, people were making overly moral arguments. A first observation about the "don't judge" theme in this context, then, is that anti-judgmentalists like this author move the framework from discussions of actual policy to questions about the tactfulness (or legitimacy) of moral arguments in general.[22]

This discursive strand involves loose phenomenological observations as well as references to more codified forms of psychological knowledge. Maja Beckers, writing for *Die Zeit* in the fall of 2020, observes a new type of sentiment in public life which she terms "*Corona-Scham*": in her perception, there are now many cases where showing symptoms such as coughing in public means "being in danger" of "being judged as not cautious enough" (*läuft Gefahr, als unvorsichtig verurteilt zu werden*) in everyday situations. This is seen as problematic and unfair; in typical fashion, the argument is supported by anecdotal narratives about the author's emotional experience.

---

21 Some of this – including Gehlen's work – goes back to the works of Carl Schmitt, the fascist legal theorist and critic of liberalism. However, there is a much longer (and international) genealogy of such arguments that involves (politically ambiguous, but often conservative) arguments such as Burke's critique of anti-traditionalist universalism and Hegel's critique of Kant's ethics.

22 On tact as a necessary suspension of moral demands, cf. Luhmann 2008b.

The term "*Corona-Scham*" (probably best translated as "Corona shame" or "embarrassment") implies both unfair judgments and a vague but powerful sense of internalized self-aggression.[23] It thereby evokes popularized psychological concepts such as ego-ideal, super-ego or the guilty conscience.

Aversions to being judged are part of a broader landscape of negative feelings that merge and articulate with "aversive sentiments" of a stronger political character. The "don't judge" theme is a specific strand here. The fact that the problem of suffering under others' moral judgments becomes assigned to all sorts of situations and groups during the Coronavirus pandemic through such narrations suggests that it is indeed part of an important contemporary (moral) *structure of feeling* (Williams 1961; 1973). Furthermore, this section has shown that the theme is not only present in everyday language and informal talk, but it is also evoked by professional intellectuals of various kinds. Specialists in "diagnostics of the present moment" (*Zeitdiagnosen*) take up this theme, and they do so in ways that often seem rhetorically and politically strategic. Their empirical claims about psychological-political dynamics are not necessarily self-evident – which is not to say that they are all-around counterfactual. What matters more here is that they potentially have performative effects, providing resources for and guiding everyday narrations. Overall, we are witnessing a process in which articulations between everyday affects, identities and political projects are being established and "common sense" is being shaped and negotiated both on a cognitive-discursive and affective-emotional level.

Critics of judgmentalism in this vein, then, depict demands for specific policies as unrealistic, hypocritical, and morally overdemanding and exhausting, and in doing so, they also claim to refer to common-sense knowledge about the proper place of morality in life.

Don't Judge Me: A Lifeworld Perspective on Anti-Judgmentalism(s) in Hedonistic Youth Cultural Contexts

In the next section, we move from public discourses to everyday experience and to common-sense narratives and reflections. How do anti-judgmentalist complaints about the "injustice" of judgmentalism during the Coronavirus pandemic resonate in life-world contexts?

To think through these questions, we draw on Julian Schmitzberger's case study about the world of club cultures among people mainly in their 20s and 30s in Berlin,

23 The article "teaser" claims very broad societal relevance for that observation: "A feeling comes to be in charge of social control" (*Zeit Online*, 13. Oktober 2020). The term is reminiscent of the neologism *Flugscham*, which refers to the feeling of guilt that is connected to air travel due to its impact on the world's climate.

Germany.[24] We chose this field for pragmatic reasons and as an exploratory case. Obviously, this scene does not represent the social attitudes of the population more broadly. However, our interest in the overall theme of anti-judgmentalism was piqued here: in interviews conducted with club-goers living in Berlin during the pandemic, research participants repeatedly brought up this topic without having been prompted by the interviewer. For exploratory research, the case is particularly interesting because of the apparent tensions between a hedonistic orientation – partying – prevalent here and the nature of the moral demands during the pandemic. As we will show, anti-judgmentalism does indeed resonate here, but in more differentiated ways than could be expected from a reading of public discourses alone. To illustrate and thickly describe these dynamics and to place them in their life-world contexts, we will introduce Fabian, a university student, Lena, also a student, and Marie, an actor.[25] As will become clear, all three perceive a pervasive societal judgmentalism and are highly critical of it – and of moralist attitudes more broadly. They tend to reflect on these matters in a searching mode that accommodates contradictions – but at times fall into a rather apodictic tone as well. While criticizing others' overreaching moral judgments in a generalizing manner, they also make highly moral statements themselves, producing an ambiguous position between moralization and anti-moralism. The implications of these statements, however, are very different – and in this, they point to different forms of anti-judgmentalism that, we suggest, contribute to the landscape of common sense in the current conjuncture.

24 As part of his ethnographic research project on club cultures and nightlife, Schmitzberger planned and conducted 25 interviews with partygoers from Berlin during the acute phase of the pandemic between November 2020 and February 2021. Due to the legal measures which banned cultural events, he contacted his research participants via social media, especially Instagram and Facebook. The interviews took place in a private atmosphere and collected data on how clubbing is experienced and thought of as well as how club-goers dealt with the COVID-19 crisis in particular. Although the conversations were based on a guideline which included a broad range of topics, they were not structured in a strict manner and must be imagined as guided but "organic" dialogues. This narrative approach is meant to guarantee that interviewees can formulate thoughts and views in an open manner; the dialogical aspect also implies that interview statements do more than "reflect" pre-formed thoughts. The following interview quotes have been translated from German by the authors.

25 We use first names here because this reflects the informal atmosphere during the interviews. Those three interviewees are not the only ones who referred to forms of (anti-)judgmentalism. The following passages must be seen as case studies that exemplify general cultural dynamics. Among the things that set these interviewees apart from many other people, however, are their age, urban residence, their high level of education and their orientation to a hedonistic lifestyle.

Fabian, the Anti-Moralist

When Fabian takes a seat on the couch for an interview about clubbing in Berlin, it is late December 2020. A lockdown to reduce the spread of COVID-19 has been in force in Germany for almost two months. Public life is heavily restricted, though the protective measures are not as severe as they had been in the first lockdown from March to May of the same year. Businesses that aren't part of the country's critical infrastructure must remain closed. Keeping physical distance remains the main goal of official epidemiological policies. According to newly introduced legislation, only two people from a maximum of two households are allowed to meet in private. In the beginning of the interview, Fabian talks about his plans for New Year's Eve. He seems to be of two minds: on the one hand, a party he's heard of – which will be in violation of the regulations – attracts him strongly. Before the outbreak of COVID-19, he went out clubbing almost every weekend. "It's going to be lit. Dancing on three floors in a squatted house, somewhere on the outskirts of Berlin," he says. "Real underground shit." On the other hand, he also points out that it is selfish and "irresponsible" to attend such an event during a pandemic that is life-threatening to some. He might go there, he ponders, but then he would feel ashamed – even if he measured his temperature in advance and did a rapid test. As the interview progresses, the self-avowedly hedonistic twenty-year-old gives a detailed and lively report on an unauthorized rave (one out of two) he hosted this year, during the pandemic, in a forest somewhere in the adjacent state of Brandenburg. He had no reservations when he was organizing the event. "After all, the case numbers were very low at that time," he says with confidence.

The second interview with Fabian takes place in January 2021, about three weeks later. The lockdown is still in effect and the COVID-19 death toll has reached its historic high. Fabian didn't go the New Year's Eve party he was speaking of the last time – primarily for pragmatic reasons. "We didn't get the GPS location until six-thirty in the evening, so we didn't feel like it anymore," he says at the beginning of the conversation. Instead, he celebrated in a small circle of good friends. He seems quite content, speaking of getting up early on New Year's Day to jog while listening to a good DJ set playing through his headphones. The pandemic has given him the chance to read more books, to get enough sleep and to cope with his everyday life, as he puts it. However, even though Fabian appears to be fine with New Year's Eve not having been a big night out, his inner turmoil has not ended. He seems to have a hard time distancing himself from the magnetic world of clubbing and claims he would spend a hundred Euros to be able to go to his favorite club if that were possible.

Then, quite suddenly, he changes the subject to the way he deals with the current situation. Fabian states that he complies with the latest government policies, at least to a large extent:

> In principle, I only see only one person at a time. I'm meeting a lot of people overall but almost everyone I know does so. All of us stick by the rules for the most part, but no one is trying to be perfect, you know. Otherwise, you'd go nuts, that's for sure. Don't get me wrong. I don't want to start a debate about righteous behavior during COVID. I just want to tell you how I do it. I won't let anybody judge me either (*Ich lass mich dafür auch nicht verurteilen*). I've already come to blows with others who'd say things like: "That's so unnecessary. Try to limit your contacts." And I was like: "Yo, sorry not sorry. Who are you to tell me how to live my life?" I keep following the rules, most of the time. Maybe not on New Year's, but nevertheless.

Fabian says that he does not want to be judged – i.e., morally condemned – for planning to invite a few friends over for his birthday this week, either, even though, strictly speaking, this would violate legal measures. Like many others, at this point in the pandemic he has established an ambiguous position towards the rules, going back and forth between rule-following and -breaking. He resents that many people consider him "egotistic" for meeting up with groups of others: "I think it's absolutely insincere that everyone is suddenly running around acting like utilitaristic do-gooders (*utilitaristische Gutmenschen*)." Reflecting on these matters in the second interview, Fabian talks himself into a rage – and begins a monologue about moral contradictions. His arguments are addressed to an undefined, imaginary counterpart (not the interviewer), switching back and forth between defending his stance and going onto the offensive, attacking others' hypocrisy. Fabian criticizes that it is considered socially acceptable to buy clothes at fast fashion brands like Primark or SHEIN: "If a garment factory in Bangladesh collapses, everyone is like 'Oh, my god!,' but two weeks later, they're walking into a store to buy a new top." Whilst others leave these everyday habits unquestioned, he claims to at least feel remorse when succumbing to them occasionally. Fabian is a vegetarian – for ethical reasons, not because he does not like to eat meat. Even if he boards a plane for a flight once a year, he at least does so having "calculated" the downside effects for the environment, he states. He argues that his conscience weighs more heavily on him when he buys ice cream at McDonald's than when he organizes an open-air rave during a pandemic. To him, any allegations in this regard seem "ridiculous" and presumptuous: "Those people wear outfits by H&M, they just had a *Wiener Würstchen* and then they judge you (*verurteilen dich*) because you did two raves. This simply doesn't add up."[26] Fabian's spontaneous rant ends with a small concession – and unexpected sympathy for those who may turn against him:

26 These are everyday consumption choices that, seen through the lens of claims to social justice and environmental protection, have long been publicly defined as morally problematic (Thompson 2012; Milkman 2017).

> It's ok if people judge me (*Ich kann es auch verstehen, wenn Leute mich verurteilen*). I get it, totally. I don't think they're stupid. Probably, they could be right, but we still live in an individualistic world – take it or leave it. I don't claim that everything I do is advisable or righteous. I just know if something's worth doing. In this respect, it's all about me and maintaining my wellbeing.[27]

Fabian's tirade and its ambiguities situate the demands for "good" behavior during this exceptional time in the context of a broader, contradictory "moralization" of everyday life – in spheres such as shopping, food, and mobility. Reflections like Fabian's are, as we have shown, enmeshed in a range of public discourses on (anti-)moralism, taking up the unclarity of the role of morality in everyday life that theorists like Grossberg and Brown see as typical for the ways in which the present conjuncture is experienced. His statements present high moral standards and a concern for global injustices on the one hand and a radically individualistic rejection of moral demands on the other. Referring to maintaining his wellbeing can be seen as a symptom of the diffusion of therapeutic self-help culture. At the same time, public debates about the effects of epidemiological policies which included social distancing measures were often also framed in terms of psychology. Commentators warned about the risks of permanently damaging the mental health of youth if they cannot meet in groups or in person – Fabian's reasonings echo these discussions as well.

Furthermore, in these arguments and narrations, he enacts a performative shift similar to what we have seen in the case of the journalist who frames public debates about COVID-19 as arguments about the status of morality in general: Instead of spelling out the potential implications of illegal raves, Fabian talked about others' hypocrisy and his own moral weariness and the societal context of individualism. His stance illustrates how such ethical "problematizations" of everyday routines (Collier and Lakoff 2005) challenge individuals and their self-image as moral beings, spur their reflexivity, and produce numerous contradictions and inconsistencies – as well as observations on and heated discussions about them. In speaking about these matters, Fabian presents himself as a reluctant individualist, a realist who understands his own needs as well as societal hypocrisy, and a reflexive, morally motivated, but also pragmatic and morally exhausted self. While he is obviously torn in

27 Fabian also claims that his social environment, by which, it seems, he primarily means his family, perceives a difference in the way the pandemic is handled between West Germans, whom he classifies as strict believers in authority, and East Germans, who rather tend to resist the legal measures, as he says. Essentially, the self should be responsible for its own actions, not the state. "You have to find out for yourself which rule to follow and which to break, but break it if you need to. We live in a free country," his East German family members allegedly instructed him.

different directions, exemplifying the heterogeneity of common sense, his admonishment that people should not pretend to have ethical ambitions beyond radical individualism, that they should "take it or leave it" (i.e., affirm individualist logics overall or reject them overall), exemplifies a – perhaps surprisingly – authoritarian variant of defensive-hedonistic anti-moralism. The stance is reminiscent of what Amlinger and Nachtwey (2021, 13) term "libertarian authoritarianism," a stance that combines individualism with an aggressive disregard for the needs of vulnerable societal groups.

In contrast to this position, our last section we will highlight another version of anti-judgmentalism that is prevalent in some club cultures. In talking about clubs and dancing and narrating its meanings for their biographies, several interviewees, predominantly women, consistently stressed the importance of not judging and not being judged. Moralistic normativity is seen as oppressive, especially in the realms of gender and sexuality, and defined as an obstacle for individual happiness and societal progress that should be overcome. In doing so, these interviewees also speak about what they were missing during the Coronavirus pandemic, and they provide another example for the prevalence of anti-judgmentalist attitudes in the present conjuncture.

Lena and Marie: Dancing without Judgments, Club Cultures as Safe Spaces

As mentioned above, the verb *judgen*, the German-language anglicism derived from "to judge," has become quite common in German-speaking youth cultures. For some clubgoers, the term is closely tied to the notion of *safe* or *safer spaces*: as something like their antonym. The contrast between those terms is key for defining the cultural norms of venues that represent a certain vision of "authentic" club culture. Many clubgoers see this ethic of clubbing as an oppositional order that stands in stark contrasts to prevailing norms of everyday life and societal normativity. As Lena, a 22-year-old social law student, puts it in an interview, a proper club is "a safe space" (*ein Safe Space*), and as such, "a place where you can be yourself and let it all out, without any restrictions – where you can be who you are without being judged" (*ein Ort, wo du dich ausleben kannst, wie du bist, ohne Restriktionen – dass man frei sein kann, so wie man ist, ohne gejudgt zu werden*). Safe spaces, seen as places where certain ethical rules of communication and behavior apply, offer a temporary "solution" to the problem of being judged by others, both on a discursive and an affective level.[28] During the

28 The history of the concept "safe space" can be traced back to gay and lesbian movements in Los Angeles of the 1960s. At that time, the expression referred to gay bars where one could seek refuge from police violence as well as spaces in which activists could gather to form political alliances to organize themselves against patriarchal and heteronormative power struc-

pandemic, it is not least these non-judgmental spaces that interviewees like Lena painfully lacked.

Club cultures in the disco, house and techno veins have traditionally been associated with freedom and mutual tolerance, especially for women and sexual minorities. One could argue that those signifiers are, amongst other things, produced and regulated by emotions such as the feeling of (not) being judged. Entering the realm of "true" club culture – rather than mainstream "discos" – for the first time is often described by afficionados as a process in which one learns to be "open minded," and break down one's own prejudices and is in turn "accepted" by others, as Lena puts it.[29] For her, the club is a safe space not only because people tolerate each other but also because she can safely consume drugs. This illustrates how the notion of safe space is not limited to "classic" forms of discrimination. On the other hand, not being judged (*nicht gejudgt werden*), which is fundamental to her vision of safe spaces, is reflected in the looks that others give her, the ways in which people dance with each other and the fact that "people simply leave you in peace." In this case, not being judged is less about verbal communication than it is about patterns of (sexualized) interaction and the perception of the gaze and the classificatory schemata and rankings of others.

Another excerpt from an interview can exemplify this dynamic. Marie, an actor in her thirties, talks about one of the first times she went to a club where a sex-positive event was taking place. She describes her experience as an epiphany: "I danced myself to ecstasy. Everyone being naked, sweaty bodies all around me. I could feel the bass, this amazing beat. I really thought, I've been enlightened (*erleuchtet*). [...] I didn't worry if my breasts are too small, if my butt is too big, no. I could let it all go, completely." Marie believes that she gained a new form of self-confidence in this moment of sudden insight. Through dancing, she explored "her sexuality" and was able to "get to know my body in a completely new way," as she says. In retrospect, it was this exact moment that helped her stop judging herself.

The atmosphere of clubbing and the pronounced non-normativity that is a norm in certain clubs can be best described by pointing to what potentially disrupts them. As Marie moves on with her story, she talks about a group of young women – "girlies"

---

tures. Early safe spaces have been described as variants of feminist consciousness-raising groups (Kenney 2001). Starting from the mid-2010s, the concept gained popularity through debates about safe spaces on college campuses, primarily in the English-speaking world (MacKinnon 2018). Academic safe spaces are safe in the sense that they are meant to be places for marginalized or vulnerable groups. They are intended to prevent acts of hate speech, but also to avoid more subtle forms of potential harm sometimes called microaggressions.

29 The distinction between the supposedly "true" club culture and mere mainstream discos is not an objective representation of the field of nightlife scenes, but rather a "partial truth" and an expression of a specific position within this field (a classic analysis of related dynamics can be found in Thornton [1995]).

(*Mädels*), she says[30] – who did not adhere to the codes of nightlife she herself has learned. Marie disapproves of them for visually "scanning" others and "comparing" themselves to these others. She interprets their looks and gestures and equates them with discriminatory behavior based on perceptions of age, physical handicaps, or body types:

> I've been observing those girls who were constantly doing this [she takes her hand and throws her hair back], clinging to their handbags, looking around – you can tell, if people are scanning you or if they compare themselves to you. I could tell by looking at them. That really bugged me. This is not a zoo! Well, there is some 60-year-old with a 60-year-old dick, yes. Deal with it. *Don't judge!* [...] I think, you should stop yourself a bit from making judgments, generally (*Ich glaube, man sollte ein bisschen die Wertung rausnehmen aus allem*). The pleasant thing about KitKat [a club] is that you see a range of people, of different bodies, young and old. For quite a while there has been a guy in a wheelchair. That's the reason why it is a *safe space*. You really shouldn't judge (*Man sollte wirklich nicht urteilen*). It's not exclusively for girls with bodies shaped like a model. [...] Once, I've met a woman, about my age, who was flirting with me that night. She must have weighted more than 200 pounds – she was so hot, so sexy, so self-confident. Somehow, I was attracted to her. I can't imagine that this is the same in other clubs where other rules apply.

Here, to judge by appearances in a conventional sense, and to value or devalue others accordingly, is equated with discriminatory behavior and "lookism" (Tietje and Cresap 2005). Marie claims that people who have learned not to judge have overcome this and have reached a higher stage of enlightenment. "Don't judge!" – spoken in English – is presented as a general maxim that helps to transcend oppressive societal norms. These norms are of different kinds, but they have a similar anti-emancipatory logic. Marie's use of the phrase and her narrative of an epiphany clearly have a feminist sound. Her narrative of her learning process was not so much about self-exploration as an active confrontation with her own personality – the dominant theme in many self-help guides. Rather, it was the sense of not being evaluated and judged (*beurteilt*, primarily) by others that opened a new space for redefining and enjoying herself. In contrast to Fabian's rejection of judgmental moralism during the coronavirus pandemic, and the rhetoric of newspaper commentary, her admonition "don't judge" is less about a rejection of potential accusations from people with whom she generally shares crucial moral norms, but about establishing an actual social and spatial figuration in which values such as tolerance and mutual respect take shape – and in which "better" moral norms prevail.

---

30 The wording – including the reference to handbags – and argument are closely reminiscent of Thornton's analysis.

While it may seem that Marie is concerned purely with rejecting (or even condemning) *aesthetic* judgments about attractiveness, a closer reading shows that moral norms in a very classic sense play a prominent role here as well: by learning not to judge others and herself, she overcomes norms restricting promiscuity and fostering heteronormativity – basic cornerstones of "traditional" morality. In that sense, she argues – in a generalized fashion, too – against judgments that adhere to a traditional morality that she sees as limiting and discriminatory, and in favor of a stance that could also be described as rationalistic, universalistic, and opposed to all forms of discrimination. There is a utopian political quality to such statements, an idea of societal progress being foreshadowed, even if it remains unclear whether the delineated sphere of nightlife with its temporary "heterotopias" (Foucault 1986) will really prefigure "better" and – in this sense – non-judgmental worlds more broadly. While there is no direct connection to public health policies during the pandemic, this kind of ethic seems to easily segue into a discourse centered around notions of mutual care.

Discussion

We do not, however, suggest making a systematic and straightforward comparison between these case studies from club culture during the COVID-19 pandemic. The frame of reference in Fabian's narration on the one hand and Marie's and Lena's on the other remains different: whereas the latter speak about certain clubs as spaces in which an egalitarian, non-judgmental ethic is lived, Fabian explicitly reflects on moral dilemmas during the COVID pandemic and everyday life in general. We also do not intend to make claims about the actual political orientations of Fabian, Marie and Lena. Rather, we have used their statements to ideal-typically exemplify different logics and for showing different ways in which subjects position themselves towards the problematic of being judged.

Fabian takes recourse to living in an individualistic society and claims his right to a "realistic," common-sense individualism ("take it or leave it") that may be harmful to others but, in his view, fits with the reality of a society whose rules are set by competitive individualism. He questions others' authority – neither do they know enough nor are they without fault. He also, importantly, points out the disconnect between "moralized" fields, especially those of consumption and social distancing, and less moralized fields, and highlights that – if one takes morality seriously – ethical-political convictions should not stop at the borders of those delineated areas. This enables him to point out others' hypocrisies. He creates a personal balance sheet of ethical decisions. While his reflections are in many ways idiosyncratic, his critique of judgmental moralism resonates with discursive interventions by journalists and public intellectuals who partake in the mediated construction of common sense.

On the other side, the two advocates for the concept of safe spaces present a stance in which traditional morality and judgments harm some, especially (historically) devalued groups, and limit others from reaching personal freedom. Therefore, judging (*urteilen, beurteilen* and *verurteilen*) is also seen as wrong in a generalized way. Overcoming this, however, can only be achieved through responsiveness to others' needs and through mutual attunement for which some club cultures offer a concrete utopia. Theirs is a stance against being judgmental that many critics of (politically progressive, universalistic) "moralism" would find *particularly moralistic*: here, not to judge demands a radical break with many aspects of traditional morality and the everyday normativity built upon it.

Conclusion

In this chapter, we surveyed anti-judgmentalism as a cultural theme that crosses different discursive fields. During the coronavirus pandemic, this took on a particular urgency: many people felt that the moral climate was getting harsher. However, as we have shown, the pandemic was neither the origin of nor the only reason for such developments. Since the term "to judge" and its German-language equivalences are semantically vague, we analyzed the components of their usage. Having identified and surveyed different strands in public discourses and the narratives of clubgoers during the Corona virus pandemic, we summarize that although these terms are semantically slippery and their usages are far from consistent, they share certain features which have become engrained in common sense ways of speaking about morality and its limits.

It is worth noting that the anti-judgmentalist reasonings presented by the people quoted here overlap with arguments made against moralism by moral philosophers, for example concerning the judgmental moralist's typical disregard for nonmoral reasons for actions and their potential legitimacy.[31] However, our exploration goes beyond this literature in a number of ways: for one, in our analysis, anti-judgmentalism is as much a heterogeneous assemblage of citations, beliefs, sentiments and interpersonal relationships – a form of common sense – as it is a set of clear-cut arguments. Its evocation blurs the distinction between ethical-political, aesthetic, performance- or conventions-related critiques – all of them are presented as illegitimate judgments from which a fragile, vulnerable self must be protected. The supposed wrongness of judging is therefore claimed to be *felt* emotionally as much as it is recognized intellectually. To put it more broadly: the discourse on anti-moralism in general and anti-judgmentalism in specific tends to contextualize political debates through a (political) psychology of morality and moral sentiments.

31 Cf. the summary in Neuhäuser and Seidel (2020).

Our survey of this cultural theme has also shown – at least in an exploratory fashion – how anti-judgmentalist attitudes are articulated with a specific sociopolitical conjuncture, and it has hinted at how they contribute to it. Our analysis thereby provides both an update and a concreteness – as a piece in a puzzle – that is lacking in larger-scale diagnoses by cultural theorists like Brown, Grossberg or Gilbert about the unclarity of the relation of ethics and politics in the contemporary conjuncture and the contradictoriness of moral rigorism and systemic complicity prevalent therein. There also is a technological side to this: social media worlds are pervaded by quick classifications, evaluations, comparisons. Platform designs afford and encourage a specific range of quasi-judgmental practices such as liking, rating, swiping, commenting. Similar tendencies pertain to the field of work, where indicators for the comparison and ranking of employee performance have in many cases been formalized electronically (Fourcade 2016; Groth 2019). Arguably, echoes of this can be heard in the interviewees' reflections on being judged.

Adding to conjunctural analysis, our investigation also shows that the anti-judging verdict has become articulated with different sociopolitical identities and projects – even if they are not fully formed and determined, which is itself an important point that suggests a certain (ethical-political) openness among people like the interviewees. Simplifying gradual matters, it can be said that the harsh and resentful rejection of moral interpellations during the pandemic *as overdemanding* tends to align with (broadly right-wing) populist and libertarian rhetoric, which can also link to seemingly anti-authoritarian subcultures and scenes (Amlinger and Nachtwey 2022), whereas the rejection of morality (and its demands) *as traditionalist morality* leans left(-liberal).

At this point, it is worth remembering that for conjunctural analysts such as Grossberg and Brown, the much-criticized "moralization" of public life – whether it is understood as an actual tendency or a discursive construction, whether it is supported or objected to – should be contextualized in a historical situation where there is wide-spread disillusion or even cynicism towards larger-scale, straightforwardly political strategies for societal transformation and emancipation. This skepticism also pertains among many people who are generally critical of the status quo. In such a situation, individualized and individualizing moral interpellations are plausible at least in part because other strategies for social transformation seem inaccessible and unrealistic. In that sense, the popularity of the "don't judge"-theme is a symptom of the uncertainties that Grossberg and Brown have written about, and it illustrates two emergent ways for navigating through these dilemmas. The immediate COVID crisis, however, represented an exceptional state of moralization where moral demands – and subsequent judgments – were less about broad questions of (in-)justice and social transformation than about a clear and limited goal of halting the virus's spread.

Bibliography

Amlinger, Carolin, and Oliver Nachtwey. 2022. *Gekränkte Freiheit: Aspekte des libertären Autoritarismus*, Suhrkamp.

Bolz, Norbert. 2021. *Keine Macht der Moral! Politik jenseits von gut und böse*, Matthes & Seitz.

Bourdieu, Pierre. 1984. *Distinction: A Social Critique of the Judgement of Taste*, Routledge.

Butler, Judith. 1990. *Gender Trouble: Feminism and the Subversion of Identity*, Routledge.

Coady, C. A. J., editor. 2006. *What's Wrong with Moralism?*, Blackwell.

Collier, Stephen, and Andrew Lakoff. 2005. "On Regimes of Living." *Global Assemblages. Technology, Politics, and Ethics as Anthropological Problems*, edited by Ai-hwa Ong and Stephen J. Collier, Blackwell, 22–39.

Crehan, Kate A. F. 2002. *Gramsci, Culture, and Anthropology*, U of California P.

Ege, Moritz. 2024. "Pop vs. the people? Spaltungsdiagnosen und Moralisierungskritiken." *"Parallelgesellschaften" in populärer Musik? Abgrenzungen – Annäherungen – Perspektiven*, edited by Ralf von Appen, Sarah Chaker, Michael Huber and Sean Prieske (~Vibes – The IASPM D-A-CH Series Vol. 3 meets GFPM | Beiträge zur Popularmusikforschung 48), transcript, 33–58.

Ege, Moritz. 2022. "Ethisierung als Diagnose und Vorwurf: Einige Dilemmata der stadtethnografischen Forschung heute." *Stadt – Migration – Moral. Analysen zur lokalen Moralisierung der Migration*, edited by Jan Lange and Manuel Dieterich, Tübinger Vereinigung für Volkskunde, 167–204.

Ehn, Billy, Orvar Löfgren, and Richard R. Wilk. 2016. *Exploring Everyday Life: Strategies for Ethnography and Cultural Analysis*, Rowman & Littlefield.

Fassin, Didier. 2015. "Troubled Waters. At the Confluence of Ethics and Politics." *Four Lectures on Ethics. Anthropological Perspectives*, Michael Lambek, Veena Das, Didier Fassin, and Webb Keane, HAU Books, 127–174.

Fassin, Didier, and Samuel Lézé, editors. 2014. *Moral Anthropology: A Critical Reader*, Routledge.

Felman, Shoshana. 2002. *The Juridical Unconscious: Trials and Traumas in the Twentieth Century*, Harvard UP.

Festinger, Leon. 1954. "A Theory of Social Comparison Processes." *Human Relations*, vol. 7, no. 2, 117–140.

Foucault, Michel. 1978. "Nietzsche, Genealogy, History." *Nietzsche*, edited by John Richardson and Brian Leiter, Oxford UP, 139–164.

Foucault, Michel. 1986. "Of Other Spaces." *Diacritics*, vol. 16, no. 1, 22–27.

Foucault, Michel 1992. *The Use of Pleasure*, reprint, Penguin Books.

Foucault, Michel 1997. "On the Genealogy of Ethics: An Overview of a Work in Progress." *The Essential Works of Michel Foucault, 1954–1984*, edited by Paul Rabinow, New Press, 253–280.

Gehlen, Arnold. 2004. *Moral und Hypermoral. Eine pluralistische Ethik*, Klostermann.

Gilbert, Jeremy, and Alex Williams. 2022. *Hegemony Now: How Big Tech and Wall Street Won the World (and How We Win It Back)*, Verso.

Gramsci, Antonio. 1971. *Selections from the Prison Notebooks of Antonio Gramsci*, Lawrence & Wishart.

Grau, Alexander. 2017. *Hypermoral. Die neue Lust an der Empörung*, Claudius.

Hall, Stuart, and Alan O'Shea. 2013. "Common-Sense Neoliberalism." *Soundings*, vol. 55, 9–25.

Hier, Sean P. 2011. "Tightening the Focus: Moral Panic, Moral Regulation and Liberal Government." *The British Journal of Sociology*, vol. 62, no. 3, 523–541. https://doi.org/10.1111/j.1468-4446.2011.01377.x.

Hier, Sean P. 2019. "Moral Panic and the New Neoliberal Compromise." *Current Sociology*, vol. 67, no. 6, 879–897. https://doi.org/10.1177/0011392119829511.

Hinrichsen, Jan. 2019. "Moralische Problematisierungen, oder: Wozu soll eine Ethnografie des 'guten Lebens' gut sein?" *Forme(l)n des guten Lebens. Ethnografische Erkundungen alltäglicher Aushandlungen von Glück und Moral*, Tübinger Verein für Volkskunde, 7–47.

Hunt, Alan. 1999. *Governing Morals: A Social History of Moral Regulation*. Cambridge Studies in Law and Society, Cambridge UP.

Koselleck, Reinhart. 1979. *Kritik und Krise: Eine Studie zur Pathogenese der bürgerlichen Welt*, 3rd edition, Suhrkamp.

Lindner, Rolf. 2003. "Vom Wesen Der Kulturanalyse." *Zeitschrift Für Volkskunde*, vol. 99, 177–188.

Hermann Lübbe, Peter von Oertzen, and Karl Teppe, editors. 1985. *Politisierende Moral, Moralisierende Politik? Ein Cappenberger Gespräch: Veranstaltet am 29. Januar 1985 in Frankfurt am Main. Cappenberger Gespräche der Freiherr-Vom-Stein-Gesellschaft, vol. 20*, Grote W. Kohlhammer.

Lübbe, Hermann. 1985. "Politischer Moralismus. Zum Komplementärverhältnis von Gesinnungsintensität und Common-Sense-Schwund." *Politisierende Moral, moralisierende Politik? Ein Cappenberger Gespräch: Veranstaltet am 29. Januar 1985 in Frankfurt am Main. Cappenberger Gespräche der Freiherr-Vom-Stein-Gesellschaft, vol. 20*, edited by Cappenberger Gespräch, Hermann Lübbe, Peter von Oertzen, and Karl Teppe, Grote W. Kohlhammer, 14–30.

Lübber, Hermann. 2019. *Politischer Moralismus. Über den Triumph der Gesinnung über die Urteilskraft (Vortrag, Gehalten 1984)*, LIT.

Luhmann, Niklas. 2008a [1997]. "Politik, Demokratie, Moral." *Die Moral der Gesellschaft*, Suhrkamp, 175–195.

Luhmann, Niklas. 2008b [1978]. "Soziologie der Moral." *Die Moral der Gesellschaft*, Suhrkamp, 56–162.

Maasen, Sabine, Jens Elberfeld, Pascal Eitler, and Maik Tändler, editors. 2011. *Das beratene Selbst: Zur Genealogie der Therapeutisierung in den "langen" Siebzigern, 1800–2000*, vol. 7, transcript.

Mieth, Corinna, and Jacob Rosenthal. 2020. "Spielarten des Moralismus." *Kritik des Moralismus*, edited by Christian Neuhäuser and Christian Seidel, Suhrkamp, 35–60.

Milkman, Ruth. 2017. "A New Political Generation: Millennials and the Post-2008 Wave of Protest." *American Sociological Review*, vol. 82, no. 1, 1–31. https://doi.org/10.1177/0003122416681031.

Neuhäuser, Christian, and Christian Seidel. 2020. "Kritik des Moralismus. Eine Landkarte zur Einleitung." *Kritik des Moralismus*, edited by Christian Neuhäuser and Christian Seidel, Suhrkamp, 9–34.

Stegemann, Bernd. 2018. *Die Moralfalle: für eine Befreiung linker Politik*, Matthes & Seitz.

Sutter, Ove. 2016. "Alltagsverstand. Zu Einem hegemonietheoretischen Verständnis alltäglicher Sichtweisen und Deutungen." *Österreichische Zeitschrift für Volkskunde*, vol. LXX/119, no. 1–2, 42–70.

Thompson, Stacy. 2012. "The Micro-Ethics of Everyday Life: Ethics, Ideology and Anti-Consumerism." *Cultural Studies*, vol. 26, no. 6, 895–921. https://doi.org/10.1080/09502386.2012.704636.

Thornton, Sarah. 1995. *Club Cultures: Music, Media and Subcultural Capital*, Polity Press.

Ticktin, Miriam. 2011. *Casualties of Care: Immigration and the Politics of Humanitarianism in France*, U of California P.

Tietje, Louis, and Steven Cresap. 2005. "Is Lookism Unjust? The Ethics of Aesthetics and Public Policy Implications." *Journal of Libertarian Studies*, vol. 19, no. 2, 31–50.

Williams, Raymond. 1961. *The Long Revolution*, Chatto and Windus.

Williams, Raymond. 1973. *The Country and the City*, Oxford UP.

Williams, Raymond. 1977. *Marxism and Literature*, Oxford UP.

Zigon, Jarrett. 2007. "Moral Breakdown and the Ethical Demand: A Theoretical Framework for an Anthropology of Moralities." *Anthropological Theory*, vol. 7, no. 2, 131–150. https://doi.org/10.1177/1463499607077295.

Žižek, Slavoj. 1999. *The Ticklish Subject: The Absent Centre of Political Ontology*, Verso.

Injustice Narratives of Vaccine Critics

Insights from German Telegram Groups

Julia Brose

Introduction

The Corona pandemic, the "mother of all crises" (Lessenich 2020, 217), has determined our global social interactions since 2020 and is still a catalyst to highlight political, social and individual grievances. In 2020 and 2021, high infection rates, lockdowns and vaccination debates shaped the public discourse in Germany and beyond. While it is widely agreed protection of health and the guarantee of health care should always be the priority of political action, the Covid-19 pandemic made global structural injustices in health care visible (Iyengar et al. 2020). Despite the global health crisis, movements manifested themselves that not only criticized anti-pandemic policies, but also rejected vaccinations in the same move: *QAnon*[1] and so called *Querdenken*[2] brought this fundamental opposition to the streets. Studies for German-speaking countries indicate that people with a critical attitude towards the state and who perceive themselves as marginalized due to political measures (curfews, lockdowns, regulations on gatherings, etc.) gather in these contexts (Frei, Schäfer and Nachtwey 2021). Not only the rhetoric of the speeches at these demonstrations, but also the attack on the Reichstag building in Berlin in August 2020 showed the radicalization of the scene. It is of particular interest to be able to understand which narratives these people use. Understanding their narrative could help in two ways: first, this could be an opportunity to trace the process of radicalization, and second, the content can make it clearer why not all adult German citizens will want to take advantage of the comprehensive vaccination offer from June 2021. By the end of the year 2021 still almost 9 million people over 18 years

1 *QAnon* is an American movement against the government and their Covid-politics. The protests became known worldwide for their march to the Capital in Washington D.C. 2020 (Conner/MacMurray 2021).

2 *Querdenken* is a German movement which was started by a small group of protesters in Stuttgart before growing into the most known Corona-politic protest movement nationwide (Plümper/Neumayer/Pfaff 2021).

in Germany have not received a first vaccination against Covid-19 (Statista 2022). The number of unreported cases is even higher due to falsified vaccination cards in Germany (Kniestedt 2021).

To understand especially these people who have decided against a Covid-19 vaccination despite its availability, recommendations of the Standing Committee on Vaccination (STIKO) and social relevance, this paper will try to elaborate their narrative of injustice. The comprehension of narratives surrounding injustice, particularly in the context of vaccine opponents, bears significance not only for comprehending the dynamics of their movement, but also holds potential utility in informing responses to future (health) crises. Given the assumption that the understanding of injustice among vaccine opponents is fundamental to the overall societal perception, it could, to some extent, contribute to tracing the rationale behind vaccine hesitancy beyond scientific evidence. The reference to injustice is relevant to make clear why these individuals sporadically perceive themselves as marginalized (Frei, Schäfer and Nachtwey 2021) when, at the same time, they have made a conscious decision not to receive the available vaccines. The content will be accessed via *Telegram*, as this messenger in particular plays a central role in the exchange and discussions of corona vaccination critics (Curley, Siapera and Carthy 2022). The three German channels and one group I selected were publicly accessible at the time of the survey between October and December 2021. Their content is primarily concerned with criticism of Covid-19 vaccines and policies against measures to contain the virus. However, during my research, one channel was deleted by *Telegram* early on and the group was removed in November 2021 due to violations of *Telegram*'s terms of service. By analyzing the virtual narratives of Corona vaccination critics, I have gained insights into their perceptions of injustice and marginalization, as well as their reasons for refusing to get vaccinated. However, to fully understand the social and political implications of vaccine hesitancy, it is important to consider the broader context in which it occurs. In particular, the Corona pandemic has triggered protests and debates about the role of the state, the legitimacy of public health measures, and the distribution of resources and opportunities in society. Examining the theoretical framing of injustice can help shed light on these complex issues and guide policy responses that promote social inclusion, equity, and resilience in times of crisis. Hence, the following key questions will also need to be asked of the generated material: how is injustice and the experience of injustice addressed? Who experiences unjust treatment as a result?

Corona Protests and Injustice

Social inequality becomes more visible during the Corona pandemic—for example the fact that people living in poorer circumstances are at higher risk of infection

(Powers et al. 2021). Populations such as single parents or students from socially deprived backgrounds are disproportionately more affected by the pandemic than others (Collins et al. 2021). But what unequal treatment were demonstrators against the Corona measures addressing? Was social injustice the basis of the argumentation or was a different starting point fundamental?

The Demonstrators

Christine Hentschel (2021) defines "corona publics" as "[...] gatherings of discontent over state policies toward the pandemic that manifest themselves in the squares and streets of German cities as well as in chat rooms or on YouTube" (ibid, 62). Hentschel explores these communities, whose common denominator is the critique of the coronavirus policy but who otherwise differ greatly in their social demographics (Frei, Schäfer and Nachtwey 2021; Reichhardt 2021). Narratives play an overriding role here, as they can be transmitted offline as well as online. Hentschel therefore also focuses on the narratives of the "corona publics" (2021, 62) which must remain vague and malleable, but nevertheless endure in order to be able to carry the consensus further (ibid, 64). Frei, Schäfer and Nachtwey's (2021) ethnographic observations, especially in relation to the speeches given, reveal the continuous use of the words "dictatorship" and "division." It also became clear that the participants perceived themselves as the "marginalized" (ibid., 254–255). In addition, it is described that the participants of the demonstrations felt as the "oppressed," who perceive a possible vaccination obligation as a threat and generally see themselves deprived of their freedom by the measures (ibid, 253). The demonstrations are predominantly organized on the messenger service *Telegram* and reach people who were not politically active before (Richter and Salheiser 2021, 80). It seems evident that an influence of injustice affects and is reproduced in the demonstrations.

The Understanding of Injustice

Preliminary considerations for such a research project reveal that understanding injustice narratives based on individual data from social media becomes more challenging due to the absence of the ability to follow up with clarifying questions. At all times, each statement made by the participants under investigation must be accepted as a subjective perception without intervention from the researchers. This realization justifies not only the need for a long data collection period, as repetitions in arguments and text fragments are relevant, but also the focus on individual statements in chats and channels, which, through their accumulation, contribute to a spectrum of subjectively shared narratives within the anti-vaccine group. Shklar's concept of the "Sense of injustice" from *The Faces of Injustice* (1990) provides a perspective on this subjective perception of injustice. It acknowledges that individual feelings of injustice can be subjective but can still point to objective injustices. When people discuss injustice on social media, they can express their sense of injustice by pointing out specific cases or systems that they perceive as unfair. Judith Shklar's concept of a *Sense of injustice* refers to an individual's ability to recognize and respond to instances of injustice in their society. According to Shklar, this sense of injustice is a crucial aspect of political liberalism and is necessary for a healthy democratic society. Shklar argues that the *Sense of injustice* is not simply an emotional response to unfair treatment, but rather a moral judgment about the legitimacy of certain social practices and institutions. It is an awareness of the ways in which power is distributed within society, and a recognition of the ways in which certain groups may be disadvantaged or marginalized. By cultivating a *Sense of injustice*, individuals can become more aware of the injustices around them and can take action to challenge and change these practices. Shklar sees this as a fundamental aspect of citizenship and a necessary condition for maintaining a just and democratic society.

Injustice is part of every (modern) society and influences it beyond the micro level: according to Shklar, perceived injustice is a personal experience caused by particular events, which can also lend to public consequences. Shklar does not propose a universally applicable framework for contrasting injustice with justice, but instead highlights the significance of moral perception and the interpretation of experiences of injustice within democratic systems. Perspectives from (political) philosophy regarding injustice connect it to factors within the economic, social, and political realms, and assume the ability to differentiate between injustice and mere unhappiness (Shklar 1990).

To provide a more comprehensive framework for contextualizing these subjective perceptions originating from the *Telegram* chats and channels, it is essential to adopt a broader perspective. This approach transcends individual evaluation and entails an examination of structural (and epistemic) injustice. By doing so, we gain a deeper understanding of injustice not only at the individual level but also within the wider context of societal and systemic dynamics. Such an encompassing approach enables us to comprehend and address injustice in a more nuanced manner. Furthermore, drawing on Miranda Fricker's (2007) work on epistemic injustice, which explores how certain individuals are systematically disadvantaged in terms of knowledge transmission and interpretation, provides a valuable framework for a more comprehensive understanding and addressing of injustice within both individual and broader societal contexts. Fricker's work on testimonial and hermeneutic injustice concerns the ways in which individuals or groups can be wronged in their capacity to communicate and have their experiences understood and acknowledged. *Testimonial injustice* refers to situations in which someone is not given the same level of credibility or respect as others when sharing their experiences or knowledge due to some prejudice or stereotype held by the listener. *Hermeneutic injustice*, on the other hand, occurs when there is a structural limitation in the shared resources of a particular community, making it difficult for a particular group to communicate their experiences effectively. Fricker argues that testimonial and hermeneutic injustices can have significant effects on individuals and groups, as they can lead to silencing, marginalization, and exclusion. She suggests that recognizing and addressing these forms of injustice is necessary for building more just and inclusive communities.

Individuals who experience hermeneutic injustice would be more likely to perceive injustice as misfortune in the context of Shklar's (1990) remarks. Fricker argues that hermeneutic marginalization results from systematic hermeneutic injustice, which is steadily reproduced in the absence of enlightenment. Thus, individuals who are systematically affected by hermeneutic injustice have "[a] more general susceptibility to different kinds of injustice" (Fricker 2007, 159). Consequently, people who are exposed to these forms of epistemic injustice are not only affected because of their statements based on social affiliation, but also marginalized because of their lack of knowledge about the injustice they face: "For something to be an injustice, it must be harmful but also wrongful, whether because discriminatory or because otherwise unfair" (Fricker 2007, 151). For Fricker, the forms of injustice are as liquid (Schicktanz 2012, 280) as Judith Shklar's (1990) sense of injustice. Both concepts are subject to commonly shared perceptual schemas of (in)justice and society's dispositions about social attributions. Central to my data is not only the subjective *Sense of injustice* (Shklar 1990) in the participants' content but it also needs to be considered whether testimonial or hermeneutic injustices (Fricker 2007) occur from the perspective of the participants, in order to assess their overall societal relevance.

Methods: Qualitative Analysis of Telegram Content

At the time of the study, *Telegram* was a central platform for German-speaking vaccine-critical communication and had 8 million active users in Germany. The platform was founded in Russia in 2013 and is currently headquartered in Dubai (Telegram 2022). The messaging app makes it possible to share text, images, files, voice messages, videos and links with up to 200,000 people in groups or with unlimited numbers in channels. It is not mobile number based, other users can also be found by their usernames. These are public as soon as they have been defined. One's own cell phone number remains hidden unless it has been changed in the privacy settings. It can be stated that the exchange on *Telegram* can be done via the cell phone number or only via the usernames. The channels and group chats available on *Telegram* can, but do not have to, be password-protected, or require an invitation from another group/channel member or are freely accessible and can thus be found via the search function on *Telegram*.

The most important difference between channels and chats is that it is not possible to write your own messages in channels per se, but links and forwardings can be collected there. However, depending on the setting, there is a comment option on these links, so that the exchange can take place there. In addition, the creators of the channels can designate admins who can not only preselect the forwards, but these can even compose messages themselves and designate other participants to whom this can also be possible. Moreover, it is also possible that in the publicly accessible channels, redirects to appropriate groups or other channels are shared (Telegram 2022).

Telegram's infrastructure and moderation practices differ from those of many other platforms, and public groups and channels can remain accessible while still being difficult to monitor systematically. It is relevant for my present work that these groups and channels are accessible and public for all *Telegram* users. For the present study, it was relevant that the selected groups and channels were accessible and public for all Telegram users. Public accessibility reduced, but did not eliminate, research-ethical concerns. Therefore, group and channel names were anonymized, usernames were not reported, and the analysis focuses on aggregated narrative patterns rather than identifiable individuals.

The search for suitable groups and channels for the first overview was carried out using the *Telegram* search function. The keywords used were combinations of "anti," "against" and "non" with "vaccination," "corona," "corona politics," and similar. The following self-defined selection criteria were applied to select the groups and channels analyzed in my research:

1. The groups and channels must be publicly accessible in order to avoid research ethics problems due to the intrusion into a private (virtual) space.
2. The news content should be 60% Corona-related. This excludes, for example, channels and groups that only offer themselves as a networking opportunity and give people a platform to find like-minded people in their own environment and then communicate with them privately.
3. The focus of the exchanged message content should be on the written word. Emojis, videos, GIFs and voice messages not only mean more data but also increase the size of the chats to be exported.
4. The groups and channels were to generate a reliable flow of messages over the entire survey period. Accordingly, groups and channels were sorted out that provided output for two weeks but were then neglected by members.

The relevant names of the group and channels were simplified to ensure anonymization to the full extent. From these points of view, the composition of the source material is as follows:

Table 1: Overview of the examined Telegram content from 11th October 2021 – 31st December 2021

Names (simplified and anonymized)	**Exchange type**	**Number of members/subscribers (At the beginning and end of the survey)**	**Messages per day (average)**
Group1	Chatgroup	6,076 members 7,023 members	750
Channel1	Admin-managed channel without the possibility of commenting	22,002 subscriptions 24,356 subscriptions	15
Channel2 (closed in the beginning of November 2021)	Admin-managed channel with possibility to comment	3,117 members 3,363 members	90
Channel3fig 1	Admin-managed channel with possibility to comment	1,329 members 1.250 members	10

The starting point of the survey was set for 11th October 2021, as from this date the Covid19-citizen tests would no longer be available free of charge. Until then, these had made it possible for German citizens to be tested free of charge for the Covid-19 virus by rapid test. Although this regulation was quickly revised, it still served as a starting point. The coding ended with the last news of the 31st of December 2021, as it was already apparent in the analysis that the patterns of argumentation and content are constantly repeated. The material comprised about 67,000 text messages for the 12-week survey period. About 20% of these are emojis, which were also sent as individual messages and were not selected by the export process. Of the remaining approximately 53,600 messages, only the required 60% are also related to Corona discourse. Thus, approximately 32,000 text messages were included in the analysis. The expected narrative units of chat messages, being relatively brief, are insufficient to fully capture the narrative on their own. However, by employing "stories that address both cognitive and emotional aspects" (Gesser-Edelsburg 2021, 2), the exchange between the individuals under investigation allows for a comprehensive depiction of information and attitudes. This approach enables a deeper understanding of relevant factors, particularly in relation to the transmission of information. The data was exported and then processed in a way that was compatible for the software *Atlas.ti 9*. Afterwards, a qualitative content analysis according to Kuckartz (2019) could be performed with the help of *Atlas.ti 9*. The deductive and inductive working method, the mixed form of category formation, and the constant reference back to the research questions is recommended above all by Kuckartz (2019) and lent itself to my software-assisted qualitative content analysis (Kuckartz 2014).

Results: Mistrust, Exclusion, Division: All Unfair?

The analysis reveals three main themes: widespread mistrust in the pandemic strategy, social exclusion and loneliness among the non-vaccinated, and a belief in underlying injustices. These findings highlight the deep-seated mistrust, divisions, and perceived injustices within the content, providing insights into the perspectives of non-vaccinated individuals during the pandemic.

Mistrust

The general criticism of the political strategy against the Corona pandemic is evident in the content studied. It is fostered by the feeling of being lied to and based on the lack of trust in the measures that were implemented by the authorities:

> So what remains is the prospect of another 6 months of sadism...and then they're guaranteed to come up with something...I don't believe ANYTHING they say anymore...[3] (Group1_P29 10/18/2021)

> For 2 years, there has been no transparency, promises are broken, people are isolated, opinion is criminalized, justice is denied, etc. (Channel1_P1 12/27/2021)

The distrust in the political authorities is initially justified primarily by the "unfair" treatment of unvaccinated persons by politicians and the resulting measures. During the survey period, this framework changes in the chat group studied. Politicians, virologists, and all related institutions are increasingly criticized for their promotion of vaccination (especially because of the discourse around booster vaccinations in October 2021). In the process, those in power are referred to as "criminal" or as "felons." This also results in the general vaccine criticism, which is subsumed by the

3 The quoted statements have been translated into English verbatim by me. No spelling errors have been included, while punctuation and capitalization have been preserved for authenticity.

lack of trust and the lack of trust is growing by their reproduction of the vaccine criticism. Here, the vaccine criticism manifests itself through the beliefs that the sampled users assume Covid-19 vaccination causes at least severe illness.

This conviction was maintained throughout the whole investigation period: the personal observations of chat and channel participants are particularly relevant to the argument about vaccine safety. For example, various participants reported knowing people affected by vaccine damage and deaths in proximity due to vaccination ("I now know of 5 [death] cases after the swamp,[4] no sick person because of this invented disease" (Group1_P46 09.11.2021). This additionally strengthens the considerations to remain unvaccinated, even if this could lead to loneliness, exclusion from the social life or job loss[5] in individual cases of the examined content.

Exclusion and Division

Loneliness and isolation from family or social environments due to non-vaccination is the result of two factors according to the subjective experience of the sample group: The non-vaccinated are excluded from social life based on various measures (test regulations; 2G rule [entry to restaurants, cinemas, events, etc. only for recovered or vaccinated]). The stigmatization by the "mainstream media" that reinforces exclusion and thus discriminates against the unvaccinated. According to the material, this leads to some participants feeling lonely and seeking understanding in the groups. This strengthens the sense of community among vaccination critics.

> I'm increasingly on my own. I'm persona non grata, so to speak. It doesn't make life any easier, but vaccination will never be an option for me. (Group1_P37 06.11.2021)

> Remember you are not alone! We are many, we hold together & do not give up! But we must be patient. (Channel_P5 08.11.2021)

The division of society is a process started by politics and its measures and driven by the reporting of the "mainstream media." They experience this division as a passive process that is primarily driven by political means and their influence on the majority society:

4 "Swamp" is used by the investigated in the chat group as a synonym for the word vaccination. This illustrates the devaluation of the vaccination.

5 Job loss is discussed at various points, as certain participants also reject any measures of testing or the process of testing itself. Conversations about the necessity of wearing masks are similar.

> […] The result of one and a half years of Corona is a split in society that is unparalleled. Public broadcasting has played a major role in this. It fulfills its responsibility to build bridges between the camps and promote exchange less and less. (Channel1_P1 05.10.2021)

What remains central in the context of felt exclusion in social life, discrimination and division by the political authorities and the media is the shared opinion that this happens unjustifiably. The blaming of the unvaccinated, which is dominated by the media, the regulations and anti-pandemic politics, reinforces the sense of unwarranted blame, especially considering the exclusion of those studied. The material makes clear that specific measures are viewed according to perspective: when it is officially argued that the incidence values are high and that it is primarily unvaccinated people who become infected this is, according to the content examined, simply due to the fact, that they have to test themselves more common. They don't see the higher risk of infection because of the non-vaccination. After their argumentation politicians and the media want to create a public image that it is only the unvaccinated people who are ill and are therefore to blame for the closures, lockdowns and 3G/2G regulations:

> The bad thing is that you are no longer heard with logical thoughts and explanations, suddenly you are even guilty as an unvaccinated person. (Group1_P4 13.12.2021)

The statements assign blame for the measures to the vaccinated because they reaffirm the legitimacy of these measures by their supposed non-questioning of the political decisions. In doing so, they also support the public blaming of the unvaccinated for the existence of the pandemic. This argument is distorted to the point that, according to the understanding of the content examined, it is not the unvaccinated who are to blame for the Covid-19 pandemic, but politicians, the pharmaceutical industry, and other policymakers. According to this understanding, the vaccinated part of the population is itself responsible for the existing measures of the pandemic, because they support them and direct the anger about it to the wrong people: to the unvaccinated instead of the politicians.

> Merkel has said that the unvaccinated will soon face severe restrictions. Starting with daily tests at the workplace. This is sick, because the vaccinated are contagious. (Group1_P9 3.11.2021)

The members of the sample groups see themselves as the healthy ones, who also want to stay healthy and accordingly do not get vaccinated. According to this understanding, the experienced exclusion becomes even more unjustified, because most of them only want to stay healthy and do not want to expose themselves to the dangers of the vaccines. Nonetheless, a vaccination pressure is exerted on them, which is reinforced by the opinion in the media. Criticism of the measures, apart from the wearing of the mask (the "rag"), is particularly evident in connection with the testing strategy:

> In this country, no restaurant can deny you access because you're black, because you're gay, or because you have red hair. Quite simply because discrimination does not work legally in this country. That's how we were taught, and because domestic law can never take precedence over fundamental rights. Except in the case of healthy people. Even if they are officially "tested" as healthy on a daily basis. From now on, every restaurant in the city is allowed to deny them access. With the express reason that they are "only healthy" [...] (Group1_P42 26.10.2021)

They describe themselves as the healthy ones, who would be "made sick" by the vaccination. In addition, they speak of a vaccination compulsion through which they feel "socially pilloried" (Group1_P34 25.10.2021): "[...] Every little restriction is now blamed on the unvaccinated" (Group1_P19 11.10.2021).

The central results of my investigation can therefore be presented in a diagram as follows. This should make the basic logic and the sense of injustice in connection with the lack of trust more comprehensible.

Fig. 1: Overview over results of the narrative of injustice from the point of view of the content studied.

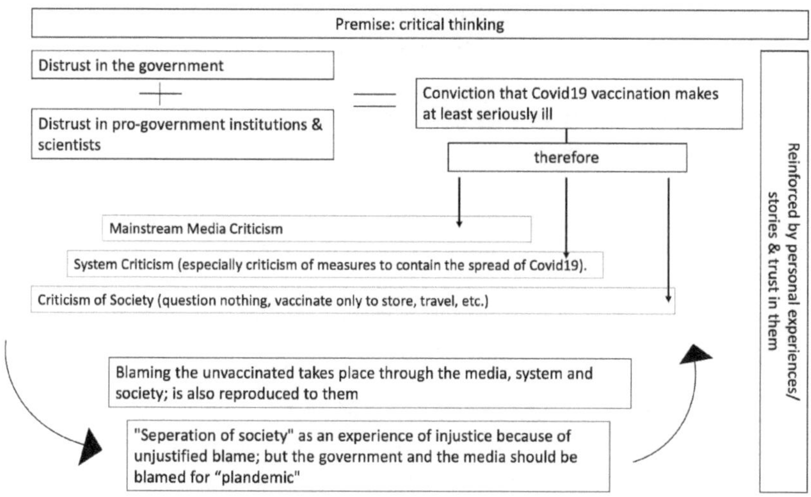

The figure shows in conclusion how the individual views of the respondents were linked, and under which premises they were consistently reproduced over the survey period. Assuming a critical thinking perspective, mistrust in the government and politically affiliated institutions is expressed. In this particular case, the dominant belief is that the recommended vaccinations not only cause severe illness but also provide no protection against Covid-19. Personal narratives, which are fully trusted, support these beliefs. As a result, discontent accumulates towards the so-called mainstream media, generating a general critique of the system and stigmatizing the majority of vaccinated German citizens as blind and obedient. The injustice that emerges as an output is primarily the unwarranted blame they experience and the division of society. This experienced injustice, in turn, reinforces the shown cycle of mistrust in politics.

The Contextualization of Injustice

> People pride themselves on their "social competence." Unfortunately, they lack the moral competence to stand up when injustice happens. (Group1_P33 10/22/2021)

> The injustice is so great and by now so clear that blind people would have to see it. (Group1_P26 12/24/2021)

The frequency of the use of "unjust" or "injustice" as explicit terms is low. However, when injustice is mentioned, it is as a comment that the majority society does not see the "Corona injustice" and does not do anything about it. According to this, injustice happens primarily under the guise of blackmail, which, however, is only perceived as such by the non-vaccinated and is not necessarily classified as unjust by the vaccinated.

Another use of "unfair" occurs sporadically when talking about what made the sample group "critical" and "awake":

> [...] I was often sick and experienced many injustices as a result. I think that makes you see a lot of things differently [...] (Group1_P9 21.10.2021)

> [...] and unfortunately it seems that previous suffering, experienced injustices open the eyes (Group1_P6 10/21/2021)

This dialogue makes clear that the *critical way of thinking* is attributed to injustices in the biography. In this context, the expressions "thinking differently" and "being awakened" are used again by "open the eyes" (Group1_P16). Other respondents also refer to a similar rationale when they talk about how they have already "been through a lot" and accordingly "don't trust anyone."

Nevertheless, across the survey period, personal narratives of injustices experienced are not common. The content studied only hints at these experiences and keeps them general. They do not see themselves fundamentally as victims of injustice, but as the *awakened* and *enlightened ones* who recognize it as such and are only waiting for everyone to understand the "agenda" behind the so-called "Plandemic." It is speculated that in the future events will occur that are supposed to justify the behavior of the unvaccinated and it is then put into perspective that one is now exposed to this exclusion: "Let's see how living together will be just THEN" (Chat1_P4 11.10.2021).

Injustice as a term is thus rarely used in context. Injustice is rather implied when it comes to the unjustified blame, the experienced exclusion and the discrimination by vaccinated people, media, and politics.

Discussion: The Perspectives of Injustice

The following remarks focus on the sample groups' own subjectively perceived *Sense of injustice* (Shklar 1990). The content analysis reveals the clash of two perspectives in our society's reality: the users in the sampled groups who refuse vaccination out of the belief that it may harm them, feeling excluded and treated unfairly, versus those who find it unfair, despite recommended vaccinations, to tolerate further restrictions due to the high number of unvaccinated people. The narrative of the unvaccinated and the way arguments are presented suggest a fundamentally different view of democracy. According to Shklar (1990), in a democratic society, people need to publicly acknowledge when something is unjust. Therefore, democracy should recognize and provide space for addressing feelings of injustice. Some users believe that democracy has become a "disguised dictatorship" due to the pandemic, rendering the elected officials irrelevant. This differing view of political structures (Koos 2021) and the desire for a new order can explain why people have different perceptions of injustice. While society observes people suffering from measurable social inequality during the pandemic, protesters spread conspiracy theories and feel they have been treated unfairly.

In essence, it can be stated that there are essential differences between the individuals affected by (measurable) injustice during the pandemic and the subjects under investigation. Firstly, there is a proactive decision against not only vaccination but also the testing strategy in the present case. Secondly, there is the non-measurable marginalization of those studied. While marginalization may affect certain populations more than others due to socio-economic factors such as income, origin, place of residence, diseases, etc., the users analyzed here perceive themselves as marginalized based on their vaccination status. Their perception of being subjected to political and democratic injustice is a result of feeling that their perspective, concerns, and criticism are not taken seriously or invalidated. This phenomenon aligns with Fricker's (2007) concept of epistemic injustice, which refers to the systematic suppression or devaluation of certain knowledge claims and experiences due to prejudice or power imbalances. Those who are vaccinated or support prevailing political and medical opinions may dismiss the concerns and experiences of the unvaccinated as unimportant or irrational, leading to epistemic injustice. The voices of the unvaccinated may not be heard or considered valid contributions to the discourse on pandemic control. This imbalance in perceiving and recognizing the experiences and perspectives of the unvaccinated can give rise to a sense of political injustice. However, reconstructing these claims through the lens of epistemic injustice does not mean that every rejected knowledge claim should be understood as epistemically unjust. Rather, the point is that the actors themselves interpret the dismissal of their concerns as a form of testimonial or hermeneutic marginalization. It creates the impression that their concerns are not adequately taken into account, resulting in their perceived disadvantage in democratic society due to their vaccination status. This perception of political injustice further reinforces the feeling of marginalization and exclusion experienced by the subjects, and this perception further reinforces distrust toward official institutions and increases reliance on *Telegram*-based counter-publics.

Discussion: The Crisis of Trust

As shown in figure 1 before, the distrust is fundamental for the understanding of injustice and the reproduced narrative. The only trust that is expressed in this communication is for those who think alike. This is particularly evident in the case of vaccine criticism: the analysis showed that official recommendations and surveys regarding the various vaccines are not trusted, but personal contributions from other people in the chat group or link channels are *never* questioned. When people report that they know of deaths after vaccination, or at least know people who have become seriously ill as a result, this is not treated with suspicion. This is mainly due to the prevailing belief that vaccination at least makes people seriously ill and that in the course of time those vaccinated will die from the consequences in a vague and unspecified future. The analysis showed that these expectations, combined with the personal stories of those negatively affected by vaccination, are fundamental to the position against pro-vaccination discourse:

> Group-based misanthropy in the service of the criminal pharmaceutical industry is fascistoid, at the latest since 11.10. we live in a 2-caste society. Unvaccinated par-

ticipation in society is now "luxury." The vaccination compulsion must go away, it divides! (Group3_P1 12.10.2021)

The "crisis of trust" in all institutions leads to official information being classified as insufficient (Goldenberg 2021, 109–111). To compensate for this, people could either continue to inform themselves until they feel they are sufficiently informed by official institutions, or they look for other sources, or they trust people to bring the content to them instead.

But those who, as in the present study, assume that they *have to* critically question everything the government and the "mainstream media" report, will not be able to restore the lack of trust, especially not if they are caught up in a feedback loop of misinformation within their social group. The reason for this distrust can only be vaguely surmised from the self-attributions of the subjects in the group. The messages reflect that the individuals already describe themselves as having "always been critical." Lack of trust in (scientific) institutions, politics and the media is not equated with mistrust but with the "ability to think critically." In this context, critical thinking about scientific content is not per se a denial of trust in science (Goldenberg 2021, 117).

Goldenberg (ibid.) suggests that many individuals who are hesitant or resistant to vaccines do not necessarily hold anti-science beliefs, but instead have concerns about the way vaccines are developed, tested, and marketed. They may feel that their voices and experiences are not being taken seriously by healthcare providers and government officials, or that they are being pressured or coerced into vaccinating themselves or their children.

According to Goldenberg (ibid.), these concerns can be seen as a response to broader forms of social and political injustice, such as systemic racism, poverty, and inequality, which have led to a general lack of trust in institutions and authorities. The anti-vaccine movement, therefore, can be seen as a symptom of a larger problem of distrust and alienation from the healthcare system. In the present work, trust shows up primarily detached from scientific data: It is most evident when the personal narratives of other group or channel members are not challenged, ensuring that the narrative of exclusionary government or harmful Covid-19 vaccination is reproduced.

Accordingly, those under investigation have "horizontal trust," not in all fellow citizens as Budnik (2021, 24) elaborates, but at least in those they perceive to be same-thinking fellow citizens. The "vertical trust" (ibid.) is no longer present, so that those under investigation long for a reboot of the system. Therefore, it is less surprising that the investigated contents finding themselves in their own representations of *injustice through division* and *unjustified blame*, withdraw more and more into the virtual spheres of action of those who are supposed to know better.[6]

As the results of the German COSMO survey (Betsch et al 2022a) indicate too, general trust in institutions and the federal government declined over the winter months of 2021, and 56.5% of respondents said in January 2022 that they tended to trust the German government less than in the months before (Betsch et al 2022b). An impact in the distrust is named as the failure of politicians to fulfill their promises contributes to a mindset of suspicion among those who I investigated. In the context of this study, the statement made by German Minister of Health Jens Spahn in a speech to the Bundestag on November 18, 2020 is particularly significant: "I give you my word: there will be no compulsory vaccination in this pandemic." Individuals who are investigated use such declarations as a basis for criticizing those in power. Despite the absence of a mandatory vaccination requirement, they believe that they are being indirectly forced to get vaccinated through various coronavirus-related measures or specific testing and 2G regulations, which they perceive as blackmail. This skepticism is reinforced by political implications that further erode trust (Shklar 1990) and even (temporary) law changes are viewed as an injustice by members of this group (Harbach 2008, 61).

The people examined in the chat groups and channels are presumably increasingly people who have not only been skeptical of political institutions since the Corona pandemic. They write about having "always been critical," which implies distrust. Relevant literature also indicates that vaccine-critical individuals tend not to trust political decision makers, scientific institutions or authorities (van Mulukom et al. 2022, 6; Schmid et al. 2017, 16; WHO 2017). Consequently, damaged trust in government and resulting conspiracy theories also have a negative impact on society as a whole and its approach to knowledge (Butter 2020; Milošević Đorđević et al. 2021). Moreover, with an increasing number of individuals being influenced by such theories, the likelihood may also rise that they will succumb to the discourse that fosters distrust.

However, conspiracy theory statements did not appear to be a determinant of distrust in politics, media, and science in the present study. In the present case, there is a correlation between distrust in politics and distrust in government-related science, which are under the influence of conspiracy theory beliefs. It is nevertheless clear where and in whom trust is placed. Trust is only placed in people and reports that share the opinions and criticisms. They are not questioned and often use

6 That could be attributed to the emerging phenomenon known as "pandemic fatigue" (Lilleholt et al 2020) which can naturally affect vaccinated individuals as well. Pandemic fatigue refers to a general weariness or exhaustion experienced by individuals due to the prolonged duration and ongoing challenges associated with a pandemic, such as restrictions on daily life and the overall impact on mental and emotional well-being.

"emotional language" (Germani and Biller-Andorno 2021, 4–14) or "emotional grip" (Hentschel 2021, 64) and focus on their own suffering:

> I just can't take it anymore. There must finally be peace and quiet again... (Chat1_P4 20.10.2021)

The literature provides evidence that people who believe in conspiracy theories are also more likely to distrust science (van Prooijen, Spadaro, and Wang 2021; Goldenberg 2021). The content studied indicated that while scientists who were closer to the government were more likely to be rejected[7] while scientists who addressed or wanted to address vaccination side effects, for example, were trusted.[8]

Trust and reputation are not turned away from science per se, but only from those scientists whose views do not conform with the ideological narratives of the sample groups. This view is biased but not apodictically anti-scientific.

Discussion: The (Postfactual) Source of Knowledge

If scientific expertise, studies and the resulting guidelines for and by politicians are not to be trusted, there are two options for those affected: they either rely entirely on themselves and their perceptions or seek and create new sources of information (Holzer et al. 2021). Such new sources of information which were dominant in the chat and channels investigated are for example German Internet magazines such as *Rubikon – Magazin für die kritische Masse*[9], *NachDenkSeiten – Die kritische Website.*[10] But also, videos by Prof. Sucharit Bhakdi, a microbiologist who has received multiple

7 For example, the German virologist Christian Drosten or the head of the Robert Koch Institute Lothar Wiehler. Both had a major media impact on the information Germans gained throughout the pandemic, especially at the beginning.

8 For example, German pathologist Peter Schirmacher (head of the pathology institute at the University of Heidelberg), who made it clear he wanted to autopsy more bodies of people who died contemporaneously after Covid19 vaccination.

9 This website (translated: Rubikon – Magazine for the critical masses) was referred to in some places by the investigators or recommended for further reading. Rubikon is basically more of a blog than a magazine where various independent journalists share their critical perspectives on current world affairs, relying more or less on official figures (e.g., those of the German Federal Statistical Office or the Paul Ehrlich Institute). Rubikon has also founded its own publishing house and distributes books that have even become German bestsellers. https://www.rubikon.news (30.10.2022).

10 This page (translated: NachDenkSeiten – the critical website) have also been frequently recommended in my analysis for gaining a "fresh" perspective. https://www.nachdenkseiten.de (30.10.2022).

awards from the scientific community who became a Covid-19 denier whose popular channel was eventually deleted from YouTube. As was evident in the previous findings, both forms of knowledge generation are found in the content studied, but they are confirmed and consolidated through personal narratives or eyewitness accounts rather than verified sources. The information of like-minded people becomes more relevant than results of science that says otherwise. In this context, Skudlarek (2021) reads this as an attempt by the individuals within these skeptical groups to regain control over their lives. For those who assume that the virus and the vaccination strategy follow a hidden agenda are better able to cope with the disarray of everyday life, since they are not made vulnerable by the mistrust they already have in the government. Neither by the virus nor by the vaccination nor by the "hypnotization" through the "mainstream media."

This myth of invulnerability is also evident in the chat and channels. The more dominant the exchange about the supposed superiority through more knowledge or critical thinking was, the stronger the perception of unjustified blame assignment became.

With this own logic, it is almost impossible to simply accept statements since the supposed critical thinking and superior knowledge obstruct the acceptance of announcements regarding the Covid-19 virus by politicians or institutions as simply true. The people in my case studies have created their own "cultural knowledges" and this conditions the reading under which they view messages (Fiske 2007). It became also clear that the members of the sample groups either do not consume any news outside their *Telegram* circle of influence or evaluate the so-called "mainstream media" from perspectives formed exclusively by their own cultural knowledge. By sharing the content within the feedback loops of their channels, the studied reproduce their beliefs through their supposed (superior) understanding and reading. This makes it difficult to access and transfer knowledge from other social groups to those of the studied.

This better knowledge and selective perception with regard to science can be subsumed under the term *postfactual*: everyone chooses the truths that best fit their own positions and goals. Postfactual phenomena are characterized by the fact that they seek to trigger emotions in those who read or listen to them instead of generating facts. Awareness of what quality and outcome certain messages want to trigger must be trained (Ferretti 2021). Accordingly, the fact that certain websites or *YouTube* videos want to generate reach and capital through clicks must be reflected on more critically.

Conclusion

The content analysis of the data collected over the period from October 2021 to the end of December 2021 was not only able to show the self-affirming structures in the arguments of the vaccination critics. It also became clear that they were motivated by a feeling of being excluded and stigmatized and that they found alternative community support in the groups and channels on *Telegram*. Through this online exchange, they are also able to repeatedly verify their own ideas regarding the vaccination as a potential threat. This is supported, on the one hand, by the idea that those in power do not act in the interests of the health of the population and only represent the interests of the pharmaceutical industry. On the other hand, the content studied points to the hope of a "new system" soon. This additionally supports the feeling of group solidarity and togetherness as a coping mechanism for the felt alienation from the majority society. Representations of the unvaccinated in official public discourse were particularly involved. Nevertheless, the vaccination critics studied distinguish themselves by describing vaccinated persons as "sheeple" and "hypnotized" by the "mainstream media."

It should be noted that the injustice narrative analyzed in my study only considers the unjustified blaming and exclusion of the vaccination critics themselves, while overlooking the fact that these opponents also reproduce similar injustices when they blame and exclude the broader society due to their non-vaccination. The argumentation logic of the persons in the chat group and the link channels is thus characterized by "emotional language" (Germani and Biller-Andorno 2021, 4–14) and focuses on their own experiences and experiences that verify their own thinking. Other ways of thinking are only included if they fit their counter-narrative, both of injustice and corona criticism. In doing so, they label those in power as criminal while pretending to only want to protect themselves from their division. Loneliness and exclusion from social life are accepted. The knowledge and reasoning they draw on seems to be primarily postfactual.

These findings do not map the full reality of corona vaccination critics' lives, but they do show how difficult it can be to reach them on a different level. Reducing social injustice, structural problems, and a more open approach on the part of policymakers without stigma may not reduce the current number of unvaccinated but could create a higher level of trust that would be essential for future crises.

As highlighted by Goldenberg (2019) in her work, it is crucial to acknowledge issues of injustice and rebuild trust in institutions and authorities in order to address vaccine hesitancy and enhance public health outcomes. By actively listening to and responding to the concerns of individuals hesitant about vaccines, healthcare providers and officials can foster stronger and more equitable relationships with their communities. In conclusion, the findings of this study underscore the imperative of confronting the fundamental social and structural determinants underpinning vaccine hesitancy, as this serves as a vital foundation for cultivating public trust and fortifying societal resilience in times of crisis. Accordingly, policymakers face the challenge of devising a more progressive and inclusive strategy that not only nurtures trust but also effectively tackles vaccine hesitancy. The challenge for policymakers is therefore not only to correct misinformation, but to address the social and epistemic conditions under which institutional distrust becomes a plausible and emotionally compelling narrative.

Bibliography

Betsch, Cornelia, and the team of the COSMO Konsortium. 2022a. *Ergebnisse aus dem COVID-19 Snapshot Monitoring COSMO: Die psychologische Lage. 61. Welle [PowerPoint]*. https://projekte.uni-erfurt.de/cosmo2020/files/COSMO_W61.pdf, last modified May 30, 2022.

Betsch, Cornelia, and the team of the COSMO Konsortium. 2022b. *Ergebnisse aus dem COVID-19 Snapshot Monitoring COSMO: Die psychologische Lage. 59. Welle [PowerPoint]*. https://projekte.uni-erfurt.de/cosmo2020/files/COSMO_W59.pdf, last modified May 30, 2022.

Budnik, Christian. 2021. "Vertrauen als politische Kategorie in Zeiten von Corona." *Nachdenken über Corona. Philosophische Essays über die Pandemie und ihre Folgen*, edited by G. Keil and R. Jaster, Reclam, 19–30.

Butter, Michael. 2020. "Verschwörungstheorien: Zehn Erkenntnisse aus der Pandemie." *Jenseits von Corona*, edited by B. Kortmann and G. G. Schulze, transcript, 225–231.

Collins, Caitlyn, Leah Ruppanner, L. Christin Landivar, and William J. Scarborough. 2021. "The Gendered Consequences of a Weak Infrastructure of Care: School Reopening Plans and Parents' Employment During the COVID-19 Pandemic." *Gender & Society*, vol. 35, no. 2, 180–193. doi:10.1177/08912432211001300.

Conner, Christopher T., and Nicholas MacMurray. 2022. "The Perfect Storm: A Subcultural Analysis of the QAnon Movement." *Critical Sociology*, vol. 48, no. 6, 1049–1071. doi:10.1177/08969205211055863.

Curley, Cliona, Eugenie Siapera, and Joe Carthy. 2022. "Covid-19 Protesters and the Far Right on Telegram: Co-Conspirators or Accidental Bedfellows?" *Social Media + Society*, vol. 8, no. 4. doi:10.1177/20563051221129187.

Ferretti, Maria Paola. 2021. "Post-Factualism, Political Communication and the Role of Citizens." *Virtues, Democracy, and Online Media: Ethical and Epistemic Issues*, edited by Nancy E. Snow and Maria Silvia Vaccarezza, 1st edition, Routledge. doi:10.4324/9781003083108.

Fiske, John. 2007. *Reading the Popular*, Unwin Hyman.

Frei, Nadine, Robert Schäfer, and Oliver Nachtwey. 2021. "Die Proteste gegen die Corona-Maßnahmen: Eine soziologische Annäherung." *Forschungsjournal Soziale Bewegungen*, vol. 34, no. 2, 249–258. doi:10.1515/fjsb-2021-0021.

Fricker, Miranda. 2007. *Epistemic Injustice: Power and the Ethics of Knowing*, Oxford UP.

Germani, Federico, and Nicola Biller-Andorno. 2021. "The anti-vaccination infodemic on social media: A behavioral analysis." *PLOS ONE*, vol. 16, no.3, e0247642. doi:10.1371/journal.pone.0247642.

Gesser-Edelsburg, Anat. 2021. "Using Narrative Evidence to Convey Health Information on Social Media: The Case of COVID-19." *Journal of Medical Internet Research*, vol. 23, no. 3, e24948. doi:10.2196/24948.

Goldenberg, Maya J. 2021. *Vaccine Hesitancy: Public Trust, Expertise, and the War on Science*, U of Pittsburgh P.

Harbach, Heiner. 2008. "Eine Soziologie der Ungerechtigkeit." *Soziologie sozialer Probleme und sozialer Kontrolle*, edited by A. Groenemeyer and S. Wiesler, Verlag für Sozialwissenschaften, 48–69.

Hentschel, Christine. 2021. "Das große Erwachen: Affekt und Narrativ in der Bewegung gegen die Corona-Maßnahmen." *Leviathan*, vol. 49, no. 1, 62–85.

Holzer, Boris, Sebastian Koos, Christian Meyer, Isabell Otto, Isabelle-Christine Panreck, and Sven Reichhardt. 2021. "Einleitung: Protest in der Pandemie." *Die Misstrauensgemeinschaft der „Querdenker,"* edited by Sven Reichardt, Campus, 125–158.

Iacoella, Francesco, Patricia Justino, and Bruno Martorano. 2021. "Do pandemics lead to rebellion? Policy responses to COVID-19, inequality, and protests in the USA." *WIDER Working Paper 2021/57*. UNU-WIDER. doi:10.35188/UNU-WIDER/2021/995-2.

Iyengar, Karthikeyan, Ahmed Mabrouk, Vijay Kumar Jain, Aakaash Venkatesan, and Raju Vaishya. 2020. "Learning opportunities from COVID-19 and future effects on health care system." *Diabetes & Metabolic Syndrome*, vol. 14, no. 5, 943–946. doi:10.1016/j.dsx.2020.06.036.

Kniestedt, Fanny. 2021. "Polizei vermutet hohe Dunkelziffer bei gefälschten Corona-Impfzertifikaten." *MDR*, Oktober 29, 2021. https://www.mdr.de/nachrichten/deutschland/gesellschaft/corona-impf-pass-ausweis-faelschung-100.html, last modified July 7, 2022.

Koos, Sebastian. 2021. "Konturen einer heterogenen 'Misstrauensgemeinschaft': Die soziale Zusammensetzung der Corona-Proteste und die Motive ihrer Teilnehmer:innen." *Die Misstrauensgemeinschaft der „Querdenker,"* edited by Sven Reichardt, Campus, 67–89.

Kuckartz, Udo. 2014. *Qualitative Text Analysis: A Guide to Methods, Practice and Using Software*, SAGE. doi:10.4135/9781446288719.

Kuckartz, Udo. 2019. "Qualitative Content Analysis: From Kracauer's Beginnings to Today's Challenges." *Forum Qualitative Sozialforschung / Forum: Qualitative Social Research*, vol. 20, no. 3, 1–20. doi:10.17169/fqs-20.3.3370.

Lessenich, Stephan. 2020. "Soziologie – Corona – Kritik." *Berliner Journal für Soziologie*, vol. 30, 215–230. doi:10.1007/s11609-020-00417-3.

Lilleholt, Lau, Ingo Zettler, Cornelia Betsch, and Robert Böhm. 2020. "Shedding Light on Pandemic Fatigue." *PsyArXiv Prepr*, 1–36. doi:10.31234/osf.io/2xvbr.

Milošević Đorđević, Jasna, Silvia Mari, Milicia Vdović, and A. Milošević. 2021. "Links between conspiracy beliefs, vaccine knowledge, and trust: Anti-vaccine behavior of Serbian adults." *Social Science & Medicine*, vol. 277, 113930. doi:10.1016/j.socscimed.2021.113930.

Plümper, Thomas, Eric Neumayer, and Katharina Gabriela Pfaff. 2021. "The strategy of protest against Covid-19 containment policies in Germany." *Social Science Quarterly*, vol. 102, no. 5. doi:10.1111/ssqu.13066.

Powers, Martha, Phil Brown, Grace Poudrier, Jeniffer Liss Ohayon, Alissa Cordner, Cole Alder, and Marina Goreau Atlas. 2021. "COVID-19 as Eco-Pandemic Injustice: Opportunities for Collective and Antiracist Approaches to Environmental Health." *J Health Soc Behav*, vol. 62, no. 2, 222–229. doi:10.1177/00221465211005704.

Reichardt, Sven, editor. 2021. *Die Misstrauensgemeinschaft der "Querdenker,"* Campus.

Richter, Christoph, and Axel Salheiser. 2021. "Die Corona-Pandemie als Katalysator des Rechtsextremismus und Rechtspopulismus in Thüringen, Deutschland und Europa?" *Wissen schafft Demokratie. Schwerpunkt Demokratiegefährdungen in der Coronakrise*, vol. 9, Institut für Demokratie und Zivilgesellschaft, 76–87. http://www.idz-jena.de/wsddet/wsd9-8/.

Schicktanz, Silke. 2012. "Epistemische Gerechtigkeit. Sozialempirie und Perspektivenpluralismus in der Angewandten Ethik." *Deutsche Zeitschrift für Philosophie*, vol. 60, no. 2, 269–283. doi:10.1524/dzph.2012.0019.

Schmid, Philipp, Dorothee Rauber, Cornelia Betsch, Gianni Lidolt, and Marie-Luisa Denker. 2017. "Barriers of Influenza – Vaccination Intention and Behavior – A Systematic Review of Influenza Vaccine Hesitancy. *PLoS ONE*, vol. 12, no. 1, e0170550. doi:10.1371/journal.pone.0170550.

Shklar, Judith Nisse. 1990. *The Faces of Injustice*, Yale UP.

Skudlarek, Jan. 2021. "Die 'Plandemie': Verschwörungserzählungen und Wahrheitsprobleme in der Corona-Pandemie." *Zwischen Wahn und Wahrheit*, edited by M.C. Bauer and L. Deinzer, Springer, 137–157.doi:10.1007/978-3-662-63641-1.

Spahn, Jens. 2020. "Bundesgesundheitsminister Jens Spahn im Bundestag bei der 2./3. Lesung des Entwurfs eines Dritten Bevölkerungsschutzgesetzes. [speech]." Berlin, November 18, 2020. https://www.bundesgesundheitsministerium.de/presse/presse/archiv-reden-19-legislaturperiode/drittes-bevschutzg-beschluss-bt.html, last modified May 30, 2023.

Telegram. 2022. "Telegram FAQ." *Telegram*. https://telegram.org/faq?setln=en, last modified May 30, 2025.

van Mulukom, Valerie, Lotte J. Pummerer, Sinan Alper, Hui Bai, Vladimira Čavojová, Jessica Farias, Cameron S. Kay, Ljiljana B. Lazarevic, Emilio J.C. Lobato, Gaelle Marinthe, Irena Pavela Banai, Jakub Šrol, and Iris Žeželj. 2022. "Antecedents and consequences of COVID-19 conspiracy beliefs: A systematic review." *Social Science & Medicine*, vol. 301, 114912. doi:10.1016/j.socscimed.2022.114912.

van Prooijen, Jan-Willem, Giuliana Spadaro, and Haiyan Wang. 2022. "Suspicion of institutions: How distrust and conspiracy theories deteriorate social relationships." *Current Opinion in Psychology*, vol. 43, 65–69. doi:10.1016/j.copsyc.2021.06.013.

World Health Organization (WHO). 2017. *Vaccination and Trust – How concerns arise and the role of communication in mitigating crises*. https://www.who.int/publications/i/item/vaccination-and-trust, last modified May 30, 2023.

Personal Responsibility and Inequality

The Anti-Vaccine Discourse in the United States

Jennifer A. Reich

Introduction

The outbreak of COVID-19, the largest pandemic in most people's lifetime, led to millions of deaths. The advent of vaccinations against the virus that caused the pandemic did not entirely eliminate infection but did a great deal to significantly reduce severity of illness and risk of death. Yet, in the United States and beyond, the introduction of vaccines against SARS-CoV-2, the virus that caused the pandemic, was met with suspicion and often passionate opposition. Although this response was baffling to many, it in fact built upon existing narratives of infection and prevention that pre-date COVID.

Almost two decades ago, I began studying why parents in the U.S. were increasingly opting out of vaccines for their children, rejecting some or all, or creating alternative schedules that do not align with any expert recommendation. I found that vaccine hesitancy and opposition represented the coalescence of individualist notions of health and parenting (Reich 2016). Parents in general, and mothers in particular, saw themselves as experts on their own children and vaccine decisions as one of a multitude of daily consumer choices they make to promote their children's health. Many considered vaccination as largely unnecessary given the range of other decisions and lifestyle choices they perceived to be adequate to protect their children's health.

As concerns about COVID-19 began escalating in Spring 2020, public health agencies increasingly focused on personal responsibility and individual behavior as decisive factors that could increase or mitigate risk of infection but also identified baseline health and underlying conditions as aspects that may increase vulnerability. Age, obesity, immune compromise, and chronic health conditions were all identified as predictive of worse outcomes of infection. As vaccines against SARS-CoV-2 eventually became available in early 2021, arguments about their safety and necessity accelerated, with many younger healthy adults insisting that their overall good health, healthy lifestyle, or lack of underlying risk factors meant that they did not need the vaccine. Rather than highlighting the unpredictability of infectious disease, COVID amplified the belief that personal behaviors, lifestyle choices, and consumer decisions can mitigate serious illness. In this chapter, I examine narratives created by vaccine opponents, that is, those who speak publicly and work to undermine confidence in vaccines, to show how their efforts rely on the belief that health lies within the individual, and is manageable and controllable through hard work, good consumption choices, and faith in the natural powers of the body.

Infectious Disease, Vaccines, and Perceptions of Risk

Narratives of health promotion often identify personal responsibility, hard work, lifestyle, and behavior as key to illness avoidance. These frames, which are often commercialized, are persuasive, but ignore the reality that most aspects of health and illness are beyond individual control and reflect complex interactions between genetics, environment, lifestyle, resources, social location, and luck. Yet they are ubiquitous in claims that vaccines are unnecessary when one has good health and health practices.

Individual decisions about whether to receive a vaccine, which is given to healthy people to prevent hypothetical harm, involves weighing a perceived risk of an adverse reaction to a vaccine against a perceived risk of a vaccine preventable disease. Notably, risk has an objective component in the calculation of the probability of a result arising from an action, but it also depends on subjective interpretation to make it socially meaningful (Douglas 1990). Pointing to the socially meaningful interpretations of risk, Horlick-Jones argues that "[a]ny assessment of risk involves, by necessity, a summation over a variety of potential harms posed by a given hazard. Such a summation involves a weighting process that either implicitly or explicitly introduces valuations of the relative importance of each harm" (1998, 80).

To be motivated to seek out health interventions, individuals must perceive they are susceptible to a particular health problem, that this health problem is a serious one, that utilization of a treatment or medication will reduce risk of that condition, and there must not be any serious barriers to accessing the treatment (Rosenstock 1966). Those who would seek out health interventions must also find ways that the prescribed treatments fit their lives and match their own goals and lifestyle as well as their perception of a negative outcome (Conrad 1985). Yet, we live at a cultural moment in which risk is most often framed within the terms of what Lupton calls "lifestyle risk discourse" which she defines as "the responsibility of the individual to avoid health risks for the sake of his or her own health as well as the greater good of society" (Lupton 2009, 463). From this standpoint, risk can be managed and mitigated through lifestyle changes, which promise to ensure good health outcomes.

Immunization is at core a risk containment technology. Unlike other pharmaceutical interventions, vaccines are given to healthy people to avoid risk, rather than to sick people to manage symptoms or cure illness. Immunizations against childhood illnesses are touted as one of the greatest achievements of modern medicine and are credited with drastically reducing, and in many cases virtually eliminating, incidences of measles, mumps, rubella, polio, diphtheria, haemophilus influenzae type b, tetanus, and whooping cough (or pertussis) in the much of the world. Vaccines for adults prior to COVID-19 were less often used, but also held lifesaving possibilities. Estimates are that without vaccines against SARS-CoV-2, there would have been approximately 1.1 million additional COVID-19 deaths and more than 10.3 million additional COVID-19 hospitalizations in the U.S. by November 2021 (Schneider et al. 2021).

Personalization of Health and the Challenges of Community Intervention

Unlike other medications, vaccines most often do not just protect the person who receives inoculation, but the disabled, the aged, the immune-compromised, those who did not gain immunity from vaccines, and the pregnant women whose fetuses could be devastated by infection. Even vaccines like those against SARS-CoV-2 that do not fully eliminate transmission of the virus do save lives and may reduce transmission (Stokel-Walker 2022). These benefits are often underestimated as potential consumers of vaccines consider the level of personal benefit rather than community benefit (Reich 2016).

Vaccines, a technology most effective as a communal rather than individual strategy, contradict the cultural logic of healthism, in which individuals are personally and morally responsible for their own health outcomes. This ideological position represents, as Crawford (1980) and others have argued, the shifting of responsibility for health from the state to the moral obligation of the individual. Drawing on a neoliberal logic, healthcare decisions, including disease prevention, medication consumption, and elective procedures, are assigned to the individual. Biotechnology has presented opportunities for lifestyle enhancement or "optimization," but also presents a highly prescriptive form of social control (Loe and Cuttino 2008; Conrad and Potter 2004). As Crawford points out,

> [t]he failure of healthist ideology to treat individual behavior, attitudes, and emotions as socially constructed reproduces the disablement fostered by medical ideology and the ideology of individualism in general. Instead of approaching the complex inter-relationship of individual characteristics, choices, and larger social structure, healthism promotes a new moralism (1980, 384–385).

The ideals of healthism are encoded culturally everywhere. In families, women are encouraged to adopt the role of advocate, researcher, and informed consumer as they navigate their family's health and healthcare, nutrition, and consumption of household products (MacKendrick 2014). More broadly, health itself has come to be defined as the outcome of personal choices and behaviors, often through consumption and risk management (Clarke et al. 2003). Individuals must actively manage their lives, work hard, behave morally, and avoid calculable risk through informed decision-making to remain healthy, the imagined state of the body without corruption (Juffer 2003). The individual in a "regime of self" is expected to actively shape her or his life through active health choices, with socially defined good choices becoming the cultural norm against which an individual's morality might be evaluated (Rose and Novas 2004). (The condemnation of smokers or overweight people illustrates this as well).

The regimes of self-governance that center on health promotion through consumer choice resonate with a range of corporate enterprises to promote health or avoid illness. Within and outside of medicine, we see heightened attention on how medical care can be personalized to meet the needs and desires of the individual. Promises of new methods of identifying individual risk of developing certain diseases, genetic tests for predisposition, or calculating risk of health challenges are advertised and sold in ways that promise individualized care and personal control. Although companies are beginning to offer racial and biological analyses of individual genetic material, and pharmaceutical companies promise to create personalized medicine that could eventually match drugs to individual personal genetic profiles, these innovations have yet to hold major practical uses or even hit the market (Hunt and Kreiner 2013). Notably, individualized care, which is often desired, does not necessarily yield better health outcomes, but it may create a more positive experience of health care (Fenton et al. 2012). Nonetheless, narratives of health as personalized, individualized, and commercialized shape perceptions and at core contradict public health logics that require uniform efforts to prevent communicable disease.

Personal responsibility and individual preference shape how individuals think of vaccine decisions. Yet, public health assumes that individuals can absorb a measure of risk to themselves (or their children) or sacrifice some freedoms in order to protect others in the communities in which they live or travel. This sometimes frustrates individuals who often insist they "should be 'empowered' to pursue their own self-interest as a condition of their rights (and obligations) as consumers of public resources," which places their desires for themselves or their children ahead of others (Wilkins 2014).

This commitment to the regime of self represents the simultaneous challenge to the role of the expert and the democratization and contestation of scientific knowledge (Barker 2008). Record profits posted by pharmaceutical companies, direct marketing to physicians, and pharmaceutical advertising have contributed to the erosion of trust in medical institutions and providers (McKinlay and Marceau 2002; Hartley and Coleman 2008). The COVID-19 pandemic, with the tight collaboration between nation-states and for-profit pharmaceutical companies, furthered this distrust. Calls to return control of health to the state after decades of public health agencies' insistence that individuals were responsible for their own health were broadly met with skepticism and likely furthered the delegitimization of expert claims on how to best promote health.

Sources of Narratives for Analysis

In order to analyze narratives of vaccine opponents during the COVID-19 pandemic, I watched streamed content and then listened to and read transcripts of that content, which were recorded in 168 audio files ranging in length from 20 minutes to three hours. These videos offered information on how to promote health without vaccines, advised on how to challenge or undermine vaccine or mask requirements in work or school environments, or encouraged audiences to view vaccines specifically and medical systems in general with suspicion.

These online videos were produced and distributed by two sources. First, a group hosted two multi-day online conferences they called the Health Freedom Summit during the COVID pandemic and posted interviews and workshops with dozens of different speakers from these virtual events. Combined, these two conferences had 72 different sessions. Some speakers returned for both events while others were only part of one conference. Second, Jonathan Otto, a self-described humanitarian documentary filmmaker, posted three to five hours of content daily for about 40–50 days throughout COVID. These long videos, ranging from one to three hours, were installments in a series that ran for 8–10 consecutive days at a time, with series titles like, "Covid Secrets Exposed," "Vaccine Secrets Reloaded," or "Unbreakable." Each of these videos was edited around a specific theme and included five to eight speakers. The content was posted for free for 24 hours and then reverted to paid subscription to access it.

I cannot provide estimates of the numbers of viewers on either of these platforms, though they often included some of the biggest names in anti-vaccine rhetoric, including Robert Kennedy, Andrew Wakefield, Mary Holland, Naomi Wolf, Joseph Mercola, and Robert Malone. More broadly, it is difficult to overestimate the reach of these narratives that seek to undermine vaccines and public health, a phenomenon the World Health Organization has termed an "infodemic." Estimates suggest that, in the American context, just twelve anti-vaccine advocates are responsible for almost two-thirds of anti-vaccine content circulating on social media platforms. Ten of them participated in these online events.

Although some members of what has been termed "the disinformation dozen" are part of this analysis, there are many self-described experts who are also included. Notably, both content creators have a monetized component to accessing content and also sell or promote products that claim will improve health, "detoxify" the negative effects of vaccination, or cure COVID. The transcripts of these webinars and video presentations were supplemented with emails and website information from the same sources. I analyzed transcripts of these videos to identify patterns in how vaccines, infection, health, and COVID were presented. The quotes provided here offer examples of the kinds of rhetoric that proliferated in these sources.

The views that health is a personal project and that individuals can control through behavior were common before COVID-19. Yet, during the pandemic, these claims were amplified as an explanation why vaccines in general – and against SARS-CoV-2 specifically – were unnecessary. These arguments seem persuasive because they align with larger cultural definitions of personal responsibility, but they ignore the reality that infectious disease is largely beyond individual control. Many were reminded during the COVID-19 pandemic that hard work and precautions alone cannot eliminate all risk of exposure to an infectious agent. Although pre-existing conditions and underlying health issues may place some individuals at greater risk of the worse outcomes of infection, it is a myth that individuals who do not have risk factors will not be significantly affected by infection. In the following sections, I examine the narratives put forward by those who oppose vaccines to show how they rely on a view of the body as naturally perfect and as able to combat infection without pharmaceutical assistance, and of disease as controllable. I then show how they explain COVID-related deaths as the result of personal failings including poor nutrition and pre-existing health conditions, rather than of the unpredictability of infection. Together, these narratives reinforce an ideology of individualism that makes public and community-level interventions more challenging.

The Body as Naturally Perfect

Much of the narrative of vaccine opposition originates from the belief that the body is naturally perfect and thus, does not require medical or pharmaceutical intervention. Vaccine decisions start somewhere on a continuum that views the body as varyingly vulnerable, at risk, or invincible. Often, those who reject vaccines see their bodies as naturally perfect, often as made by God, and able to handle infection which at times leads them to the conclusion that vaccines undermine the body and can be harmful.

Vaccine opponent and microbiologist Christina Parks explains on one of the videos produced by Otto, how those who promote immunization do not understand that the body is perfectly designed to fight infection without vaccines:

> we are fearfully and wonderfully made, and...we're being told all you know, we need something manmade, that man is the measure of all things. Not God. He didn't design you, right? We've got to fix it. And so there's so much so that we don't know, but what we do know is that what God designed is always superior to what man designs and so we need to bolster the body, build it up.

Parks continues, explaining that illness results from toxic exposure, which the body can also handle, noting,

> [y]ou know, we talked about all the contaminants, right? And so that's what's predisposing us to all this illness. And so yes, we are in a toxic soup, but even still, the fact that any of us are healthy, God has designed us to be able to heal always to be able to heal, and it's the lie that we are dependent on something a man has created in order to heal and move forward or protect ourselves.

Like Parks and others, Daniel Nuzum, a naturopathic physician who sells supplements and offers telehealth consultations, explains on one of Otto's videos how illness only emerges when the body is undermined, noting, "I approach healing from the standpoint that God designed us perfectly. If we're not functioning perfectly, there's just there's something causing that." That "something" is seldomly identified as simply an infection or development of illness but more often as exposure to or failure to consume adequate nutrition.

The body, as it is imagined here, sometimes requires intervention to return it to health through "natural" interventions. Notably, the false dichotomy between natural and artificial is unacknowledged. Much like Bobel found in her research: "When mothers spoke of nature, they spoke of a monolithic and static concept, the one true thing that predates humankind and remains pure and unadulterated. To them, nature is the perfect model for human behavior because it is separate from and unpolluted by human manipulation" (2002, 127).

Mark Sherwood, another naturopathic doctor, who, with his wife, runs a clinic, records a podcast, and sells supplements insists his practice works to "lead people down a pathway of true healing," which includes helping their patients "to eradicate all self-imposed, choice driven disease conditions" (FMI 2023). In his clinic, he follows an approach to care that asks individuals to optimize their health through changes in personal behavior. As stated on his website and on his publicity materials, "[e]ach person will need to make their own decision, and carefully weigh the risks versus benefits. In our clinic, every person that we have dealt with has done very well on natural therapies to optimize function – whole body in general. In our belief, God created the body in His own image. Every system in the body – including the immune system." Substantiating his health views within a religious frame,

Sherwood explained to Otto: "[h]uman beings are the only ones made in his image. Jesus did not spend his time on earth worrying about being sick."

Seeing the body as naturally perfect allows for a narrative that insists that health and illness avoidance are within individual control. Often referenced in terms of intelligent or godly design, vaccine opponents present a narrative of the body as naturally healthy and only sick when undermined through poor lifestyle or poor decision-making. At core, the worst outcomes of infection, they insist, can be combatted by allowing the body to return to a natural, superior state, which may include improved nutrition, better feeding practices, consumption of supplements, or treatments that many of these speakers sell.

The Healthy Body's Power to Heal Itself

This myth of natural perfection feeds the assumption that the body can heal itself from infection or illness when it is in an ideal state of baseline health. Within these narratives, vaccines are at best an underestimation of the body's abilities and at worse, a chemical exposure that undermines them. Illustrating this, Jenny Crane, a self-described "medical freedom advocate, top network marketing leader, boy mom & chef wife," points to how the pandemic and insistence on vaccines subverts confidence in the body. She explains,

> I always say the pandemic is a pandemic of fear, right. That's the problem. That's the virus. But if you think about it, we're being fed this information and it's all doom and gloom and they want to think that the only way to get healthy is by getting healthy with a needle in a bottle. And that is simply not the case. We know that when the body is working properly. And when it's empowered, the body is the miracle.

The insistence that individuals can control disease hinges on a belief that the body can successfully manage infection so long as it has not been weakened by "harmful" behaviors or lifestyles. Andrew Kaufman, a psychiatrist and COVID denier explains,

> [w]hat really results in us being ill are things that we can actually control 100%. Like what we put in our body, when we put synthetic chemicals and toxins in our body. So once you understand that actually, all the real causes of disease are things that we have the ability to influence and change and allow our bodies to either maintain health or restore to full health, then the fear of a mysterious invader from beyond is not present. And this is something that makes me really sleep well at night not only for my own health and safety, which is really secondary. It's mostly about my children. That I know that if they have an illness is very easy to

> correct and it very seldom occurs because we try to do those things that I described to keep ourselves healthy from the beginning.

This is another example of how the narratives to undermine vaccines rely on the claim that personal behaviors prevent or cause disease. An espoused commitment to natural living – through superior nutrition, and lifestyle – is key to this. Weakness in the body, in immunity, manifests by becoming sick, and therefore reflects individual failures. Once the body is imagined to be self-curing, any inability to recover from illness represents an underlying failure.

This logic underpins how vaccine opponents explain why most people recover from COVID without medical intervention, but a high number of people require medical care and even succumb to infection. Henry Ealy, another naturopathic doctor and founder of the Energetic Health Institute, argues that those who are healthy do not need to worry about COVID infection:

> The data is very clear. The high percentage, the insanely high predictions, insanely, a significantly high percentage – 99 percentile of people recover without really any help or any assistance. Yes, some people have severe symptomatology from infection. Some people require hospitalization. Some people require a lot of intervention and typically those people have, are entering into these situations, these infections, with a severe nutrient deficiency status and a severe number of comorbid pre-existing conditions. The data is very clear on which groups, what age groups in which health groups are succumbing to the infection. And it's very clear it's not a young and it's not the people who are in a good state of health. So, this is where we come in and we say that old adage still holds true. An ounce of prevention is worth a pound of cure.

Jonathan Murphy, an integrative medicine physician, also highlights how the body's perfect design can heal itself when not overwhelmed with toxins or pollutants:

> I think that the body heals and is very well designed, and we have the most perfect design... I think healing – pull a splinter out of the thumb, you know, don't put a splinter in the mouth of the root canal too. Let's try to minimize our exposure to toxins by trying to eliminate as much as possible unneeded pesticides, unneeded plasticizers and other pollutants. But the body can heal if we nourish it and detoxify it.

Rather than seeing infection as sometimes random and unpredictable, these narratives frame lifestyle and personal resolve as key to mastery over disease. The vaccine, they suggest, erroneously and immorally promises illness avoidance without the hard work required to truly be healthy. As Mark Sherwood, who calls vaccines "symptoms of science," explains,

> [t]here's a lot of ignorance around people being manipulated, conned, bribed, scared into taking the vaccine and a lot of people listening right now are right there... We need to understand that the concept of self-governance and self-responsibility must not be eliminated.

These narratives are linked by a shared assumption that vaccines inevitably and unavoidably compromise health. Attendees of the online live forums Otto and his invited "experts" would host understood this, but faced with vaccine requirements for work, school, or travel, would ask for advice on which is the least toxic COVID vaccine to take. For example, one woman asks, "My daughter, 24, is getting the vaccine to take a cruise with her boyfriend's family. Which one does the least damage?" In response, chiropractor and vaccine opponent Bryan Ardis, replies, "We get this a lot. People want to, want us to determine, a lot of us health professionals, they want us to declare which one is safer than the others. None of them are safe. None. None of them are safe. There's not even a discussion about which one's safer than others."

Should someone get a vaccine anyway, Ardis and others typically suggest supplements and self-designed protocols to heal what they insist are inevitable vaccine-caused injuries. Illustrating this, Ardis answers another question with a recommendation for his own concoction, ironically named after the National Institutes of Health, the research arm of the U.S. federal government:

> This is Susan. She says due to mandates I may be forced to get the shots. I'm in Canada. What can I do to protect myself from the spike proteins before and after?... I actually created a list. I called it the disease prevention cocktail for the last 10 months. The boards for the state and the NIH didn't like that so they reached out to me and wanted to try to destroy my rights to create a disease prevention cocktail. So if you go [online] right now, it's actually listed as the NIH cocktail. I abbreviated NIH because if the NIH can put in drugs to kill you and hurt a whole lot of people and cause disease, I decided I can create the NIH cocktail to help reverse it toward their agenda. NIH on my site stands for Natural Immune Health cocktail. There's four primary nutrients that everyone should consider to try to protect against the shedding of vaccines and then if you're going to get the vaccines or gotten the vaccine. Those four are vitamin C at high doses I would say orally 5000 milligrams a day work up to 10,000 a day consistently. And then magnesium at 500 milligrams everyday minimum selenium at 200 micrograms and then apple pectin powder at 700 milligrams twice a day. I hope that answered that for you. That's what I would do.

While some, like Ardis, try to sell their own protocols or products to manage what they insist are the ways the body is undermined by vaccines, others insist the damage is long-lasting. Jonathan Murphy argues that COVID vaccines for children are especially problematic and likely permanently compromise children's health:

> It just seems almost evil to me. It's either idiocracy [sic] or some type of authoritarian evil that were perpetrating on children with this jam. I can't say strongly enough, and yet I realized that because of mass formation psychosis, that there's a lot of parents out there who say, "When can I get my child a vaccine? When can I get the child a vaccine?" But if you put a revolver with a single bullet in it, they wouldn't let their child playing with it. It's a Russian roulette of a vaccine. One of a 1000 is totally disabled the rest of their life… "Oh, but you know, thinking of the people they're saving because of the vaccine." Now it's not saving the children because of the vaccine. There's no proof of that. We haven't seen massive amounts of deaths in children from Corona. It does sometimes complicate asthma. Certainly, it's a complication of obesity and diabesity. But you know, this is not the way to deal with it.

Identifying vaccines as a source of harm lies in relation to the view that illness is remediable or preventable without pharmaceutical intervention. Trust that the body is able to heal itself presents a positive view of the immune system, which indeed is quite often able to fight infection. Yet, this view situates personal behavior as able to shape immune response and draws causal relationships between behavior and disease outcome that are not supported by scientific evidence (Offit 2013). Rather, these claims draw on a class-based logic of wellness that sounds intuitive and is thus believable. Despite ample evidence that toxic exposures and pollutants are beyond individual control (MacKendrick 2014), this rhetoric continues to dangerously prioritize self-regulation and rejection of fear of infection as key to health. It also frames vaccine decisions as a choice between health through self-regulation and faith (vaccine rejection) or cynicism, laziness, and susceptibility to fear (vaccine acceptance).

Frankenfoods and Immune Harms

As individuals are urged to live healthy and without vaccines, food was most frequently referenced as the best sources of health prevention among vaccine opponents. Michele Sherwood, a doctor of osteopathic medicine and wife of the aforementioned Mark Sherwood with whom she runs a "Functional Medicine Clinic," explains how nutrition is more important to disease prevention than vaccines: "If you think about nutrition being the number one most important medical decision that you make every single day, and you make that three times a day, sometimes three times a day and two snacks over 365 days a year. It's either toxic, nutrient void, or calorie insufficient."

Fast food held a particular place of suspicion in this discourse but lack of nutrients generally – which led to calls for supplements – were also invoked to explain illness. Daniel Nuzum cautions that

> [i]f you're eating the standard American diet, it's only supplying seven essential nutrients you need at very, very bare minimum 73 nutrients. So what that is is...about 20% of 73. If we went to your car and randomly removed 80% of the nuts and bolts from your car, how well would it operate if you went [and] tried to turn it on? It's not going to operate probably won't even operate. Right? So it's [sic] let's say your brain is missing 80% of the nutrients okay? How is it supposed to operate properly?

Although there were frequent recommendations for fasting, coffee enemas, and cleanses, which purportedly could eliminate toxins from the body and return it to a healthier natural state, poor food choices were seen as undermining these interventions. Illustrating this, Jonathan Murphy explains how the benefits he believes exist in taking an anti-parasitic medication like Ivermectin to combat COVID may be less effective with fast food or other inferior nutritional choices:

> Think about the food as a base layer, and that is going to be helpful and critical. For example, someone's taking an anti-parasitic, like Ivermectin, and then they're eating McDonald's. It's going to create some problems for them in getting rid of the toxic waste and you want to keep the bowel movements going while you're doing parasite cleanses. You want to get rid of that junk and you want to have a high fiber diet, which you're going to get the more plant-based you eat. For example, the more greens you have, the more raw food you eat, the more fiber you're going to get. And so that's a great way to approach it.

Of course, excellent nutrition is no guarantee that a person can avoid illness, which at times led to more complicated conversations between vaccine opponents. Jonathan Otto discusses with Daniel Nuzum how those who promote nutrition as the key component sometimes misunderstand the health issues a person is facing. Drawing on an example of a woman with a rheumatoid arthritis and Hashimoto's thyroiditis, two autoimmune diseases, he highlights how supplements are not adequate without understanding the root cause of what he assumes inevitably must be malnutrition. He explains,

> [s]he was a good girl... Do you know how many times this woman ate at McDonalds? I mean she had a lot of conditions. She probably looks like she probably abused herself. It doesn't surprise you to know that she in her whole life has only eaten McDonald's once. This is not somebody that tried to destroy their body. I'm sure you've seen cases like this.

Otto's explanation presumes that illness would be explicable in someone who was not "a good girl," in other words, someone who ate fast food often. He identifies others who have worked hard and still experienced illness:

People get blamed, blame people and assume that it was because they ate bad. I get upset about that because I know that a lot of the people that are even watching this right now feel upset that that has always been the thing, and they've tried so many different diets and they've stuck to it. And then their practitioner often says, I mean this happens often, "Well, you're not sticking to it strong enough" even though they completely stuck to it, or they cheated once, but it doesn't explain why they're not better than when they started.

Rather than using this example as evidence that disease is not individually manageable or that the body's susceptibilities are complex, sometimes unpredictable, or not shaped by food alone, Otto and Nuzum invoke this and other exceptions to reinforce the myth of the naturally healthy body that is undermined by toxins in and beyond food. Nuzum reflected on his own practice, noting, "I've seen people that were, you know, ate pretty clean their whole life, never smoked, never drank. Never, never did all this stuff. And the thing is we are in an environment that is toxic. We have toxins around us." Even when evidence points to the fallacy of assuming that the body is naturally healthy, vaccine opponents blame the environment in ways calculated to confirm their rhetoric of personal choice. In other words, choice remains the cure no matter the cause.

Counting COVID Deaths and Comorbidities

COVID-19 has killed an estimated 6.9 million people as of June 2023 (Worldometer 2023). By December 2021, unvaccinated Americans had 53 times the risk of death as vaccinated Americans (Johnson et al. 2022). To explain these excess deaths, vaccine critics argue that data have been misreported and that COVID-related deaths are due to pre-existing conditions and comorbidities, not the virus (Reuters Fact Check 2022). Longtime vaccine opponent Robert Kennedy, prior to becoming the U.S. health secretary, insists COVID kills very few without comorbidities, defined as one or more health maladies in addition to COVID infection. Acknowledging that he does not know how many people the disease has killed, he explains,

CDC data showed that it was only 6% of the people who died from COVID-19 that were reported as COVID deaths that had no comorbidities, are the only cause of death. Everybody else, there were other either accidents or comorbidity and those people we don't know whether they died of COVID... COVID clearly kills people. We don't know, we have very very poor data as to how many people are actually being killed.

Henry Ely has repeatedly made similar claims and even filed a lawsuit in an effort to expose what he insists are changes in the reporting of deaths in the U.S. Early claims that the federal government incentivized states to report COVID as the cause of death, even when other health issues existed. For example, he explains that when someone dies with influenza, the death certificate would "be properly reported and the cause of death would be considered to be chronic obstructive pulmonary disease, COPD, since in this case example this is the oldest comorbidity." However, Ely insists that "if this same 77-year-old person instead of it being influenza H1N1, it was SARS-CoV-2 virus, COVID, what would happen is COVID-19 would be listed as the cause of death. And all the comorbidities that had been going on for 10 years-plus would be listed in part two as contributing and that's how you start manipulating data. Because these roles, this change only applies to COVID. It doesn't apply to any other cause of death. So COVID has its own unique rules."

In claiming that comorbidities account for COVID deaths rather than the infection itself, vaccine opponents argue the disease is not serious unless one has suboptimal personal health. Illustrating this, Ely insists "[b]y and large, the common experience from COVID is not death, is not hospitalization. It's recovery. The numbers don't lie, and this is all again CDC data."

These narratives serve to underscore claims the vaccines are not important, and that underlying health is key. They thus support an ideological commitment to personal responsibility for health that holds individuals accountable for health outcomes and further translates infectious disease into an individual problem with individual solutions.

The focus on "self-responsibility" and "self-governance" ignores that some vulnerabilities require community support and that infectious disease containment relies on widespread prevention. Author Naomi Wolf has become outspoken against the public insistence that vaccines are safe and effective against COVID and require widespread use. Calling claims that vaccines protect others false, she explains how vaccines are entirely a personal choice for possible personal benefit:

> [It's] your decision whether or not to get vaccinated. Really, maybe it's a good decision, maybe it's a bad one. But it only affects you. It doesn't affect anyone else around you. However, one of the kinds of impressively great lies of all time was told at around this time over and over and over again, with sound bites like, "You need to get vaccinated for yourself, your loved ones and your community," or the way President Biden put it that fall, "You will see a winter of severe disease and death. Oh you unvaccinated, for yourselves, your loved ones, and your community." Well, all of that was an outright lie.

In rejecting the logic of community intervention, Wolf and others dismiss the role of governments and agencies in helping those who are most vulnerable to the worst outcomes of infection. Instead, the privileged views of wellness, which transform disability into a personal failure, persists, often with an accompanying marketing strategy for blogs, supplements, consultations, or even trainings on how to undermine public schools or public health.

Conclusion

Imagining health and illness as manifestations of hard work, nutrition, and self-control ignores the reality that infectious disease often does not choose its victims based on these factors. Yet the claims resonate with larger cultural trends that commercialize and prioritize individualism and promise that health is earned and rewarded.

On the surface, these claims draw on a kind of class privilege that defines health and wellness in expensive terms. The relationship between health and wealth has long been established, with lower mortality, higher life expectancy, and decreased risks of obesity, smoking, hypertension, and asthma consistently appearing for those with resources (Pollack et al. 2007). Yet, the costs associated with high quality, nutrient-dense foods and access to exercise and safe environments remain beyond reach for many. One 2021 poll found that 59% of Americans report that "the high costs get in the way of them maintaining a healthy lifestyle." That number rises to 68% in urban areas (Melore 2021). From the perspective of these narratives, successful performance of commitment to one's health requires resources of money, time, and geography.

The relationship between immunity and lifestyle is less clear. Having a diet that is lower in sugar and higher in nutrient-dense foods is associated with better immune system functioning and lower rates of diabetes and other chronic diseases that can in turn affect the immune system as well as other systems in the body (Kubala 2021). A recent study found that those with the worst diet and highest levels of social deprivation had the worst outcomes of COVID infection (Merino et al. 2021). Rather than finding a dose-response to food and supplements, where the amount consumed would lead to a commensurate improvement in health, the authors caution that "[i]ndividuals who eat healthier diets are likely to share other features that might be associated with lower risk of infection such as the adoption of other risk mitigation behaviours, better household conditions and hygiene, or access to care" (Merino et al. 2021, 2103).

The relationship between supplements and infection is also unclear. Vitamin deficiency can lead to worse outcomes, but there is no evidence that supplements can entirely solve this (Vlieg-Boerstra et al. 2022; Israel et al. 2022). What is clear is that high doses or chronic use of supplements commonly claimed to be COVID cures have been linked with adverse effects, including "vitamin D with muscle pain and loss of bone mass; vitamin A with elevated liver function tests and blurred vision; vitamin E with bleeding risk; plant extracts, magnesium with gastrointestinal effects; and selenium with hair loss and brittle nails" (McGuire 2022).

Despite the lack of scientific evidence, the supplement industry is estimated to have grown by 20–25 percent during COVID, with vitamins C, D, and zinc seeing the greatest increase in demand. The largely unregulated supplement business is estimated to be a $36 billion industry (Roedel 2022).

These claims take a toll as the narratives of infection that insist that disease is containable, controllable, and unlikely to affect individuals who take personal responsibility for their health are profitable. They also serve to undermine community solutions that protect those who are most vulnerable. This rhetoric ignores social inequality and instead blames those who, despite their best efforts, are significantly impacted by infection due to factors beyond their control. Throughout, vaccines, which have been proven to significantly lower risk of death and serious illness and to reduce the spread of diseases like COVID, are undermined and even framed as harming those they can help.

Bibliography

Barker, Kristin K. 2008. "Electronic Support Groups, Patient-Consumers, and Medicalization: The Case of Contested Illness." *Journal of Health and Social Behavior*, vol. 49, no. 1, 20–36.

Bobel, Chris. 2002. *The Paradox of Natural Mothering*, Temple UP.

Clarke, Adele E., Janet K. Shim, Laura Mamo, Jennifer Ruth Fosket, and Jennifer R. Fishman. 2003. "Biomedicalization: Technoscientific Transformations of Health, Illness, and U.S. Biomedicine." *American Sociological Review*, vol. 68, no. 2, 161–194. doi: 10.2307/1519765.

Conrad, Peter. 1985. "The Meaning of Medications: Another Look at Compliance." *Social Science in Medicine*, vol. 20, no. 1, 29–37.

Conrad, Peter, and Deborah Potter. 2004. "Human growth hormone and the temptations of biomedical enhancement." *Sociology of Health & Illness*, vol. 26, no. 2, 184–215.

Crawford, Robert. 1980. "Healthism and the medicalization of everyday life." *International Journal of Health Services*, vol. 10, no. 3, 365–388.

Douglas, Mary. 1990. "Risk as a forensic resource." *Daedalus*, vol. 119, no. 4, 1–16.

Fenton, J.J., A. F. Jerant, K. D. Bertakis, and P. Franks. 2012. "The cost of satisfaction: A national study of patient satisfaction, health care utilization, expenditures, and mortality." *Archives of Internal Medicine*, vol. 172, no. 5, 405–411. doi: 10.1001/archinternmed.2011.1662.

FMI. 2023. Functional Medical Institute. https://fmidr.com/.

Hartley, Heather, and Cynthia-Lou Coleman. 2008. "News media coverage of direct-to-consumer pharmaceutical advertising: implications for countervailing powers theory." *Health*, vol. 12, 107–132.

Horlick-Jones, Tom. 1998. "Meaning and contextualisation in risk assessment." *Reliability Engineering & System Safety*, vol. 59, no. 1, 79–89. doi: https://doi.org/10.1016/S0951-8320(97)00122-1.

Hunt, Linda M., and Meta J. Kreiner. 2013. "Pharmacogenetics in Primary Care: The Promise of Personalized Medicine and the Reality of Racial Profiling." *Culture, Medicine, and Psychiatry*, vol. 37, no. 1, 226–235. doi: 10.1007/s11013-012-9303-x.

Israel, A., A. Cicurel, I. Feldhamer, F. Stern, Y. Dror, S. M. Giveon, D. Gillis, D. Strich, and G. Lavie. 2022. "Vitamin D deficiency is associated with higher risks for SARS-CoV-2 infection and COVID-19 severity: a retrospective case-control study." *Intern Emerg Med*, vol. 17, no. 4, 1053–1063. doi: 10.1007/s11739-021-02902-w.

Johnson, Amelia G, Avnika B. Amin, Akilah R. Ali, Brooke Hoots, et al. 2022. "COVID-19 incidence and death rates among unvaccinated and fully vaccinated adults with and without booster doses during periods of Delta and Omicron variant emergence – 25 US Jurisdictions, April 4–December 25, 2021." *MMWR. Morbidity and mortality weekly report* 71.

Juffer, Jane. 2003. "Dirty diapers and the new organic intellectual." *Cultural Studies*, vol. 17, no. 2, 168–192. doi: http://dx.doi.org/10.1080/0950238032000071686.

Kubala, Jillian. 2021. "How and why does diet influence immune function?" *Medical News Today*. https://www.medicalnewstoday.com/articles/how-and-why-does-diet-influence-immune-function#Adverse-effects-of-unhealthy-diets, last modified April 9, 2021.

Loe, Meika, and Leigh Cuttino. 2008. "Grappling with the Medicated Self: The Case of ADHD College Students." *Symbolic Interaction*, vol. 31, no. 3, 303–323.

Lupton, Deborah. 2009. "Risk as Moral Danger: The Social and Poltical Function of Risk Discourse in Public Health." *Sociology of Health and Illness*, edited by Peter Conrad, Worth Publishers, 460–467.

MacKendrick, Norah. 2014. "More Work for Mother Chemical Body Burdens as a Maternal Responsibility." *Gender & Society*, vol. 28, no. 5, 705–728.

McGuire, Treasure. 2022. "Can taking vitamins and supplements help you recover from COVID?" May 9, 2022. https://theconversation.com/can-taking-vitamins-and-supplements-help-you-recover-from-covid-182220.

McKinlay, John B., and Lisa D. Marceau. 2002. "The End of the Golden Age of Doctoring." *International Journal of Health Services*, vol. 32, no. 2, 379–416.

Melore, Chris. 2021. "3 in 5 Americans think it costs too much money to live a healthy life." *Studyfinds.org*, last modified Sept 8, 2021. https://studyfinds.org/healthy-life-costs-too-much-money/.

Merino, Jordi, Amit D. Joshi, Long H. Nguyen, Emily R. Leeming, Mohsen Mazidi, David A. Drew, Rachel Gibson, Mark S. Graham, Chun-Han Lo, Joan Capdevila, Benjamin Murray, Christina Hu, Somesh Selvachandran, Alexander Hammers, Shilpa N. Bhupathiraju, Shreela V. Sharma, Carole Sudre, Christina M. Astley,

Jorge E. Chavarro, Sohee Kwon, Wenjie Ma, Cristina Menni, Walter C. Willett, Sebastien Ourselin, Claire J. Steves, Jonathan Wolf, Paul W. Franks, Timothy D. Spector, Sarah Berry, and Andrew Chan. 2021. "Diet quality and risk and severity of COVID-19: a prospective cohort study." *Gut*, vol. 70, no. 11, 2096–2104. doi: 10.1136/gutjnl-2021-325353.

Offit, Paul A. 2013. *Do You Believe in Magic?: The Sense and Nonsense of Alternative Medicine*, Harperwor.

Pollack, C. E., S. Chideya, C. Cubbin, B. Williams, M. Dekker, and P. Braveman. 2007. "Should health studies measure wealth? A systematic review." *Am J Prev Med*, vol. 33, no. 3, 250–264. doi: 10.1016/j.amepre.2007.04.033.

Reich, Jennifer A. 2016. *Calling the Shots: Why Parents Reject Vaccines*, NYU Press.

Reuters Fact Check. 2022. "Fact Check-Why those with comorbidities are still counted as COVID-19 deaths." *Reuters Fact Check*. https://www.reuters.com/article/factcheck-comorbidities-coviddeaths/fact-check-why-those-with-comorbidities-are-still-counted-as-covid-19-deaths-idUSL1N2TU22X, last modified January 14, 2022.

Roedel, Kaleb. 2022. "Pandemic boosts U.S. vitamin and supplement industry." *Marketplace*.

Rose, Nikolas, and Carlos Novas. 2004. "Biological Citizenship." *Global Assemblages: Technology, Politics, and Ethics as Anthropological Problems*, edited by Aihwa Ong and Stephen J. Collier, Wiley-Blackwell, 439–463.

Rosenstock, Irwin M. 1966. "Why People Use Health Services." *The Milbank Memorial Fund Quarterly*, vol. 44, no. 3, 94–127.

Schneider, Eric C., Arnav Shah, Pratha Sah, Seyed M. Moghadas, Thomas Vilches, and Alison Galvani. 2021. "The U.S. COVID-19 Vaccination Program at One Year: How Many Deaths and Hospitalizations Were Averted?" *Commonwealth Fund*.

Stokel-Walker, Chris. 2022. "What do we know about covid vaccines and preventing transmission?" *bmj*, vol. 376.

Vlieg-Boerstra, B., N. de Jong, R. Meyer, C. Agostoni, V. De Cosmi, K. Grimshaw, G. P. Milani, A. Muraro, H. Oude Elberink, I. Pali-Schöll, C. Roduit, M. Sasaki, I. Skypala, M. Sokolowska, M. van Splunter, E. Untersmayr, C. Venter, L. O'Mahony, and B. I. Nwaru. 2022. "Nutrient supplementation for prevention of viral respiratory tract infections in healthy subjects: A systematic review and meta-analysis." *Allergy*, vol. 77, no. 5, 1373–1388. doi: 10.1111/all.15136.

Wilkins, Andrew. 2014. "Affective Practices and Neoliberal Fantasies: Mothers' Encounters with School Choice." *Mothering in the Age of Neoliberalism*, edited by M. Vandenbeld Giles, Demeter Press.

Worldometer. 2023. "Covid-19 Coronavirus Pandemic." https://www.worldometers.info/coronavirus/.

Intergenerational Solidarity
The Normative Significance of Narratives in the Corona Pandemic

Niklas Ellerich-Groppe, Mark Schweda

Introduction[1]

"Live in a way that the old can survive" – with this phrase, the German journalist Samira El Ouassil summarized the "new categorical imperative" of the COVID-19 pandemic and subsequently spelled out the implicit moral expectations towards the younger generations: "To protect the old, the young should now show what they were expecting from the old regarding climate change: sacrifice" (El Ouassil 2020 [own translation]).

This comment not only illustrates the prominence of moral appeals for solidarity between generations in public debates about the pandemic in Germany (Ellerich-Groppe et al. 2020; Ellerich-Groppe et al. 2021). By connecting the COVID-19 crisis with previous inter-generational controversies on global warming, it also shows how such appeals are frequently intertwined with narrations of biographical and historical processes intended to substantiate the accompanying normative claims. At closer inspection, El Ouassil's appeal is carried by a "contractualist" narrative of mutual reciprocal concessions between members of different, yet interdependent age groups faced with fundamentally different risks and challenges at different points in time. However, other contributions to the debate conveyed much more partisan and conflict-ridden storylines. For example, the "Boomer-remover" hashtag surfacing in early 2020 alluded to the previously popular narrative of a selfish cohort who had recklessly ruined the planet for future generations and therefore

1 This chapter is a slightly revised English version of the following article: Ellerich-Groppe, Niklas, and Mark Schweda. 2025. "Die normative Bedeutung von Narrativen in den Debatten um intergenerationelle Solidarität in der COVID-19-Pandemie." *Narrativität und Medizin. Interdisziplinäre Zugänge*, edited by Christian Hißnauer and Claudia Stockinger, transcript, 211–235. The research was funded by Volkswagen Foundation. Project: The Public (Re-)Negotiation of Intergenerational Solidarity and Responsibility in the Corona-Pandemic – Media Discourse Analysis and Ethical Evaluation (PRISMAE) (Az.: 99340).

could not expect their compassion or support in the face of the pandemic (Elliott 2022). By contrast, in a German TV-report from December 2021, an elder interviewee voiced a different, discursively well-established storyline about his own age group in order to justify claims to priority of the older generation in the context of COVID-19 vaccination: "In vaccinating, we started with the elders, who have accomplished a certain life's work and thus have done a lot to ensure that the younger generation is doing so well today" (Stumpf 2021 [own translation]).

These examples already highlight that "the public ethics narrative" (Samuel and Lucivero 2022) regarding the pandemic comprises a whole polyphony of storylines that suggest different, competing, and at times outright contrarian moral or political claims (Pedersen 2020). Against this backdrop, this chapter explores the normative significance of narratives in the German public media discourse about intergenerational solidarity during the COVID-19 pandemic. The focus is on the questions which narratives became salient in the discourse and what argumentative function they fulfilled, that is, how they were used to shape, contextualize, and substantiate specific normative claims. To this end, we first provide a brief overview of the public discourse about intergenerational solidarity in the context of the pandemic and outline our theoretical perspective by reference to the concept of "justification narratives" (Forst 2013 [own translation]). On the basis of a comprehensive media discourse analysis of leading German newspapers between March 2020 and July 2021, we then consider exemplary contributions to the debate and highlight three types of narrative elements: (a) *expository narratives* that serve to define and frame the problem at hand, (b) *identificatory narratives* that help construct and specify the collective identities of generations as subjects or objects of solidarity, and (c) *explanatory narratives* that lend plausibility to normative claims regarding solidarity between generations. In light of the concept of justification narratives, we finally discuss the normative significance of these kinds of storylines as well as criteria of their acceptability and critical evaluation. In doing so, we also address the relevance of public media and art forms like literature and film for shaping and conveying common cultural narratives, thus pointing out perspectives for fruitful collaboration between ethics and literary or cultural studies.

Background: Discourses on Intergenerational Solidarity in the COVID-19 Pandemic and the Role of Narratives

Given the lack of knowledge about – let alone therapies and vaccines against – SARS-CoV-2 at the beginning of the pandemic, the slogan "all together now" appeared to define the public and political maxim of the day (e.g., Ellerich-Groppe 2023; Zimmermann et al. 2023). Calls for social cohesion and cooperation were particularly pronounced with regard to intergenerational relations. Heads of governments and international organizations frequently addressed the issue of solidarity with older people as a particularly vulnerable group in the pandemic. In spring 2020, 36 members of the European Parliament published an open letter to the presidents of the European Commission and the European Council demanding that "solidarity between generations must guide the EU response to and recovery from COVID-19" (Brglez et al. 2020). The WHO Regional Director for Europe urged the public to "act in solidarity" and be "supporting and protecting older people" (Kluge 2020). Similar appeals were also trending in public media and civil society discourses. Numerous commentaries stressed the vital importance of solidarity of the young with the old (cf. Haan 2020; Seyffarth 2020). Adolescents were asked to stay at home and young families were admonished not to visit the grandparents or draw on their services as babysitters. In many public pleas, residents were called upon to help older people (e.g., BAGSO 2020).

Over time, however, these attitudes were countered by an increasing number of voices that reversed the direction of solidarity between generations. Discussions about a possible triage of scarce intensive care resources like respirators were replete with suggestions for age-based rationing (Rueda 2021). In light of the persistence of far-reaching infection control measures like social distancing or complete lockdowns that meant substantial restrictions of individual liberties and socioeconomic welfare, the older generation was frequently called to responsibility, to put aside their own needs and to isolate themselves so that the younger generations could reclaim their freedom and the public and economic life could continue. "The expensive protection of the old" was discussed controversially (John et al. 2020 [own translation]) and different measures for different generations were brought into play (Fifka 2020). Appeals for more solidarity of the old with the younger generations accrued (e.g., Ahrens 2020). Also, many seniors themselves expressed the wish not to burden the younger generations and, hence, pleaded for voluntary self-isolation (Haarhoff 2020). There were even suggestions that the old should sacrifice themselves for the sake of their descendants and future economic welfare (Barret et al. 2021).

In the further course of the COVID-19 pandemic, the public discourses about intergenerational solidarity took several more turns. When effective vaccines came into sight in the second half of 2021, the question of which population groups should have access first was already discussed controversially (Russel and Greenwood 2021). In many countries, age was eventually used as a decisive criterion for vaccine prioritization, spurring debates about distributive justice, the perceived privilege of older people, and the unrecognized and unrequited solidarity of the young throughout the pandemic (Allen et al. 2021). This line of argument was considerably reinforced once the detrimental consequences of pandemic policies for the mental health, psychological wellbeing, and personal as well as socioeconomic development of children, adolescents, and young adults came into the focus of public awareness in the course of the following year (Hafstad and Augusti 2021). Accusations about a preferential treatment of the older generations and a continued disregard, neglect, and discrimination of younger people throughout the pandemic became more prominent and calls for increased societal solidarity with the shaken "generation corona" began to spread (German Ethics Council 2022).

As these examples already make clear, discourses on intergenerational solidarity in the pandemic were broad, diverse, and dynamically changing over time. In this course, also the term "solidarity" itself was far from being uncontested. From a moral philosophical perspective, contributions differed with regard to at least three elements of solidarity (Ellerich-Groppe et al. 2021; cf. also Ellerich-Groppe et al. 2024). First, they varied regarding the *groups* that were addressed as the respective subjects and objects of intergenerational solidarity. Thus, the old were initially often broadly labelled as a vulnerable group in need of care and support by seemingly more resilient younger people. However, they later found themselves addressed as equal members of a citizenry with mutual solidary responsibilities or even as autonomous and privileged subjects of a selfless solidarity with the young. Secondly, the contributions to the public debate about the pandemic differed in view of the *commitments*, that is, the specific moral bonds that were assumed between these generational groups. For example, while some seemed to presuppose asymmetrical relations of unidirectional gratitude of the young towards the old, others started from the opposite notion of guilt or indebtedness of the older generation vis-à-vis the young. Thirdly, the *costs* involved for those called upon to show intergenerational solidarity also varied. Especially in the first wave of the pandemic, younger people were expected to accept considerable sacrifices in terms of individual liberties, personal wellbeing, and socioeconomic welfare in order to protect the lives and health of the old. At the same time, the old were repeatedly called upon to withdraw from public life and sometimes even asked to give their lives to save the future of the younger generations.

Despite their heterogeneity, the different appeals to intergenerational solidarity voiced throughout the German public discourse on COVID-19 have one thing in common: they are deeply intertwined with narratives, that is, stories that help to shape, specify, and substantiate the normative claims made. Indeed, an important function of narratives "is their ability to transform something given into something justifiable" (Arnold 2012, 18 [own translation]). Thus, they can introduce identity-creating origins, draw morally relevant connections between seemingly isolated events, and frame future-directed plans as a continuation of past endeavors. They also address an emotional level and can evoke a feeling of coherence and consistency. In this way, they can contribute to the justification of current moral or political claims. This normative significance of narratives has been captured in the concept of "justification narratives" (Forst 2013 [own translation]) that underpin practical claims and lend them normative force in public discourse. For example, myths of origin like the story of Romulus and Remus substantiate claims about the supreme nature and special entitlements of a political community by delineating its distinctive historical provenance (Darshan 2023). Tales about divine mandate played an important role in the justification of medieval sovereigns' claims to legitimate political rule (Burgess 1992). And the narrative of a continuous historical progress of mankind provided a basis for the justification of political battles of progressive social movements (Gröbl-Steinbach 1992).

The concept of justification narratives can also be made productive to analyze the role of narratives in the ongoing public discourses about intergenerational solidarity in the COVID-19 pandemic. The following considerations are based on a moral philosophical media discourse analysis of German newspapers between March 2020 and July 2021 (cf. Ellerich-Groppe et al. 2024). The sample consisted of 149 articles that were published in the newspapers *WELT*, *Süddeutsche Zeitung* and *taz.die tageszeitung* (print or online).[2] These media were chosen for several reasons. First, they reflect the continued importance of leading media in general. The pandemic has underlined that especially large high-quality newspapers remain an important and trusted source of information and persuasion as "key players in public health" (De Coninck, d'Haenens, and Matthijs 2020; cf. also Zimmermann et al. 2021, 4; Boeff and Kirfel 2020). The second reason is the attempt to represent the public discourse in Germany in the best possible way. Thus, newspapers "can serve as a proxy for reporting across other channels" (Amann, Sleigh, and Vayena 2021). Furthermore, the newspapers chosen here represent a scope of different political orientations and a heterogeneous readership. Therefore, they appear suitable to gain a first comprehensive insight in the public discourse. Finally, the media selected for our analysis provide a combination of daily news and more elaborated, reflexive articles on intergenerational solidarity in the COVID-19 pandemic. This makes it possible to trace the dynamics of the discourse in general and the development and argumentative function of narratives in particular in a differentiated way.

The Argumentative Function of Narratives in Public Debates on Intergenerational Solidarity during the COVID-19 Pandemic

As the cursory overview of the debate already indicates, the public media discourse on intergenerational solidarity in the pandemic was replete with a great variety of storylines right from the start. A closer inspection of the respective contributions through the lens of moral philosophy reveals at least three different argumentative functions of such narratives: (a) *expository narratives* define the problem at hand in the

2 All source material in the analysis stems from the German media discourse and has been translated by the authors.

context of overarching historical processes and thus set the stage for the discussion of intergenerational solidarity, (b) *identificatory narratives* specify the collective identities of generations as subjects or objects of solidarity by recounting shared experiences, situations, or goals, and (c) *explanatory narratives* lend plausibility to normative claims regarding intergenerational solidarity by (re-)constructing morally relevant previous interactions and entanglements between generations.

(A) Expository Narratives: Setting the Stage for the Intergenerational Drama

One important function of narratives in public discourses about intergenerational solidarity is the historical localization of the present situation. Solidarity has been described as a concept for the "state of moral emergency" (Derpmann 2013, 209 [own translation]) that is invoked when ordinary moral orientations or political institutions are called into question. Accordingly, appeals to solidarity frequently start with the diagnosis of such an exceptional state of moral or political emergency, a fundamental crisis that challenges previous certainties and thus requires an extraordinary degree of social cohesion and cooperation. This also holds true in the context of the COVID-19 pandemic.

From the onset, the pandemic was framed as a watershed moment – "a universal shock to civilization" and a "turn of times" (Selge 2021). This expository narrative emphasizes discontinuity. The pandemic appears as an incisive event that divides history in a "before" and an "after." The resulting rift between experience and expectation creates uncertainty and disorientation: Experiences made in the past may no longer be valid and applicable for a fundamentally different present and future. Thus, in an interview in the *taz* in spring 2020, Germany's former Minister of Foreign Affairs, Joschka Fischer, emphasized the historically unprecedented situation: "This is about the consequences of a fundamental, global crisis, as we have not yet experienced. [...] I know that in history such severe shocks have never remained without consequences, also for the political system" (Fischer 2020). The statement sheds light on an interesting ambivalence of this narrative: on the one hand, it stresses the historical singularity of the present situation and the corresponding uncertain consequences ("as we have not yet experienced"). On the other, Fischer – in the role of an experienced "elder statesman" – draws a parallel to other "severe shocks" to estimate expectable political consequences. In such contexts, solidarity often appears as a coping strategy in the midst of disruption and uncertainty.

Another expository narrative also highlights the historical singularity of the pandemic but frames it in terms of a *challenge*. One article states: "The corona-crisis is a challenge for the solidarity between the generations" (Laschet 2020). Elsewhere, there is even talk of a test that the whole country is facing (Wernicke 2020). By comparison, this narrative of challenges transports a more conservative historical perspective oriented towards preservation and persistence despite all ruptures. The focus lies on maintaining historical achievements and the present status quo in an existential crisis. Solidarity has a twofold role to play in this context: on one hand, it is the means to "tackle the challenge we are facing" (Dahme 2020), a collective effort to preserve valuable resources and structures. On the other, it is itself a valuable resource and structure that must be preserved. In this sense, the pandemic must not result in a loss of solidarity but rather in stronger collective efforts to sustain it. Thus, the conservative German politician Armin Laschet claimed in the face of the first pandemic wave: "Retreat into one's own four walls must not be accompanied by a retreat of humanity [...]. We must make a start now for unprecedented solidarity" (Wernicke 2020).

By contrast, a third form of expository narratives rather articulates a progressive view of history that highlights the future perspectives and the consequences of the pandemic. Thus, the crisis is framed as a chance and a possibility for collective change and learning. This is particularly evident in the following commentary: "This pandemic has taken too much from us to simply put it behind us now, without understanding it as an opportunity for change" (Behbehani 2021). The statement acknowledges the perceived historical uniqueness of the crisis but directly connects it to a positive outlook on potentials for the future. According to another commentary, the COVID-19 pandemic sheds light on social grievances, which "can also open up the opportunity to organize the economy and society differently if we draw the right conclusions" (Von Hirschhausen et al. 2020). In this context, there is sometimes a reference to further impending crises like global warming which are to be prevented or at least mitigated with what will have been learned in the pandemic (Fischer 2020). Thus, this narrative is oriented toward a positive turn that calls for a collective effort of solidarity to overcome existing social grievances and build a better future.

(B) Identificatory Narratives: Casting the Dramatis Personae of Generations

Generations are elusive entities. Their identity as collectives is usually based on the perception of some shared cultural imprint of their members. In this sense, they do not exist independent from the way they are interpreted (or interpret themselves). Narratives can have a constitutive function in this context. By articulating a common experience or outlook, e.g., a joint fate or historical mission, they help to construct and specify the collective identities of generations as (potential) subjects or objects of solidarity. Such identificatory narratives are often closely connected to age stereotypes that seem to give a concrete face to the respective generational group. This also applies in the context of public debates on intergenerational solidarity in the pandemic that were replete with age stereotypes (cf. also Steckdaub-Muller et al. 2026).

While older people were immediately detected and protected as a particularly vulnerable group during the first wave of the pandemic, this sweeping and ultimately biologistic stereotype of the "vulnerable old" was soon challenged by more specific narratives that cast the respective age group as a specific generation with a distinctive history and characteristic sociomoral features and achievements. One of these narratives was the story of the "oldest old" who had experienced the end of the war and the collapse of Nazi-Germany as children and adolescents. The respective narrative encompassed the survival of World War II and the ensuing profound upheaval with existential hardships while rebuilding a functioning and prosperous democratic community out of ruins. Accordingly, it countered the image of the vulnerable old with an epic storyline that attributed virtues of self-restraint and heroic sacrifice, e.g., strength, wisdom, and resilience, to the members of this age group, thus portraying them as role models for younger generations in a time of crisis:

> Those over 80 today, […] belong to the post-war generation that was brought up not to be weak and to cope by themselves at all costs. Gritting one's teeth, not letting on, trusting in oneself – that was the maxim throughout one's life. Even more so in old age, they do not want to be a burden to anyone. Asking for something and simply taking it without anything in return, "outing" oneself as weak and in need of help, does not fit in with the mindset of this generation. It is neither learned nor wanted. (Kutz and Haist 2020)

Another prominent but more ambivalent identificatory narrative targeted the subsequent younger segment of the old as the "baby boomer generation" at the center of intergenerational debates. Frequently portrayed as a generation who had grown up in a historically unprecedented era of political stability and economic growth in the Western world, they had long been characterized as a spoiled and egocentric age group, largely focused on individual fulfilment and excessive consumerism, e.g., in debates about intergenerational conflicts in the context of the welfare state or global warming. "They got the economy humming and developed a cracking lifestyle: big cars, big houses, big trips. Unfortunately, also: big ecological footprint. […] There are eco-social outrages, but the parents' generation was good at hiding them on the way up" (Balbierer 2021). Thus, cast as the self-centered, presumptuous, and reckless generational no-good at the center of many contemporary intergenerational conflicts, they suddenly found themselves in the role of a vulnerable group in need of protection and support. "The 'golden agers,' with their supposedly generous pension entitlements throughout and their supposedly cross-class lust for pleasure, have suddenly become frail people in need of protection, sitting frightened in their apartment waiting for their neighbors to help them with their shopping and only a face mask away from almost certain virus-related demise" (Lessenich 2020). Accordingly, reactions ranged from petty satisfaction to calls for magnanimous forgiveness. A younger commentator declared: "Now my generation must show greatness" (Seyffarth 2020). Either way, the storyline of the baby boomer generation got a new narrative twist in the pandemic: the dethronement and humbling of its previously larger-than-life protagonists.

Eventually, a third identificatory narrative takes the pandemic itself as the collective experience that is shaping a new generation. In accordance with the idea that collective generational experiences usually affect individuals of a similar birth cohort during the formative years of their personal biographies, the target group are the children and adolescents that lived through almost two years of pandemic emergency. They are the "generation corona" for whom the pandemic and its aftermath will mark the decisive imprint of their collective identity (Behbehani 2021). This narrative is particularly interesting as it is clearly interwoven with two other kinds of pandemic storylines. On the one hand, it is embedded in the expository narrative of an unprecedented and at the same time still ongoing crisis with unclear outcomes. The young are "a generation [...] growing up in crisis mode" (Laskus 2020). Accordingly, the generational identity of the "generation corona" is not yet fully visible and determinable. It is only just emerging, and its future shape will ultimately be the crucial touchstone of our present management of the crisis. At the same time, the storyline is linked to another kind of pandemic narratives that delineates morally relevant entanglements between generations. The "generation corona" is described as a forgotten and disregarded generation who had to carry an unproportionate share of the physical, mental, and social burden of infection control measures for the sake of other age groups and without receiving appropriate attention or later reciprocal solidary support. Nobody "sacrificed as much of life as the young: school, training, studying, rock concerts, soccer practice, birthdays, bonfires, dancing, dreaming, making out. It's a stolen time, and yes: it hurts" (Balbierer 2021). In this sense, they often appear as a betrayed generation, the "big loser[s] of today" (Matzig 2021) who now deserve special attention and maybe even compensation.

(C) Explanatory Narratives: Tracing the Dramatic Conflict between Generations

We usually do not count on solidarity from complete "moral strangers." Instead, the expectation of attitudes and actions of solidarity seems to presuppose some preexisting moral bond or relationship. Narratives can play an important part in this context. They recount past interactions and entanglements, for example, a shared history of mutual support or, on the contrary, unilateral failure and abandonment. In this way, they can help to substantiate current moral claims and liabilities among or between the respective individuals or groups. Such *explanatory narratives* were also pervasive in the public discourse on intergenerational solidarity in the COVID-19 pandemic.

One prominent explanatory storyline from the first year of the crisis was a narrative of incrimination and reprehension of the younger generation. Alluding to reports of violations of infection control measures and so-called "lockdown-parties" among adolescents, it condemned the behavior of the young as carefree and reckless, thus driving the pandemic at the expense of vulnerable groups as well as the general public. From this perspective, they appeared largely "inconsiderate and lacking solidarity" since they only took into account their own risks and benefits, thus provoking further pandemic waves and being held responsible for the ensuing infection control measures:

> It is their fault that we all have to go back into lockdown. Because they didn't want to give up partying and traveling, even for a few months, we all have to suffer now. Because they themselves felt safe from severe disease trajectories due to their youth, they did not keep to the rules of social distancing, did not wear a mask and thus endangered older people and other risk groups. (Friedrich 2020)

From the point of view of many younger commentators, however, an opposing explanatory narrative of intergenerational entanglement suggested a completely different allocation of moral praise and blame between the generations that became apparent especially in the further course of the pandemic. Based on the story of a collective sacrifice of personal freedom and wellbeing of younger people for the sake of the protection of the older, more vulnerable generation, it brought to bear an expectation of gratitude and reciprocal solidarity that was subsequently frequently disappointed, e.g., in the context of the age-based prioritization of vaccines: "The latest outrage: while vaccinated people, so far mainly the older ones, are now allowed to celebrate birthdays and coffee parties again, the young continue to wait in isolation for their vaccination" (Balbierer 2021).

This narrative of unrequited support could ultimately nurture fundamental doubts about the overall state of intergenerational solidarity: "It is wonderful that life is gradually returning. But as a young person, one wonders what has become of the politicians' appeals for more solidarity: Did they only apply in one direction?" (Balbierer 2021).

By expanding the temporal horizon of the narrative explanation, some older commentators actually arrived at a similar moral assessment of the situation and behavior of younger people in the pandemic. Assuming and at least tacitly regretting that the younger generations had long been economically disadvantaged and exploited as low-priced and fungible workforce in a precarious German labor market, these commentators now almost expected some form of (appropriate or at least understandable) retribution in the form of disregard and abandonment in the face of the COVID-19 crisis:

> Now the "generation internship"[3] is taking back what we stole from them, I thought. Now they are occupying the streets, the professions, the stores, locking us older people in our living rooms and putting food in front of our doors. This was followed, as if to prove it, by the horror images of overcrowded intensive care units and locked-up nursing home residents, cut off from the love of their relatives. (Selge 2021)

This type of explanatory narrative appears particularly interesting as it seems to be able to draw connections and conduct "moral accounting" across completely different crises at different points in time, thus (re-)constructing a morally charged intergenerational history that may span years or even decades. Thus, in an early contribution to the debate, a member of the older generation drew a connection between the assumed failure of his age group with regard to the prevention of global warming and the feeling of a moral indebtedness vis-à-vis the younger generation in the context of the pandemic: "He knows […] that his decision is also about shame, he now sounds thoughtful: 'Shame for a hardship, even if one is not to blame'. Of course, neither he nor anyone else can be ashamed of the pandemic, but he can be ashamed of the state in which he and his generation left the planet to those who came after them" (Haarhoff 2020). Such narratives can also have important implications for the moral justification of present decisions and future plans. Thus, a sense of shame for past moral failure and the wish for due exculpation can motivate actions aimed at restoration, compensation, and rehabilitation for those wronged:

If he had his way, those old people who can afford it thanks to their wealth should voluntarily make a financial contribution to mitigate the economic catastrophe that the young in particular will suffer after the pandemic. "I'm thinking of a foundation, 'Old for Young after Corona,' or perhaps a fund that could then be used to invest in training, education, and employment." (Haarhoff 2020)

Discussion and Conclusion: The Coronavirus Pandemic as a Justification Narrative in Progress

With its reference to exceptional situations, specified social collectives, and reciprocal interactions between them, the concept of solidarity seems to have a particular affinity to narrative elements. Accordingly, the public discourse on intergenerational solidarity in the face of the COVID-19 pandemic is replete with a great variety of narratives. They help to shape, contextualize, and plausibilize the normative,

3 The term "generation internship" refers to young people who, around the turn of the millennium in Germany, had difficulties to obtain a permanent position due to the labor market situation despite their good education and were therefore shuttled from one internship to another.

moral or political claims articulated in the pertinent discussions about solidarity between generations. Starting from the concept of "justification narratives" (Forst 2013 [own translation]), we could distinguish at least three general types of such narratives according to their respective argumentative functions: expository narratives, identificatory narratives, and explanatory narratives.

Expository narratives offer a comprehensive historical classification and interpretation of the present situation. By drawing connections between events and integrating them into an overarching storyline, such narratives can generally provide traceability, orientation, and normative significance (Viehöver 2011). In the case of the pandemic, the definition and framing of the given situation in terms of a fundamental historical crisis thus frequently sets the stage for normative appeals to intergenerational solidarity as a (more or less) necessary and adequate response. Sometimes these expository narratives transport a whole implicit philosophy of history, some notion of the nature, structure, and direction of the historical process that also has implications for the ensuing conceptualization of the solidarity needed. For example, the narrative of the pandemic as a rupture emphasizes the discontinuity of the historical process and the openness and unpredictability of the current situation that necessitates standing together in the midst of fundamental uncertainty. The narrative of the pandemic as a challenge often rather expresses a conservative sense of history in terms of heritage and tradition that is accompanied by a communitarian understanding of solidarity as the collective preservation of past achievements in the face of destabilizing new developments. By contrast, the narrative of the crisis as a chance rather conveys a progressivist idea of history in terms of constant renewal and improvement. From this perspective, the pandemic uncovers the flaws and insufficiencies of the existing society and motivates a collective endeavor to overcome or optimize given institutions or structures. All in all, the relevance of such expository narratives for framing public debates about intergenerational solidarity must not be underestimated and therefore calls for critical analysis. After all, they can help clarify what is historically at stake in an imminent crisis, but also contribute to its trivializing appeasement or alarmist exaggeration and polarization (Roitman 2013).

Furthermore, *identificatory narratives* construct generations as subjects or objects of intergenerational solidarity by reference to shared experiences, situations, or goals. The potential to shape personal or collective identities has often been connected to narrative approaches (Viehöver 2011, 195; Forst 2013, 11; Lübbe 2012). In the pandemic, different kinds of such narratives were taken up and further developed in order to specify the identities of the different generations involved. Often starting from the recollection of joint historical experiences and employing generalized images of age(ing), more or less clearly defined and homogeneous generational groups were (re-)constructed, for example, the battle-tried, wise and resilient veterans as a virtuous role model in times of crisis, the spoiled and self-indulgent baby boomers who become dethroned and humiliated in the pandemic, or the "generation corona" whose future collective identity is at stake and will be decisively affected by our ability to cope with the pandemic. In light of such identificatory storylines, it is crucial to distinguish between those who narrate stories and those who are the subject matter of these stories. While the narrative (re-)construction of generations is often an act in which groups reassure themselves about their own collective identity by telling a shared storyline, the pandemic discourse was quite often dominated by external attributions which are prone to ageist stereotypes and stigmatization. Polemical generational caricatures like the needy or demanding old or the reckless young ignore individual differences and instead reinforce problematic othering, scapegoating, and discrimination (Meisner 2020; Vervaecke and Meisner 2021). Moreover, a simplistic view on generational relations during the pandemic may ultimately overlook the relevance of other intersecting social categories, such as class, race, or gender, as roots of social disadvantage and conflict (Rueda 2021).

Finally, *explanatory narratives* can serve to lend plausibility to normative moral or political claims regarding intergenerational solidarity by outlining relevant previous entanglements and interactions between generations that are envisioned in stories of achievement, gratitude, failure, guilt, indebtedness, forgiveness, exculpation, rehabilitation, etc. These narratives can reinforce mutual bonds and support between different generations but also bring to bear "open accounts" (Müller-Salo 2022 [own translation]) that need to be settled. For example, they comprise the incriminatory storyline of the reckless youths and their blameworthy misconduct in the pandemic that deserves reprimand and punishment, as well as the heroic narrative of a collective solidary sacrifice of the younger generation that remained largely unacknowledged and unrequited and now calls for due reparations. At the same time, there are more encompassing explanatory stories about the failure of older generations in previous crises connected to excessive capitalism, unrestricted industrialization, environmental pollution, and impending global warming that suggest a historical guilt and responsibility vis-à-vis subsequent and future generations that needs to be paid off. Of course, such explanatory narratives as well as their societal consequences are always in need of closer examination. Storylines about past entanglements between collectives have a notorious tendency to become biased, ideological, and instrumentalized political myths or conspiracy narratives that serve to "other," scapegoat, and ultimately fight or suppress individuals or whole groups (Bergmann 2018). The emotional charge of narratives can complicate a rational discussion, here, but at the same time motivate it. Therefore, it is of crucial importance to critically assess such narratives with regard to their historical accuracy and balance in order to evaluate the plausibility of the moral or political claims derived from them.

The closer inspection of these different kinds of storylines thus shows that such "narratives are by no way innocent, they can contribute to the solidification of repressive domination and inequality as ideologies [...], they can justify discrimination, prosecution, hate and violence" (Forst and Günther 2021, 15 [own translation]). Under these circumstances, the critical appraisal of pandemic narratives on intergenerational solidarity clearly is a necessary and important task. This first and foremost concerns the epistemic quality and weight of the respective stories as well as the moral value of the justified notions of solidarity between generations. However, while there is a large variety of accepted theories and criteria regarding the evaluation of moral arguments, it seems much less clear how narratives are to be assessed from an epistemological and moral philosophical point of view. Criteria like historical correctness and normative acceptability (Forst 2013) appear obvious but remain vague and controversial. For example, stories obviously always leave space for various legitimate interpretations of events, and it is not clear *prima facie* how to decide between these different narrative versions of the past. Apparently, additional aspects like authenticity or coherence must be taken into consideration in order to judge the plausibility of narratives. At the same time, the normative force of narratives is not just a matter of their internal validity but also of their actual external impact. Therefore, the ethical discussion of the plausibility and persuasiveness of pandemic narratives has to be complemented by the critical analysis of the social effectiveness and influence they unfold. This also solicits further analyses of the role of art forms like film and literature in shaping and reproducing narratives, as well as an investigation of media like TV, print, or social media that amplify their impact and extend their social reach (Venkatesan et al. 2022; Nulman 2021).

Such a critical examination of justification narratives in a time of crisis can ultimately provide important insights into the fundamental moral constitution of our society – also for the future. Although pandemic narratives have turned out to be quite diverse, many of them have one thing in common: they assign a singular historical significance to the present moment in time. Such developments are predestined to become the starting point for new overarching justification narratives themselves (Forst and Günther 2021). Hence, the different narratives in the pandemic as well as the narrative of the pandemic itself will go on in one way or another and will play a role in future debates, for example, regarding our response to climate change. It is still open which of these narratives will persist and develop. In this sense, a commentator asked at the begin of the pandemic:

> Will people later tell stories of us as a society that took care of its weakest members in a time of greatest need and not only made a charitable daily or weekly project out of it, but also learned the lesson that it can't work any other way than together? Or will they report of cold, inhuman considerations according to which an old human life counted less than a small business? (Klute 2020)

Not least due to the fact, that "narratives (including those in the public arena) have an important role to play in creating and shaping moral futures through social processes" (Samuel and Lucivero 2022), it will also be an ethical task to analyze and criticize the COVID-19 pandemic as a narrative in progress.

Bibliography

Ahrens, Lukian. 2020. "Corona-Krise. Wir brauchen jetzt Solidarität mit der jungen Generation." *Hamburger Morgenpost*, May 26, 2020. https://www.mopo.de/hamburg/corona-krise-wir-brauchen-jetzt-solidaritaet-mit-der-jungen-generation-36748854/

Allen, Laura D., Idalina Z. Odziemczyk, Jolanta Perek-Białas, and Liat Ayalon. 2021. "We should be at the back of the line: A frame analysis of old age within the distribution order of the COVID-19 vaccine." *The Gerontologist*, vol. 61, no. 8, 1317–1325. https://doi.org/10.1093/geront/gnab094.

Amann, Julia, Joanna Sleigh, and Effy Vayena. 2021. "Digital contact-tracing during the Covid-19 pandemic: An analysis of newspaper coverage in Germany, Austria, and Switzerland." *PloS ONE*, vol. 16, no. 2, e0246524. https://doi.org/10.1371/journal.pone.0246524.

Arnold, Markus. 2012. "Erzählen. Die ethisch-politische Funktion narrativer Diskurse." *Erzählungen im Öffentlichen. Über die Wirkung narrativer Diskurse*, edited by Markus Arnold, Gert Dressel, and Willy Viehöver, Springer, 17–63.

BAGSO (Bundesarbeitsgemeinschaft der Seniorenorganisationen). 2020. "Protecting human life – strengthening cohesion. BAGSO recommendations in times of the spread of the coronavirus." https://www.bagso.de/fileadmin/user_upload/bagso/06_Veroeffentlichungen/2020/Statement_Protecting_human_life.pdf.

Balbierer, Thomas. 2021. "Danke für nichts." *Süddeutsche Zeitung*, May 14, 2021. https://www.sueddeutsche.de/projekte/artikel/gesellschaft/warum-deutschland-einen-generationenkonflikt-braucht-e388419/?reduced=true.

Barrett, Anne E., Michael Cherish, and Irene Padavic. 2021. "Calculated ageism: Generational sacrifice as a response to the COVID-19 pandemic." *The Journals of Gerontology: Series B*, vol. 76, no. 4, e201-e205. https://doi.org/10.1093/geronb/gbaa132.

Behbehani, Sara Maria. 2021. "Wir, Generation Corona." *Süddeutsche Zeitung*, May 29/30, 2021, 11–13.

Bergmann, Eirikur. 2018. *Conspiracy & Populism: The Politics of Misinformation*, Springer International.

Boeff, Melanie, and Gudrun Kirfel. 2020. "Mit Corona schlägt die Stunde der Qualitätsmedien." *NDR ZAPP*, March 18, 2020. https://www.ndr.de/fernsehen/sendungen/zapp/Mit-Corona-schlaegt-die-Stunde-der-Qualitaetsmedien,coronavirus620.html.

Brglez, Milan, Jaroslaw Duda, Ivars Ijabsb, Irena Joveva, Dietmar Köster, Elena Yoncheva, Alexis Georgoulis et al. 2020. "Solidarity between generations must guide the EU response to and recovery from COVID-19." *Letter*, May 28, 2020. https://towardsanagefriendlyep.files.wordpress.com/2020/05/letter-to-ec-and-council_solidarity-between-generations.pdf.

Burgess, Glenn. 1992. "The Divine Right of Kings Reconsidered." *The English Historical Review*, vol. CVII, no. CCCCXXV, 837–861. https://doi.org/10.1093/ehr/CVII.CCCCXXV.837

Dahme, Ulrike. 2020. "Wir werden alle lernen müssen, wieder unter Menschen zu sein." *SZ Magazin*, April 7, 2020. https://www.sueddeutsche.de/magazin/coronatagebuch/corona-seelsorge-einsamkeit-szm.88620

Darshan, Guy. 2023. *Stories of Origins in the Bible and Ancient Mediterranean Literature*, Cambridge UP.

De Coninck, Davide, Leen d'Haenens, and Koen Matthijs. 2020. "Forgotten key players in public health: News media as agents of information and persuasion during the COVID-19 pandemic." *Public Health*, vol. 138, 65–66. https://doi.org/10.1016/j.puhe.2020.05.011.

Derpmann, Simon. 2013. *Gründe der Solidarität*, mentis.

Ellerich-Groppe, Niklas, Mark Schweda, and Larissa Pfaller. 2020. "#StayHomeForGrandma – Towards an analysis of intergenerational solidarity and responsibility in the coronavirus pandemic." *Social Sciences & Humanities Open*, vol. 2, no. 1, article 100085. https://doi.org/10.1016/j.ssaho.2020.100085.

Ellerich-Groppe, Niklas, Larissa Pfaller, and Mark Schweda. 2021. "Young for old – old for young? Ethical perspectives on intergenerational solidarity and responsibility in public discourses on COVID-19." *European Journal of Ageing*, vol. 18, 159–171. https://doi.org/10.1007/s10433-021-00623-9.

Ellerich-Groppe, Niklas. 2023. "Mit Bluetooth ein Signal der Solidarität senden? – Eine medizinethische Analyse der öffentlichen Debatte über die Corona-Warn-App." *Ethik in der Medizin*, vol. 35, 265–283. https://doi.org/10.1007/s00481-023-00751-z.

Ellerich-Groppe, Niklas, Irmgard Steckdaub-Muller, Larissa Pfaller, and Mark Schweda. 2024. "Moral Paradigms of Intergenerational Solidarity in the Coronavirus-Pandemic." *Analyse & Kritik*, vol. 46, 85–119. https://doi.org/10.1515/auk-2024-2010.

Elliott, Rebecca. 2022. "The 'Boomer remover.' Intergenerational discounting, the coronavirus and climate change." *The Sociological Review*, vol. 70, no. 1, 74–91. https://doi.org/10.1177/00380261211049023.

El Ouassil, Samira. 2020. "Lebe so, dass die Alten überleben." *Spiegel Online*, March 12, 2020. https://www.spiegel.de/kultur/coronavirus-lebe-so-dass-die-alten-ueberleben-a-98f668c8-4f36-4a24-afd5-5e2d7ac12d48.

Fifka, Matthias. 2020. "Jüngere wollen in Zukunft andere Corona-Maßnahmen als Alte." Interview by Jan Petter. *Spiegel*, May 26, 2020. https://www.spiegel.de/panorama/wissenschaftler-zu-corona-krise-juengere-menschen-machen-sich-sorgen-um-ihre-zukunft-a-b5e6289b-bd88-4d6e-b786-807c6fb20b15.

Fischer, Joschka. 2020. "Die Frage ist: Was kommt danach?" Interview by Peter Unfried. *Taz. Die Tageszeitung*, April 5, 2020. https://taz.de/Joschka-Fischer-ueber-Corona-Krise/!5675233/.

Forst, Rainer. 2013. "Zum Begriff des Rechtfertigungsnarrativs." *Rechtfertigungsnarrative. Zur Begründung normativer Ordnungen durch Erzählungen*, edited by Andreas Fahrmeir, Campus, 11–28.

Forst, Rainer, and Klaus Günther. 2021. "Normative Ordnungen. Ein Frankfurter Forschungsprogramm." *Normative Ordnungen*, edited by Rainer Forst, and Klaus Günther, Suhrkamp, 9–24.

Friedrich, Jörg Phil. 2020. "Wir sollten weniger zornig auf die Jugend sein." *Die Welt*, November 10, 2020, 22.

German Ethics Council. 2022. *Pandemic and Mental Health. Attention, Assistance and Support for Children, Adolescents and Young Adults in and after Societal Crises*. https://www.ethikrat.org/fileadmin/Publikationen/Ad-hoc-Empfehlungen/englisch/recommendation-pandemic-and-mental-health.pdf.

Gröbl-Steinbach, Evelyn. 1994. *Fortschrittsidee und rationale Weltgestaltung. Die kulturellen Voraussetzungen des Politischen in der Moderne*, Campus.

Haan, Yannick. 2020. "Solidarität der Generationen ist notwendig." *Deutschlandfunk Kultur*, April 22, 2020. https://www.deutschlandfunkkultur.de/millennials-und-die-coronakrise-solidaritaet-der.1005.de.html?dram:article_id=475123.

Haarhoff, Heike. 2020. "Sperrt uns ein!" *Taz. Die Tageszeitung*, April 11, 2020. https://taz.de/Isolation-in-der-Coronakrise/!5675306/.

Hafstad, Gertrud Sofie, and Else-Marie Augusti. 2021. "A lost generation? COVID-19 and adolescent mental health." *The Lancet Psychiatry*, vol. 8, no. 8, 640–641. https://doi.org/10.1016/S2215-0366(21)00179-6.

John, Gerald, Andreas Schnauder, and Selina Thaler. 2020. "Der teure Schutz der Alten." *Der Standard*, May 24, 2022. https://www.derstandard.de/story/2000117640844/der-teure-schutz-der-alten.

Kluge, Hans Henri P. 2020. "Statement: older people are at highest risk from COVID-19, but all must act to prevent community spread." *WHO*, April 3, 2020. https://www.who.int/europe/news/item/03-04-2020-statement-older-people-are-at-highest-risk-from-covid-19-but-all-must-act-to-prevent-community-spread.

Kutz, Susanne, and Karin Haist. 2020. "Hilfe? Nein Danke!" *Taz. Die Tageszeitung*, May 12, 2020. https://taz.de/Ehrenamt-in-Zeiten-von-Corona/!5681769/.

Klute, Hilmar. 2020. "Der große Stillstand." *Süddeutsche Zeitung*, March 28, 2020. https://www.sueddeutsche.de/projekte/artikel/gesellschaft/corona-krise-der-grosse-stillstand-e782749/

Laschet, Armin. 2020. "So viel Zuspruch und Ermutigung wie noch nie in meinem politischen Leben." Interview by Ulf Poschardt. *Welt*, April 25, 2020. https://www.welt.de/politik/deutschland/plus207490875/Armin-Laschet-zum-Corona-Exit-So-viel-Zuspruch-wie-noch-nie.html.

Laskus, Marcel. 2020. "Der Staat vergisst die Jungen." *Süddeutsche Zeitung*, December 1, 2020. https://www.sueddeutsche.de/politik/corona-krise-der-staat-vergisst-die-jungen-1.5133466.

Lessenich, Stephan. 2020. "Verwundbar ist, wer zu uns gehört." *Süddeutsche Zeitung*, May 6, 2020. https://www.sueddeutsche.de/kultur/coronavirus-vulnerabilitaet-triage-1.4897768.

Lübbe, Hermann. 2012. *Geschichtsbegriff und Geschichtsinteresse*, Schwabe.

Matzig, Gerhard. 2021. "Kinder, auf die Barrikaden." *Süddeutsche Zeitung*, June 23, 2021, 11.

Meisner, Brad A. 2020. "Are You OK, Boomer? Intensification of Ageism and Intergenerational Tensions on Social Media Amid COVID-19." *Leisure Sciences*, vol. 43, no. 1–2, 56–61. https://doi.org/10.1080/01490400.2020.1773983.

Müller-Salo, Johannes. 2022. *Offene Rechnungen. Der kalte Konflikt der Generationen*, Reclam.

Nulman, Eugene. 2021. *Coronavirus Capitalism Goes to the Cinema*, Routledge.

Pedersen, Frode Helmich. 2020. "A Pandemic of Narratives." *In the Realm of Corona Normativities*, edited by Werner Gephart, Klostermann, 409–418.

Petter, Jan. 2020. "Generationenkonflikt in der Pandemie: Jüngere wollen in Zukunft andere Corona-Maßnahmen als Alte." *Spiegel*, May 26, 2020. https://www.spiegel.de/panorama/wissenschaftler-zu-corona-krise-juengere-menschen-machen-sich-sorgen-um-ihre-zukunft-a-b5e6289b-bd88-4d6e-b786-807c6fb20b15.

Roitman, Janet. 2013. *Anti-Crisis*, Duke UP.

Rueda, Jon. 2021. "Ageism in the COVID-19 pandemic: age-based discrimination in triage decisions and beyond." *History and Philosophy of the Life Sciences*, vol. 43, article 91.

Russell, Fiona M., and Brian Greenwood. 2021. "Who should be prioritized for COVID-19 vaccination?" *Human Vaccines & Immunotherapeutics*, vol. 17, No. 5, 1317–1321. https://doi.org/10.1080/21645515.2020.1827882.

Samuel, Gabrielle, and Federica Lucivero. 2022. "Framing ethical issues associated with the UK COVID-19 contact tracing app: exceptionalising and narrowing the public ethics debate." *Ethics and Information Technology*, vol. 24, article 5. https://doi.org/10.1007/s10676-022-09628-z.

Selge, Edgar. 2021. "Der Schock muss wirken." *Süddeutsche Zeitung*, June 24, 2021. https://www.sueddeutsche.de/kultur/corona-edgar-selge-was-folgt-1.5332254?reduced=true.

Seyffarth, Moritz. 2020. "Nun muss meine Generation Verzicht lernen und Größe beweisen." *Die Welt*, March 14, 2020. https://www.welt.de/wirtschaft/article206538483/Corona-Krise-Die-junge-Generation-muss-Groesse-beweisen.html.

Steckdaub-Muller, Irmgard, Larissa Pfaller, Mark Schweda, and Niklas Ellerich-Groppe. 2026. "Age stereotypes in appeals for intergenerational solidarity: disentangling the paradox." *Humanities and Social Sciences Communications*, vol. 13, article 234. https://doi.org/10.1057/s41599-025-06113-y

Stumpf, Marie. 2020. "Senioren und die Corona-Freiheiten. 'Wir haben viel dafür getan, dass es der jungen Generation gut geht.'" *RBB*, May 12, 2021. https://www.rbb24.de/studiofrankfurt/panorama/coronavirus/beitraege_neu/2021/05/corona-senioren-lockerungen-impfung-privilegien.html.

Venkatesan, Sathyaraj, Antara Chatterjee, A. David Lewis, and Brian Callender, editors. 2022. *Pandemics and Epidemics in Cultural Representation*, Springer.

Vervaecke, Deanna, and A. Brad Meisner. 2021. "Caremongering and Assumptions of Need: The Spread of Compassionate Ageism During COVID-19." *The Gerontologist*, vol. 61, no. 2, 159–165. https://doi.org/10.1093/geront/gnaa131.

Viehöver, Willy. 2011. "Diskurse als Narrationen." *Handbuch Sozialwissenschaftliche Diskursanalyse. Band 1: Theorien und Methoden*, edited by Reiner Keller, Andreas Hirseland, Werner Schneider, and Willly Viehöver, Verlag für Sozialwissenschaften, 193–224.

Von Hirschhausen, Eckart, Lucie Hammecke, Stefan Kluge, Katharina Wagner, Heinz Bude, Fritz Joussen, Janine Wissler, Leander Haussmann, Burkhard Jung, and Leoobalys. 2020. "Was erhoffen Sie sich von 2021? (III)." *Die Welt*, December 24, 2020, 23.

Wernicke, Christian. 2020. "Die Krise als Kanzler-Test." *Süddeutsche Zeitung*, March 23, 2020, 5.

Zimmermann, Bettina Maria, Amelia Fiske, Barbara Prainsack, Barbara Nora Hangel, Stuart MCLennan, and Alena Buyx. 2021. "Early Perceptions of COVID-19 Contact Tracing Apps in German-Speaking Countries: Comparative Mixed Methods Study." *Journal of Medical Internet Research*, vol. 23, no. 2, e25525. https://doi.org/10.2196/25525

Zimmermann, Bettina M., Alena Buyx, and Stuart McLennan. "Newspaper Coverage on Solidarity and Personal Responsibility in the COVID-19 Pandemic: A Content Analysis from Germany and German-speaking Switzerland." *SSM – Population Health*, vol. 22, article 101388. https://doi.org/10.1016/j.ssmph.2023.101388

A Concluding Remark

Injustice in Pandemic Narrations

Philosophical Reflections

Silke Schicktanz

Introduction

When can we consider a pandemic to be a mere misfortune and when can we see it as an injustice? Like any other natural disaster, a pandemic can be understood as an unavoidable calamity, with no one – no human, no god or devil – being responsible for its occurrence (cf. Shklar 1990). The fact that human activities can influence natural events – the current climate change may serve as the prime example here – raises the question of how the consequences of this agency affect our understanding of (in)justice. Rendering the experience of a pandemic in narrative form allows us to address these moral problems in various ways. Factional pandemic narratives may, in a similarly way as fictional ones,[1] exclude one or more relevant social groups or present a one-sided perspective, e.g., by focusing only on health policy issues only the suffering of an affected patient. Thus, the "morality" within a narrative depends on the perspective and the persuasive motivation of the narrator (Davis and Lohm 2020, 31).

As a moral philosopher, I typically seek to move beyond the subjective limitations inherent in a particular point of view. However, it is the premise of my approach that such a move does not entail abandoning narrative as such. Analyzing pandemic narratives, especially factual ones, from a meta-perspective allows one to analyze the causal chain of events: what is the source of the harmful infection? Did a virus escape from a laboratory as a biotechnological modification? Has it been deliberately or inadvertently introduced into an indigenous population by settlers and colonialists, as in the case of smallpox in Native Americans and Aboriginal peoples?

Analyzing various narratives through such a broad lens allows for the identification of potentially responsible actors (individuals and institutions) and the consid-

1 For the difference between factional vs. fictional, cf. Schaeffer (2009). I am here mainly in favor of the pragmatic definition in which a factual narrative advances claims of referential truthfulness, whereas fictional narrative advances no such claims.

eration of existing structural injustices that manifest themselves in the context of a pandemic event, sometimes against our former assumptions.

As this volume illustrates, fictional scenarios can serve as normative thought experiments for best- or worst-case scenarios regarding pandemic times. A novel such as Albert Camus' *The Plague* addresses social harms (a whole city is under quarantine and excluded from socio-political welfare politics), misbehavior (some protagonists try to benefit economically from the crisis), and advocates humanitarian action (the doctor must decide to stay or flee, and finally decides to stay at a great personal cost). This story is a fiction, but it has practical dimensions as people in pandemic situations always face similar dilemmas and must make similar choices.

Specific reflection on the moral implications of actions is needed for health policy considerations. This is because in health policy discourses the factual, the non-factual, and sometimes even the fictional come together. For example, health policies focus on measures for infection reduction which are backed by factual knowledge on transmission risks. But they also draw on non-factual, anticipated assumptions regarding the future ("X will flatten the curve"). Embedded stories and anecdotes about patients, often used as illustration in public health communication, finally can be seen as the fictional element. The epistemic dimension of infection might be framed in fictional narratives in a way that allows to demonstrate the possible consequences of human actions, often in moral categories such as good/bad, and in relation to stories about the probable causes. Such narratives involving an epistemic and a normative dimension can be understood as "mixed judgments." The combination of both premises, namely about how the world is and how the world should be, stresses the fact that both dimensions are object of our social deliberations. Narratives are part of our social discourse, especially when we debate over real pandemics. For example, a policy proposal about whether to declare a vaccination mandate or to put infected people under quarantine gives rise to normative conclusions about which intervention is justified for which reasons (e.g., to reduce the number of cases by interfering with the right to bodily self-determination or even with the right to freedom).

During the COVID-19 pandemic, charges of "injustice" were frequent – especially in the media. For example, issues of social inequality between the global south and north were discussed with regard to the access to vaccines; there were also controversies on how particular treatments discriminated against particular social groups, e.g., the elderly or children (cf. Schweda & Ellrich-Groppe's contribution in this volume). Some claimed that people who did not believe in the pandemic or in its harms were treated in a discriminatory way.[2]

---

2 German media were full of headlines using terms such as "injustice" or "unjust." Some examples (my translations): "Survey: Children consider Corona measurements as unjust" (*Telepolis* 3.5.21); "Double injustice. Corona increases social injustices worldwide" (*gruene-bundestag.de*),

What does "injustice" mean in these competing claims? In the following, I will parse several meanings of the term, relative to the scenarios in which it is deployed, and argue for the importance of a nuanced consideration of the concept of injustice in relation to the narrative. Narrative, it will be claimed here, helps to bring together competing claims of and multiple perspectives on injustice in a way that help us to de- and reconstruct injustice conceptually.

First, the concept "injustice" needs to be subjected to a more detailed and contextualized explanation to unfold its powerful normative meaning. My first aim is thus to contribute to an ethically informed analysis of current discursive practices and to suggest a more differentiated description of what is at stake in various uses of the term. Secondly, I want to show how different philosophical-conceptual considerations of injustice can allow direct and indirect forms of criticism by outlining selected philosophical theories in a sorting scheme. This is meant to show both the existing philosophical discussions can inform narratives and how a philosophically informed analysis can be used to bring together the multiple perspectives always involved in narrative claims of injustice.

Injustice as Ubiquitous Moral Experience

Justice is a central but multi-layered concept in moral philosophy. Since Greek antiquity, ethical theories have approached it in different ways. In modern ethics as well as in current legal and political philosophy, theories of justice have moved to the center of debates on morality, whereas questions of personal conduct (e.g., what is a Good Life) and values have been relegated to the more subjective domain of individual ethics. As a modern guiding principle of democratic welfare systems, justice is understood as justificatory principle for any legal order and of the distribution of material and immaterial goods (e.g., by John Rawls). Justice, as a normative concept, is relational, as it always requires an intersubjective justification of how others are treated in a system. As a concept, justice provides a positive, idealistic, and normative definition. The common term for designating a deviation from this norm is "injustice" as a negation, understood as normative critique of reality. But what does this negative definition mean in concrete terms?

Interestingly, the language of injustice shows a long pre-theoretical or everyday list of usages – the term is already used by young children long before they have a more developed theory of what justice means. For example, we use the term unjust to address unequal treatment (e. g. when others are favored), but do we use it also

---

"Easing restrictions for vaccinated people? This is unfair. Poessel explains" (*BR.de*, April 4, 2021).

when we are favored over others? It is used to describe unfair treatment when something we feel entitled to is withheld from us or when we do not have the same chances to achieve something in a self-declared egalitarian society. However, the term unjust is also used in reference to claims such as "you don't follow the rules"; "I cannot assert my interests"; "my benefit is less (than desired or that of others)"; or, "I am not respected, my self-esteem is undermined." This scope already gives an idea of how complex our understanding of (in)justice actually is.

Philosophical approaches that focus on injustice (rather than justice) are rare but have received more attention in recent years. Injustice has been described as one of the "epiphenomena" in moral debates, namely as the absence or counterpart of *justice*, a concept more commonly addressed in ethical theories (Flügel-Martinsen/Martinsen 2016, 53; Shklar 1990). But of course, in many normative definitions of justice, one can also discern basic assumptions about what injustice is. For the purpose of thinking about pandemic injustices, it may be productive to review and compare different definitions to ensure that they are applicable to address the complex situation of a pandemic: one should consider the relationship between the health care system and state politics, the context of professional care where resources among different needy individuals are allocated, as well as the role of scientific knowledge production to justify infection containment measures. It is also important to consider counter-pandemic measures that can impact everyday life and small social interactions between citizens or within families.

The Many Philosophical Faces of Injustice and Their Relevance for Pandemic Narratives

I have therefore deliberately selected different approaches, which are neither exhaustive nor without alternatives.[3] However, they are very well suited for capturing and exploring different dimensions of the pandemic and the emerging debates on injustice related to it. Some authors have already briefly addressed a short list of different approaches to injustice, e.g., a "plural theory of justice" (Axel Honneth). My attempt here is not to analyze these debates in light of their terminological or philosophical-conceptual differences. I am also not providing a detailed analysis of which theory is better, more convincing, or more or less consistent. My main intention is to give a conceptual overview and to show how each approach is suitable for analyzing various dimensions of pandemic injustice through narrative.

3 The overview here cannot and will not do justice to all details of each philosophical approach. My main aim here is to bring some philosophical concepts in conversation with other disciplines.

Maldistribution: Unequal Allocation of Resources between Few and Many

In general, theories of injustice struggle over the specific object of justice that we want to have organized in a just, fair way. The object can be of distributive, material nature that requires redistribution (e.g., material goods such as food, water, money), or is it of a procedural, abstract nature (e.g., political rights of participation or rights of socio-cultural recognition). Many contemporary philosophers accept both definitions, but that raises questions of prioritization. A very common understanding of social injustice involves "maldistribution." As Bufacchi explains (2012, 1), maldistribution describes an unequal allocation of social or natural benefits and/or burdens which are distributed according to criteria on an institutional or inter-individual level that not everyone – especially those who receive less than others – could reasonably accept (Bufacchi 2012, 9). In a pandemic, maldistribution does normally not address the spread of the infectious agent as we are "all in the same boat" in terms of susceptibility, as the factory worker in Laura Bäumel's contribution to this volume argues. But when it comes to the allocation of resources that can protect or minimize effects of infection, then maldistribution becomes an issue. In a comparison of experts' observations regarding the ethical challenges of the COVID-19 pandemic on a global scale, a research team of which I was a member found big differences between high-, middle-, and low-income countries (Vonderschmitt, Wöhlke, Schicktanz 2023). In low- and middle-income countries, the effects of pandemic containment measures as well as access to vaccines or other protective material was distributed unequally (often extremely so) between people of poorer and better incomes. While poor people did not necessarily suffer more from the infection, they did suffer disproportionally from socio-economic effects.

Structural Oppression: How some Social Groups Suffer more than Others in Pandemic Times

Young (1990) has proposed the concept of "oppression" as an adequate way of addressing the various forms of structural injustice in political discourse. The term describes how some social groups "suffer some inhibition of their ability to develop and exercise their capacities and to express their needs, thoughts and feelings" (38), "not because a tyrannical power coerces them but because of the everyday practices of a well-intentioned liberal society" (39). She differentiates between exploitation, exclusion, powerlessness, cultural imperialism, and violence. Not all five characteristics may be directly relevant or specific to the pandemic context. However, it seems helpful to briefly describe them. Exploitation, according to Young, enacts a structural relationship between social groups (e.g., class or gender) where power and inequality determine what work is, who does what for whom, and how it is rewarded. This structural system leads to the fact that a few people accumulate while others lose out. Exploitation is therefore related to what Bufacchi (2012) calls maldistribution (cf. above), but Young emphasizes the relevance of the structural power of the institutions in place. Thus, redistribution of goods alone cannot eliminate exploitation. Exploitative structures in health care work, for example, can be seen in the hierarchies between nurses and doctors. During the pandemic, nurses invested a great deal of emotional and personal resources in caring for patients, and often for their own family members, but received less social recognition and economic benefits, at least in comparison with doctors. Studies suggest that the structural effects of working conditions before and after COVID-19 led to an immense turnover of labor, moral distress, and burnout, especially in this group (Kurtzman et al. 2022). Nevertheless, there is a great deal of reluctance to address the hierarchy between nurses and doctors.

The second concept, marginalization, is defined by Young as the structural and material deprivation of a group of people from meaningful participation in social life. A third form is powerlessness. Young describes it as a lack of authority status (1990, 53) associated with absent or very low occupational status (e.g., professor versus factory worker). She observed that norms of respectability in our society are associated with professional cultures. The emerging role of experts in policymaking and the proximity of some experts to political power during the COVID-19 pandemic can be seen as an example of this, while others – non-experts as well as academics from areas considered less important (e.g., humanities and social sciences) – have often suffered a loss in status. Cultural imperialism, the next concept in Young's typology, goes beyond the economic and material parts of our social lives. It refers to the ways in which a dominant group's experience and culture is seen as universal and normative. Culturally dominated groups, on the other hand, are problematically stereotyped through their social practices, becoming "marked" and singled out as behaving in abnormal ways, or they become invisible. In pandemic times this may become relevant when cultural views on the body, illness, or health-related issues are dominated by the perspectives of a powerful group, which interprets the body and illness in a very one-sided way. Cultural views can clash with scientific facts and well-examined studies. Hence, not all cultural views might be justified, valuable, or deserve protection. However, the basis of scientific facts regarding contagious diseases can be very thin, especially in the early stages of emergence or discovery. Therefore, it would be morally sensible to respect the co-existence of pluralistic cultural views on illness as long as they do not lead to other forms of marginalization or stigmatization.

The fifth dimension addresses physical violence, cases in which members of one group are beaten, killed, or raped by members of another group. The Black Lives Matter movement, whose activities overlapped with the COVID-19 pandemic, made clear how police brutality is normalized in the U.S. and goes hand in hand with the everyday material deprivation of people of color. Violence has accompanied pandemics in many historically documented cases – anti-Jewish pogroms during plagues in the Middle Ages serve as a prominent example here (Cohn 2007). HIV-positive patients, who are often victims of violence, regularly report physical abuse both within and outside the health care system (Dlamini et al. 2007, Zierler et al. 2000), but the number of such studies is scandalously small.

Political Unfairness: How Quarantine Can Harm Political Participation

In John Rawls's *A Theory of Justice*, western philosophy's perhaps most influential study of justice (published first in 1971), there are only few direct hints related to injustice. According to Rawls the unjust man must be distinguished from a bad or an evil person. Rawls describes an unjust person as somebody who strives for excessive power and "dominion for the sake of aims such wealth or security which when appropriately limited are legitimate" (1971, 439). As this definition is very general, one can try to define injustice more precisely by reinterpreting the definitions and conditions of justice as political fairness based on what would be agreed to by rational persons in an "original position"[4] of equality – as provided in Rawls's theory. This approach suggests that injustice exists when there is no egalitarian distribution of primary goods. Such primary goods range from political rights, liberties, and opportunities (political participation through freedom of speech, assembly, and political association etc.), but also material goods such as income and wealth. Hence, injustice exists if the distribution of social material goods does not benefit everyone, especially those who are worst off. Furthermore, a social situation or system would be called unjust if the opportunities to access offices and decision-

4 The original, ideal position is Rawls' thought experiment is the veil of ignorance (Rawls 1971, 136–138): this is a thought experiment in which persons have no information about their personal place in society or about particular circumstances of their society. The assumption is that such people would rationally choose those principles for allocating rights and resources that offer the same opportunities as well as same social safety structures to all people. Obviously, this ideal position contrasts with existing social inequalities of "knowing" where one stands and how existing structures are. However, its charm lies in its rational abstraction of a moral ideal. Furthermore, in a crisis such as a pandemic, evidence and certitudes regarding our own lives and society become shaky and might remind us of the fragility of social advantages.

making positions are limited to the naturally or socially privileged. Finally, a process is unjust if it is biased or based on selective participation. Rawls's approach is procedural and contractualist. It complements the distributive approach to justice by focusing more on *how* procedures and institutions create justice; distributive theories, by way of contrast, point to *which* resources or goods are distributed in *what* quantities.

Procedural injustice during pandemics can occur in manifold ways. Persons in quarantine are often robbed of their basic political rights: they cannot naturally participate in many political and public events due to limited mobility. During the COVID-19 pandemic, various governments restricted the right to meet in large groups, even outdoors. This resulted in bans on public demonstrations and street protests – which are normally legitimate and important means for expressing views and concerns in modern democratic societies. Restricting mobilization thus limited opportunities to protest publicly against COVID-19 measures or against other political decisions that happened in parallel. The social media channels increasingly used to express public concerns regarding the (in)appropriateness of pandemic measures led to more extreme in- and out-group effects (cf. the contribution of Julia Brose in this volume), questioning the democratic potential of such virtual alternatives. The concept of political unfairness or injustice thus enables an in-depth discussion of how the right to political participation is relevant, especially in times of restricted physical mobility.

Struggle for Recognition: HIV Patient Expertise and the Fight against Homophobia and Undertreatment

Axel Honneth's theory of the struggle for recognition (2003; 2004) is also relevant when discussing participatory injustices in the context of pandemics. His approach provides a sense of injustice as a driving force for social movements in times of social conflicts – and does not start from a hypothetical perspective of an original position, but from a history of real struggles between social classes and other groups. The political struggle for recognition arises through the moral experience of injustice and previously endured humiliation. Injustice is related to the threat to physical or social integrity or dignity of persons as a collective and not exclusively in terms of individual experience. The experience of disregard as a "typical key experience of an entire group" needs collective semantics to bridge the gap between individual experience and to form collective identity (2003, 260–262). In Honneth's terms, the shared experience of misrecognition provides the motor of new social movements. Forms of social resistance, revolutions, and strikes form communities which themselves develop new insights, social bonds, and organizations to support members of marginalized social groups. If the struggle for recognition is successful, it can contribute to the moral development of society as it comes closer to common notions of a good or just society. The focus on social movements and struggle for recognition allows us to shed light on particular forms of social exclusion that often occur in pandemics.

An outstanding historical example for the struggle for recognition is ACTUP, or the AIDS Coalition to Unleash Power, an activist group that emerged during the 1980s HIV pandemic. The documentary film *How to Survive a Plague*, directed by David France (2012), narrates how patient activists and the gay community struggled against dying of HIV and stigmatization at the same time. In the film, the group fought against the lack of health care by collectivizing political agency, it became "experts" on treatment drugs, and finally forced the US health care administration and pharmaceutical companies to develop new, efficient treatments. The film's narrative focuses on the ACTUP, which was founded in 1987 in New York City as a grassroots movement to help people living with HIV get access to care and treatment. The group organized effective public demonstrations and protests at the Federal Drug Administration (FDA) in 1988, at the National Institute of Health (NIH) in 1990, and at the 6th AIDS Conference in San Francisco in 1990, which ended as a joint action of activists and scientists. These protests contributed significantly to a change in public recognition of the situation of living as a homosexual person, with or without HIV (cf. Epstein 1996). A subgroup of ACTUP, the split off organization TAG (Treatment Action Group), developed into a kind of patient-expert community who collaborated with scientists, pharmaceutical companies, and the NIH to accelerate and transform research on HIV treatments. In my opinion, this is an impressive narrative of patient-activist empowerment, but of course does not cover all dimensions of people s affected in the 1980s and afterwards by HIV policies.

Epistemic Injustice: How some Knowledge is Overheard or Ignored

The experience of social disregard also plays an important role in what Miranda Fricker (2007) calls "epistemic injustice." Her argument, based on speech act theory, focuses on inter-individual situations between a speaker and a listener, but it also considers power as implicit in such discursive settings. Epistemic injustice and its various dimensions have become a major topic in the philosophy of science (Koskinen and Rolin 2021). The academic world (but also other institutions such as courts, clinics, parliaments, and the media) are settings where knowledge and facts form the basic condition for our self-understanding and orientation for acting. In pandemic situations, facts and knowledge about developments are highly relevant. What kind of infectious agent is transmitted in what way? What is an efficient vaccine? How to treat symptoms? The epistemic dimensions of pandemics are manifold and impact communication channels and relations between the authorities and the public, regardless if the specific case is syphilis (cf. the contribution by Victoria Morick in this volume) or leprosy (cf. the contribution by Richard Hölzl).

According to Fricker, power relations and stereotypes shape communicative practices and therefore define what counts as factual knowledge. She distinguishes between testimonial and hermeneutic injustice. Testimonial injustice can be also understood as the unfair assessment of credibility: it is the underestimation of a person's capacity to provide adequate or relevant knowledge due to social stereotypes. Such stereotypes are ubiquitous in the health science context, where patients are often seen as too health-illiterate to give evidence of their condition (Schicktanz 2018). However, also the overestimation of a person's credibility – such as the supposed rationality, neutrality, or objectivity of experts – in such settings can be problematic. Indeed, the under- and overestimation of specific groups is often relational in systems of power. The above-mentioned example of the ACTUP narrative can also be discussed from an epistemic injustice perspective, because in the beginning, the testimony of HIV patients about their symptoms and experiences with the (illegal) combination of different treatment[5] was ignored as "unscientific," but later contributed to a revised clinical trial scheme which was then successful (cf. Schicktanz 2015).

A second form of epistemic injustice is hermeneutic. Here Fricker refers to the exclusion of certain social experiences from the pool of accepted facts due to a lack of opportunities for naming. Such hermeneutic injustice can occur in a pandemic if, e.g., rare long-term effects of the disease or some side-effects of countermeasures, such as pharmaceutical treatments or vaccines, are not named properly by affected patients due to the social power of expert discourse. Framing long-COVID as something purely "psychological," for instance, can discredit patients' experiences as well as limit their ability to observe and register the symptoms and to receive relevant care or social support in a timely manner. In colonial or postcolonial contexts, indigenous knowledge systems for dealing with infectious diseases are often discredited, although they can provide important insights into how to deal with infectious agents. These insights are often well-adapted to socio-economic conditions, even if they use nominally unscientific formulations or explanations. Epistemic injustice, however, affects not only health or science topics, but also the social realm. Consider the possible negative effects of pandemics on poorer citizens, whether directly

5 The movie *The Dallas Buyers Club* (2013, dir: Jean-Marc Vallée) tells the story of a straight, homophobic worker who after being diagnosed with HIV and suffering from AIDS, does not give up. Instead, he travels to Mexico and benefits from alternative, illegal or yet not clinically tested treatments. He then starts a business to import such drugs from Mexico to the US to offer to HIV patients who experiment on themselves with different treatments, after paying a monthly sum of $400.

or indirectly through disease management. These include economic deprivation, increased risk of socio-economic harm and unemployment, and the effects of mobility restrictions due to fewer social and economic resources, coupled with increased risk of stress, violence, or social isolation. How do these facts become facts? When structural inequities disfavor social science and related fields during a pandemic, as was particularly evident during the first two years of the COVID-19 pandemic, these epistemic inequities lead directly to social inequities.

Everyday Injustices

Legal-anthropological work focusing on neglected everyday injustice has been done by anthropologist Laura Nader. Nader (1980) documented the experienced injustice of disappointed consumers who complain about defects in purchased items or about miserable public services that interfere with life-as-usual in the United States. She calls such cases "little injustices" as they are normally too insignificant to be recognized by the law. According to Nader, ignoring these little injustices increases distrust in the legal system; this, in turn, can encourage criminal behavior, as people who feel ignored by the law are more likely break it. Over-bureaucratic or overly slow and inadequate responses contribute to the general sense of injustice. There is evidence that the "jailbreaking" behavior evident during the COVID-19 lockdown was understood by protestors as acts of resistance against unjust measures (cf. the contribution of Böhrer et al. and of Ege/Schmitzberger in this volume).

This is not to say that all acts of lawbreaking can be justified from a moral philosophical point of view. On the contrary, protests against perceived injustice often result in counter-injustices that should also be subjected to review. In her analysis of Telegram conversations among vaccine sceptics, Julia Brose (cf. this volume) explores how those who ignore mask mandates etc. sometimes feel stigmatized by other people, including their own family members. At the same time, some of those who feel stigmatized are capable of doing the same, for instance by calling the vaccinated and those who observe rules "smurfs" and "silly sheep." Where to draw the line between acceptable and non-acceptable injustices, even when they are small, requires important procedural consideration in civic society. This links Nadler's observation to Judith Shklar's (1990) attempt to differentiate between misfortune and injustice. She draws on Cicero to provide a normative look at so-called passive citizens (40). She focuses on citizens who turn away from actual or potential victims and, by doing so, contribute in a small way to the harms done to third persons. These small non-interventions occur in situations that have hardly any influence on life chances (in contrast to cases involving social inequality or political unfairness); they sometimes involve trivial, everyday situations such as rudeness or impertinence (e.g., someone who lifts his or her mask to sneeze in a public space). Passiveness in such cases means not raising one's voice in protest. Of course, there are always good reasons for not getting involved: people are in a rush, do not feel well, prefer to stay out of trouble, or simply respect the liberty of others. According to Shklar, we tend to frame such situations as misfortunes, as minor calamities that cannot be corrected, even when they are actually minor injustices. However, passivity helps injustice flourish, as Shklar argues, when we simply "mind our own business," as the saying goes. Also, misfortunes of these types are actually injustices when they are structurally embedded in the inequalities of the labor market, the shape of public space, or the rituals of politics and commerce. Nadar and Shklar both argue that passivity in the face of injustice – even when we mistake injustice as misfortune – can lead to "hard feelings" that influence fundamental attitudes towards society and the political-legal system. Thus, the little injustices that can and do occur during pandemics require our special attention, especially at a time when pandemics may become normalized and chronic. While glaring injustice may be obvious, we may become insensitive to the everyday injustices against vulnerable people. Here is where the elements of storytelling – narrative perspective, characterization, the different points of view – become increasingly relevant to moral thought and vice versa. Engaging with various pandemic narratives can prevent us from becoming too ignorant of the little and big injustices. Some injustices already exist, and a pandemic just makes them bigger and more visible; however, some injustices are created by the way we deal with a pandemic and how we have not learned from the past.

Some Concluding Remarks

Moral and political philosophers have long debated over how best to develop a consistent and practicable theory of justice. Combining various approaches may offer the best solution by allowing us to take different levels of interaction and interdependence into account on a case-by-case basis. We need to be able to think about the relation between citizens and the state, between social groups, between particular institutions and social groups, between particular institutions and individuals or social groups, and between citizens. Table 1 is an attempt to schematize the various considerations and perspectives summarized above.

Pandemics force us to rethink the relations of separate actors and spheres because vectors of infection can cross social barriers and distinctions. Whereas analytical ethical thinking may have trouble accounting for the confusion attending times of crisis, a narrative approach offers the possibility of bringing together separate perspectives in intersecting storylines. Comparing narrative and exploring new ways to braid them into multivalent stories may help us develop more comprehensive understandings of the (real-world) injustices involved. The new picture will not answer the futile question of which injustice is more unjust – that is not the primary goal of this volume. Our more modest goal is to sharpen our perception and description of injustice. A detailed and appropriate description of a problem can be a first step to tackling it.

Table 1: Approaches to injustice

Concept	Setting	Acts
Oppressions: exploitation exclusion powerlessness cultural imperialism violence	Social groups in a liberal-capitalist democracy	Material deprivation in work contexts Limiting participation of social life Missing social status by professional hierarchies Non-dominant culture is marked or made invisible Physical attacks or abuse
Political unfairness	State institutions vs. citizens (e.g., laws, courts)	No fair access to basic rights/primary goods because of some person's egoism or their taking advantage of already privileged positions
Maldistribution	State vs. social sub-groups	Unequal distribution of socially relevant goods (material and immaterial) resulting in structural inequalities
Struggle for recognition	Social sub-groups/working class in a social conflict/crisis	Missing recognition, no respect of dignity, or harming physical integrity
Epistemic Injustice	Knowledge production and fact exchange	Disregarding/excluding epistemic competency of some members due to social stereotypes and hence excluding persons from making epistemic contributions
Little injustices	Individuals vs. bureaucracy	Often underrated misbehavior (ignorance, complicity) in everyday contexts of consumerism
Passive injustices	Between citizens in a liberal, civic state	Intentional ignorance or unwillingness to make use of leeway in everyday context of civil society

Bibliography

Bufacchi, Vittorio. 2012. *Social Injustice*, Palgrave Macmillian.

Coen, Sharon, Vezzoli Michela, and Zogmaister Cristina. 2022. "Theoretical and methodological approaches to activism during the COVID-19 pandemic—between continuity and change." *Frontiers in Political Science*, vol. 4. https://doi.org/.3389/fpos.2022.844591.

Cohn Jr, Samuel K. 2007. "The Black Death and the burning of Jews." *Past and Present*, vol. 196, no. 1, 3–36.

Davis, Mark, and Lohm Davina. 2020. *Pandemic, Publics, and Narrative*, Oxford UP.

Dlamini, Priscilla. S., Thecla W. Kohi, Leana R. Uys, René D. Phetlhu, Maureen L. Chirwa, Joanne R. Naidoo, and Lucy N. Makoae. 2007. "Verbal and physical abuse and neglect as manifestations of HIV/AIDS stigma in five African countries." *Public health nursing*, vol. 24, no. 5, 389–399.

Epstein, Steven. 1996. *Impure Science: AIDS, activism, and the politics of knowledge*, vol. 7, U of California P.

France, David, director. 2012. *How to survive a plague*, IFC films.

Fricker, Miranda. 2007. *Epistemic Injustice: Power and the Ethics of Knowing*, Oxford UP.

Honneth, Axel. 2003. *Kampf um Anerkennung*, Suhrkamp.

Honneth, Axel. 2004. "Recognition and Justice: Outline of a Plural Theory of Justice." *Acta Sociologica*, vol. 47, no. 4, 351–364.

Koskinen, Inkeri, and Kristina Rolin. 2021. "Structural epistemic (in) justice in global contexts." *Global Epistemologies and Philosophies of Science*, edited by David Ludwig, Inkeri Koskinen, Zinhle Mncube, Luana Poliseli, and Luis Reyes-Galindo, Routledge, 115–125.

Kurtzman, E. T., L. V. Ghazal, S. Girouard, C. Ma, B. Martin, B.T. McGee, and H. L. Germack. 2022. "Nursing workforce challenges in the postpandemic world." *Journal of Nursing Regulation*, vol. 13, no. 2, 49.

Nader, Laura. 1980. *No Access to Law: Alternatives to the American Juridical System*, Academic Press.

Rawls, John. 1979. *Eine Theorie der Gerechtigkeit*, Suhrkamp.

Schaeffer, Jean-Marie. 2009. "Fictional vs. factual narration." *Handbook of Narratology*, edited by Fotis Jannidis, Matías Martínez, John Pier, and Wolf Schmid, de Gruyter Brill, 98–114.

Schicktanz, Silke. "The ethical legitimacy of patients' organizations' involvement in politics and knowledge production: epistemic justice as conceptual basis." *The public shaping of medical research*, edited by Wehling Peter, Willi Viehöder und S. Koenen, Routledge, 246–265.

Shklar, Judith. 1980. *The Faces of Injustice*, Yale UP.

Vallée, Jean-Marc, director. 2013. *The Dallas Buyers Club.*

Vonderschmitt, Jane, Sabine Wöhlke, and Silke Schicktanz. 2023. "Scare Resources, Public Health and Professional Care: The COVID-19 pandemic exacerbating bioethical conflicts. Findings from global qualitative expert interviews." *BMC Public Health*, vol. 23, 2492. https://doi.org/10.1186/s12889-023-17249-4

Young, Iris Marion. 1990. *Justice and the Politics of Difference*, Princeton UP. https://doi.org/10.2307/j.ctvcm4g4q. [2012 reprint with a foreword by D. Allen].

Zierler, Sally, William E. Cunningham, Ron Andersen, Martin F. Shapiro, Terry Nakazono, Sally Morton, and Sam A. Bozzette. 2000. "Violence victimization after HIV infection in a US probability sample of adult patients in primary care." *American Journal of Public Health*, vol. 90, no. 2, 208–215.

List of Contributors in Alphabetical Order

Laura Bäumel is a lecturer and PhD researcher in Cultural Studies at the University of Zurich, Switzerland. Her research focuses on working-class cultures, materialist feminisms, and the contemporary appeal of the far right.

Annerose Böhrer is a sociologist working in the field of history and ethics of medicine at the University of Würzburg, Germany. Current research focuses on the material cultures of medicine and biomedical futures.

Julia Brose is a research associate at the International Center for Higher Education Research (INCHER) at the University of Kassel, Germany. Her research focuses on higher education research, knowledge transfer in higher education, social inequalities in education, and mixed-methods approaches.

Marie-Kristin Döbler is a postdoctoral scientist at the ISF Munich – Institute for Social Science Research. Current research foci are presences and (mediated) social interactions; loneliness; autonomy and freedom; changing forms and organizations of work.

Moritz Ege is a professor for Every Day Life and Popular Culture Studies at the Department of Social Anthropology and Cultural Studies at the University of Zurich, Switzerland. His research areas include the links between popular culture and politics, ethnographies of social inequality, and conjunctural analysis.

Niklas Ellerich-Groppe is a research associate at the Division of Ethics in Medicine at the Carl von Ossietzky University of Oldenburg, Germany. His current research foci are intergenerational perspectives in bioethics as well as ethical questions of digitalization and diversity in healthcare.

Andrew S. Gross is a professor of American literature at the University of Göttingen, vice president of the German Association of American Studies, and editor-in-chief of the New American Studies Journal. He writes about American poetry and post-WWII American literature and culture.

Jan Hinrichsen is postdoctoral researcher at the Institute for History and Ethics of Medicine at the University Medical Center Göttingen. He is an anthropologist of knowledge and science. He currently works on the practices of producing valid data on the immunogenicity of mRNA vaccines against COVID-19.

Richard Hölzl is researcher at the Museum Fünf Kontinente in Munich and teaches at the Seminar for Medieval and Modern History, University of Göttingen. His research focuses on environmental history, history of missions, and material cultures of colonialism.

Franziska Meier is a professor of French and Italian Literature at the University of Göttingen, Germany. Current research is focussed on Dante and Boccaccio Studies.

Pierre-Héli Monot is a professor of Transnational American Studies at the Ludwig Maximilian University of Munich. He is the Principal Investigator of the ERC Starting Grant "The Arts of Autonomy: Pamphleteering, Popular Philology, and the Public Sphere, 1988–2018."

Victoria Morick is a historian at the Department of Medieval and Modern History at the University of Göttingen, Germany. Her research focuses on the history of knowledge, the history of the body, the history of public health, as well as visual and material cultures of disease and medicine.

Jennifer A. Reich, Ph.D. is Professor of Sociology at the University of Colorado Denver. Her research examines how individuals and families weigh information and strategize their interactions with the state and service providers, particularly as they relate to healthcare and welfare.

Silke Schicktanz is a professor for Ethical and Cultural Studies of Biomedicine at the University Medical Center, Göttingen, Germany. Current research foci are cross-cultural bioethics, stakeholder engagement, as well as collectivity and responsibility.

Julian Schmitzberger is an associate researcher at the Department of Social Anthropology and Cultural Studies, University of Zurich, Switzerland. His research focuses on pop and popular culture, the study of emotions and affects, and urban anthropology.

Mark Schweda is a professor for Ethics in Medicine and Health Care at the Carl von Ossietzky University of Oldenburg, Oldenburg, Germany. Current research focuses on ethical aspects of aging and intergenerational relations in medicine and health care.

Yvonne Völkl is a literary and cultural studies scholar in the field of Romance studies. Her research focuses on 18th-century literature and press, French-Canadian literature and contemporary crisis narratives.

13809202
9841402